OCCUPATIONAL THERAPY
Practice skills for physical dysfunction

OCCUPATIONAL THERAPY

Practice skills for physical dysfunction

LORRAINE WILLIAMS PEDRETTI, M.S., O.T.R.

Associate Professor, Department of Occupational Therapy,
San Jose State University, San Jose, California

with 302 *illustrations*

The C. V. Mosby Company

ST. LOUIS • TORONTO • LONDON   1981

MOSBY

1906 **75** 1981
YEARS

A TRADITION OF PUBLISHING EXCELLENCE

Editor: Don Ladig
Manuscript editor: Ivie Lewellen Davis
Design: Jeanne Bush
Production: Stella Adolfson

Printed in the United States of America

The C.V. Mosby Company
11830 Westline Industrial Drive, St. Louis, Missouri 63141

Library of Congress Cataloging in Publication Data

Pedretti, Lorraine Williams, 1936-
    Occupational therapy.

    Revision of a manual printed and distributed under
the title: Basic practice skills in occupational
therapy for physical dysfunction.
    1. Occupational therapy.   2.   Physically handi-
capped—Rehabilitation.   I. Title. [DNLM: 1. Occupation therapy.   WB   555 P371o]
RM735.P34   1981   615.8'5152   81-11076
ISBN   0-8016-3772-4   AACR2

GW/VH/VH   9   8   7   6   5   4   3   02/B/294

Preface

This book was designed for use by students of occupational therapy at the baccalaureate level. Its purpose is to help prepare the student for entry-level practice in occupational therapy for adults with acquired physical disabilities.

The arrangement of content is based on the occupational therapy process. Methods of evaluation and treatment planning and descriptions of frequently used treatment methods are presented. This foundation is followed by chapters on the application of occupational therapy to several specific physical disabilities. These were selected because they are often encountered in practice, and each is considered representative of a major classification of physical dysfunction. A chapter that includes principles of hand splinting and a self-instruction program on splint construction is designed for independent study. Its purposes are to introduce students to the elements of hand splinting and to direct them in the construction of a basic splint. Each chapter concludes with review questions to assist the student to master content, achieve learning objectives, and prepare for evaluation of learning.

Congenital and acquired physical disabilities of childhood have not been included. The sample case studies and treatment plans presented are not intended to present the only approach to the treatment of the particular dysfunction. Rather, they are designed to provide students with guidelines to treatment from which to build diverse and more specific treatment plans for hypothetical or real clients encountered in their academic preparation.

For clarity and ease of reading in this book clients or patients will be referred to in the masculine gender and therapists in the feminine gender.

This book evolved out of a manual that was first printed in 1972 as a collection of teaching materials and lecture outlines for use in the occupational therapy curriculum at San Jose State University. The original manual underwent several revisions and in 1977 was printed and distributed under the title *Basic Practice Skills in Occupational Therapy for Physical Dysfunction.*

It is assumed that the readers of this text have prior knowledge of anatomy, physiology, kinesiology, neuroanatomy, neurophysiology, orthopedic and neurological dysfunctions, medical terminology, human growth and development, and basic occupational therapy theory.

It is the nature of human beings to be active. Mental and physical activity is essential to personal health and to the health and progress of the culture or society in which individuals exist. Conversely, inactivity can lead to mental or physical deterioration and can be a deterrent to the progress of the culture or society in which human beings live.

At any age or stage in a person's life there is a desirable pattern and balance of optimum occupational performance for the maintenance of the health of the individual and the society. Disruptive forces, such as illness, injury, developmental disorders, and genetic defects, can alter the pattern and balance of occupational performance and place the organism in a state of disorder or imbalance so that it cannot achieve or maintain a desirable balance and pattern of occupational performance.

On these premises occupational therapy is viewed as an intervention agent whose roles are as follows:

1. Assess past and present patterns of occupational performance
2. Identify dysfunctions in occupational performance
3. Identify the dysfunctional performance components and their effect on occupational performance
4. Remedy or compensate for dysfunctions in occupational performance and performance components
5. Facilitate the structuring or restructuring of a pattern and balance in occupational performance that is suitable and optimal for the age, stage, and current life roles of the individual.

Occupational therapy uses standardized testing procedures, clinical observations, and purposeful, goal-directed activity to achieve these objectives.

The chapter contributors, Mary C. Kasch, Jan Zaret Davis, Guy L. McCormack, Gregory Stone, Barbara A. Baum, and Diane L. Meeder, are gratefully acknowledged for their willingness to share in the production of this text. My appreciation is extended to Linda Higgins for the cover design and illustrations and to Bart Favero for the photographs.

My gratitude is extended to those who modeled for photographs—my students Catherine Oberschmidt and

Marianne Woodall, my niece Ramona Fournier, and my colleagues Morag Paterson and Gregory Stone, San Jose State University—and to Jana Hostetter, Rehabilitation Center of Los Gatos–Saratoga, for the loan of assistive devices to be photographed.

Manuscript reviewers and consultants to whom I wish to express my personal appreciation are Joyce Gorham, Santa Clara Valley Medical Center; Amy Killingsworth, Associate Professor, San Jose State University; Dr. William Lages, Santa Clara Valley Medical Center; and John G. Russell, Jr. Carol Feinour is gratefully acknowledged for typing the manuscript so expertly and for accommodating to my schedule and special needs.

All of my colleagues in the Department of Occupational Therapy at San Jose State University, especially Amy Killingsworth, Associate Professor, and Gregory Stone, Lecturer, are acknowledged with appreciation for their support and encouragement.

Last but not least, my husband Robert Leland Pedretti is lovingly appreciated for his unending patience, assistance, support, and encouragement. I thank my son Mark Samuel Pedretti, age 4, who frequently wondered when the "book" would be finished, for never touching my materials, and for waiting patiently for my attention.

Lorraine Williams Pedretti

Contents

OCCUPATIONAL THERAPY
Practice skills for physical dysfunction

Chapter 1

Psychosocial aspects of physical dysfunction

PSYCHOSOCIAL CONSEQUENCES OF PHYSICAL DYSFUNCTION

The experience of loss of any physical part or function involves not only the painful distortion of body image and the image of oneself as a physical being but also the image of self as a social being whose family and social roles and vocational and leisure occupations may be unalterably changed. Independence, self-sufficiency, and autonomy may have to be given up partially or totally, temporarily or permanently.[2]

The onset of physical dysfunction necessitates a sudden change in daily life. The individual is likely to be thrown into the new world and life-style of a health care facility where there is enforced passivity and dependence. He must adapt to a new environment, new personnel, new food, and new time schedules. Privacy must be surrendered and virtual strangers must be allowed to probe the body. The person may be devastated by the drastic interruption of familial, occupational, and social roles.[5] Previous roles may be slightly changed, seriously impaired, or completely eliminated as a result of the disability. The damage to previously held roles may be due directly to the disability or may indirectly result from changed life circumstances brought about by the disability.[8]

The onset of physical disability affects the person who has the disability and all of those with whom he comes in contact. The individual's particular response and the responses of others to the disability will have a significant impact on rehabilitation personnel and on the rehabilitation process.[10] The disabled adult is confronted with the task of survival, first, then with regaining essential physical skills, and finally, the greater goals of resuming meaningful life roles. These are monumental and formidable tasks that require managing many overwhelming personal problems and overcoming external blockades to readjustment.[8]

Personal reactions to physical dysfunction

As a result of the major life changes brought about by the onset of physical dysfunction, the individual's de-fense mechanisms are highly taxed as he attempts to deal with the changed social interactions and sexual patterns and the ability to direct his own life and to control the environment through physical action. Concomitantly he is dealing with fears, realistic and unrealistic, physical pain and suffering, and the symbolic meaning of the physical dysfunction. Changed attitudes of family and friends may provoke stress, fears, and expectations that others will react differently and reject him.[5,13]

Individual reactions to physical dysfunction depend on the previously held body image and compromise body image and the psychological meaning of the specific dysfunction in relation to the individual's personality.[13] Paraplegia may have a very different meaning to an athlete who defines self-worth in terms of physical performance and physique than to an office worker whose sense of self may be defined more in terms of use of head and hands, for instance.

Although it is commonly believed that physical dysfunction generates only negative and disruptive psychological reactions, it has been found that opportunities and gratification may be generated as well.[11] The dysfunction may be regarded as a well-deserved punishment, especially if it is associated with an unsuccessful suicide attempt, asocial behavior, or the death of another. This attitude could gratify masochistic wishes and paradoxically lead to a greater sense of well-being.[5,13] The dysfunction may be seen as the final confirmation of a lack of self-worth and could precipitate a suicide or psychotic reaction.[13] The gratification of longed for dependency on a caring person leading to relative comfort may be satisfied by the dysfunction. Conversely the reawakening of intolerable dependency longings and rage related to a lack of satisfaction of early dependency needs can result in marked anxiety or a paranoid reaction.[5,13] Exhibitionistic wishes and the need to manipulate and control others may also be satisfied through the physical dysfunction. The dysfunction may be used as a means of expressing hostility or avoiding responsibilities by some individuals.[5] Conversely the onset of dysfunction may lead to constructive, alternative life roles and offer social and career opportunities that were not contemplated by the individual prior to the onset of the physical dysfunction.

Our culture places great emphasis and value on productivity and on physical attractiveness. To not have achieved them or be in the process of achieving them may evoke feelings of self-devaluation. Feelings of low worth tend to be all-or-none in quality. They may be evoked by consideration of only one characteristic out of many by the disabled person, yet he may conceive of self as all worthless. The feelings of low self-worth also tend to extend into the past and into the future so that the person can neither conceive of self as ever having been productive or attractive nor contemplate the possibility of future change.

The conclusions of worthlessness are in a sense true, since they are based on a self-definition in terms of degree of productivity and attractiveness. This is a distortion, since it bases the self-worth on deficits and overlooks the remaining assets and intrinsic worth. Although the concept of intrinsic worth, that is, the person is valued for self alone without external comparisons, is desirable and ideal, it is probably difficult or impossible to achieve for most people. In general, people in American society value themselves according to external standards of attractiveness, productivity, and achievements.

Disabled persons may conclude that they are worthless and of negative value and therefore that they are "awful" as well. They may expect and think that they deserve the rejection of others based on that notion. If they are not of any value to themselves, then others will not see them as valuable and therefore will reject them. This kind of thinking can persist for long periods of time and may account for withdrawal behavior or an intense search for approval and love. Some persons will draw this thinking process to what seems like a logical conclusion, which is they are worth nothing to self or to others, therefore life is meaningless and empty and they should not exist. This feeling may be especially strong in those who have intense guilt feelings.[3]

It has been assumed by many that a certain type of personality or adjustment pattern is associated with a specific physical disability or that the degree and type of dysfunction will cause psychological maladjustment. These premises have been refuted by research. It has been concluded that particular personality types or characteristics are not associated with specific dysfunctions nor is there evidence to support the notion that the severity or type of disability is correlated with the degree of psychological adjustment.[11]

Societal reactions to physical dysfunction

Attitudes of others toward physical disability affect attitudes toward oneself. A physically handicapped individual reflects attitudes of self-depreciation. In the newly disabled, devaluing attitudes toward the disabled, once an out-group, may now be directed to the self with very serious consequences.[11] Physical dysfunction was once considered divine punishment or evidence of sinfulness. This is still the belief of some individuals. It is more likely to be viewed as ugly, loathsome, or, at the very least, discomforting. Few people are really comfortable with disabled or deformed individuals. Their presence constitutes a threat to the nondisabled about their own vulnerability. To avoid the threatening feeling the nondisabled reject or avoid disabled or deformed persons.[13] The appearance of the injury or disability also engenders nonacceptance. If the disability is unsightly, this tends to be overestimated by the nondisabled and is a factor that prompts rejection or avoidance. The nondisabled may display unwarranted pity or excessive curiosity. The disabled person feels set apart from most "normal" people and is constantly striving to fight the negative implications of the physical dysfunction and gain genuine social acceptance. Nonacceptance resides in the nondisabled and stems from negative attitudes. It is a resistance or a reluctance to enter into various degrees of social interchange with the disabled person and carries an aura of ostracism.

Disabled individuals perceive a lack of patience on the part of the nondisabled toward performance ease and speed. Whether this attitude is maintained by the nondisabled or is projected by the disabled, it engenders the same feeling of nonacceptance in the disabled person.

The disabled person may perceive an apparent rather than a genuine social acceptance by the nondisabled. The latter may be perceived as motivated by pity or duty and may offer empty gestures of acceptance devoid of meaning or real pleasure in the interchange. Apparent acceptance is not more desirable than nonacceptance. In each the disabled see the underlying inability or unwillingness on the part of the nondisabled to know them as they really are.

Another tendency of the nondisabled is to judge the disabled not only in terms of the apparent physical limitation but also in terms of psychological factors assumed to be concomitant to the disability.[9] The nondisabled may treat the physically disabled as if they were limited mentally and emotionally as well.[1] The evaluation of the visible disability is spread to other characteristics that are not necessarily affected. The frequent assumption that a person who has cerebral palsy is also mentally retarded and the practice of speaking loudly to a blind person as if also deaf are examples of this phenomenon. It is generally a devaluing process, and the disabled person is thereby stigmatized and considered of lower social status and unworthy of acceptance.[9]

Words exist in the language of American culture that have a stigmatizing effect on the disabled. Expressions such as "retard," "crip," and "psycho" are examples. Within the language of the medical and allied health professions these terms become formalized to "mentally retarded," "physically disabled," and "mentally ill." These terms have value for the classification of persons into diagnostic categories, but they stigmatize as well.[1] It follows that when rehabilitation workers refer to their clients as a diagnosis or disability (for example, "quad" or "hemi"), they are contributing to the stigmatization of those who they set out to help.

Stigma may be considered as negative perceptions or behaviors of normal people toward the physically disabled or toward all persons different from themselves. Physically disabled persons are regarded in much the same way as other minority groups in the population. They are subject to stereotyping and a reduced social status. Stigmatization is a basic fact of life for nearly all disabled persons. Interpersonal relationships between the nondisabled and the disabled tend to follow a superior-inferior pattern or to not exist at all. The nondisabled tend to demonstrate stereotyped, inhibited, and overcontrolled behavior in interactions with disabled persons. They tend to show less variable behavior, terminate interactions sooner, and express opinions less representative of their actual beliefs.

There is a substantial amount of segregation of the physically disabled. Although some of this segregation is necessary (for example, institutionalization or special schools) and designed to assist disabled persons, it nevertheless sets them apart psychologically and evokes feelings of inferiority in relation to nondisabled peers. This kind of segregation should be minimized. The fact that restrictive legislation exists in reference to disabled persons testifies to the systematized stigmatization of the disabled within American society.[1]

ADJUSTMENT TO PHYSICAL DYSFUNCTION

Since there is no direct relationship between the type of physical dysfunction and personality structure, physical injury or illness resulting in disability should be regarded as one of several life stresses to which the individual brings his unique repertoire of coping mechanisms and response patterns.[12] There is usually little or no prolonged effect on personality that results from physical dysfunction. Personality structure may be temporarily disordered by the crisis of physical change but appears to be capable of drawing on its resources and integrating the crisis experience into the self to become reestablished.[11]

The individual with physical dysfunction is faced with the problem of coping with his fears and anxieties and maintaining a balance between conflicting needs and tendencies at a time when it is most difficult to cope and defenses are weakened. These anxieties may be dealt with by using a variety of defense mechanisms. Denial may be manifested by cheerfulness and an unrealistic lack of concern about the disabling condition. Undue involvement in hospital routines may be a sign of overactivity used to cope with underlying anxiety. Overdependency may be manifested by keeping family and personnel close by and having more attendant care than is realistically needed.

Bravado and aggressiveness may be used to cover helplessness and dependency and to hide deep fears and anxieties. Excessive talking may be a mechanism used to discharge emotional tension. Some individuals may be unusually cooperative and demonstrate considerable interest in details of the illness and treatment as a means of coping with fears and anxieties. Most of these defense mechanisms are not in the conscious awareness of the person employing them.[5]

According to Simon[13] the ultimate adjustment to the physical dysfunction is intimately related to the process of developing a new "compromise body image." The body image consists of multiple perceptions about the body based on past experience, current sensations, and one's personal investment in the body. The development of the body image is influenced by the attitudes and values of the culture and the views, values, and fantasies of the significant others in one's life. Parental attitudes about body parts and body functions are important factors in the development of the body image. All of the experiences and attitudes may result in an overvaluation of particular body parts and the perception of the body as good or bad, handsome or repugnant, lovable or unlovable. One may compare one's body to the bodies of others and develop derogatory attitudes toward the body or its parts. One may also develop mechanisms of compensation to obscure perceived stigma.

The ego may feel anxiety, shame, or disgust in relation to the body image and may develop defenses to avoid the unpleasant effect of an unacceptable body image. By using such defenses as denial, sublimation, repression, and overcompensation the person comes to accept the "compromise body image" that incorporates and modifies some of the unacceptable features. The compromise body image is an important factor in considering the emotional effects of physical dysfunction.

Most people who incur physical disability will initially experience worry and anxiety about the dysfunction. Old anxieties and fears about illness and disability will be evoked. The individual will experience realistic fears about the loss of security or loss of love from spouse, family, and friends. There is a loss of the fantasied future and a serious concern that the future may be dramatically altered.

Sadness and depression are to be expected for periods as long as 1 year. Depression is a mourning for the lost part or function. The lost part, function, and former body image are gradually surrendered, and there is resolution of anger. Psychic energy can then be freed for new activity, often for wholehearted involvement in rehabilitation efforts. The individual may compensate or even overcompensate for the loss in a healthy manner, and a new compromise body image emerges.[13]

Stages in adjustment to physical dysfunction

Kerr[7] described the adjustment to physical dysfunction as progressing through five stages. It is necessary to remember that the stages are points on a continuum and that all stages are not inevitable for all disabled persons. It is also important to understand the adjustment process, since there appears to be a relationship between the person's attitude toward the physical disability and the success of rehabilitation.

The stages are identified and described as follows:
1. Shock: "This isn't me."
2. Expectancy of recovery: "I'm sick but I'll get well."
3. Mourning: "All is lost."
4. Defensive A—healthy: "I'll go on in spite of it." Defensive B—pathological: Marked use of defenses to deny the effects of the disability.
5. Adjustment: "It's different but not bad."

Shock. The shock stage occurs during the early diagnostic and treatment period. The person lacks understanding that the body is ill or of the extent of the seriousness of the illness or injury. Because of these factors there may be an apparent lack of anxiety that appears to be unrealistic. As the reality of the situation becomes more apparent to the person, the reaction is "This can't be me. It's a bad dream. I'll wake up, and this will all be gone." The disabled person is likely to blame the hospital and medical personnel for the lost ability to function. The feeling is "If I could only get out of here, I'd be all right." Psychologically the person is still a normal, able-bodied person, pursuing the same goals and doing the same things as before the onset of the disabling condition.

There is an incompatibility between the person's real physical situation and the mental image. This incompatibility may account for the person's apparently inappropriate references to the disability, situation, recovery, and future performance. At this stage body image is more potent than perceptions. Perceptions that are incompatible with the self-image are rejected.

There is also an inevitable testing of reality that occurs after the onset of disability, and when the fact of changed function comes into focus, the psychological situation changes. A pathological "denial of illness" may

occur and some persons previously considered psychologically healthy remain in this stage.

Expectancy of recovery. In this stage the person recognizes that he is ill but believes he will get well. Initially he *knows* he will recover. He may make frequent references to getting well or being whole again and may discuss future plans in which full recovery or a normally functioning body is essential.

The individual's only goal is to get well. This may lead to the search for a cure and "shopping" from one physician or health agency to another. There is a preoccupation with the physical condition. Small improvements may be overestimated or misinterpreted. The person will do anything perceived as aiding recovery, since this is the primary goal. To the extent that it is believed that recovery will take place, motivation toward learning to function with a disability will be minimal.

The person believes realistically that the disability is a barrier to everything in life that is important and worthwhile. A whole body is needed to attain important personal goals. Therefore full recovery must be achieved before anything else can be undertaken.

A change in this belief system or movement toward the next stage comes about when the person is moved toward a condition more similar to normal living than to the state of being temporarily ill. Being transferred from an acute care setting to the rehabilitation unit, being sent home in a wheelchair, having therapy terminated, redirecting therapy to teaching the person to live with the disability, or being told that full recovery will not occur are some of the events that may precipitate mourning.

Mourning. Mourning occurs when there is a shift from expectancy of recovery to the realization that the disability is permanent. This realization may be overwhelming and may require the intervention of specialists in psychiatry or psychology.

This stage is one of acute distress. All seems lost, and all former goals seem unattainable. Motivation to cope with the disability is gone. The person wants to give up and may contemplate suicide. If the individual is not allowed to express grief for the lost function or part because of the reprimands and attitudes of rehabilitation personnel and significant others, discussion of these feelings may be avoided and hostility toward those who forbid the expression of feelings may be demonstrated. The result is a "problem patient" who will not work and who spends much time complaining about the health agency procedures and personnel.[7]

The person may become resigned to this fate, believing that he is worthless and inadequate, and may remain at this stage in the process. The person may adopt the role of the invalid and become a permanent resident of a health care institution.[8] He simply lives and remains dependent and possibly hostile.

The disability is now seen as an impenetrable barrier to important life goals, and unlike the hope for recovery that characterized the previous stage, the goal of recovery is now seen as unrealistic.

To effect progress to the next stage the barrier imposed by disability must be decreased. To the degree that this is possible progress in adjustment and rehabilitation can be made. It may be possible to create situations in which previously held goals can be attained. However, since self-care activities were probably taken for granted, their accomplishment may not be seen as a positive goal by adults.

The person in this stage may also begin to mourn the loss of some psychological characteristics. He may believe he has lost his "fight," "pride," or "faith," which can be more distressing than the physical loss. When this occurs it may be important to expose the person to situations in which disabled persons can be observed demonstrating these qualities. The person can then begin to realize that the disability is irrelevant for the attainment of some more basic goals.

Defensive A—healthy. The defensive stage may be considered healthy if the person begins to deal with the disability and goes on in spite of it. Motivation to learn to function with the disability increases significantly. The person is pleased with his accomplishments and takes an active interest in being as normal as possible.

The disability barrier is being reduced and becomes less impenetrable. The person realizes the attainment of some goals he held as a normal person. Some treasured experiences, albeit small, are still possible. The barrier is still present, however, but there is the discovery of ways to circumvent it. The person learns to achieve previously held goals by other routes. Other goals may remain unattainable, and the person may remain distressed by the areas perceived to be unachievable.

The movement toward adjustment comes through a changed need system. The need for a whole or normal body may be relinquished when important goals can be attained in spite of the disability. The goals are attainable, therefore the disability becomes less relevant. When physical impairment does in fact interfere with goal attainment, the person must relinquish the goals and discover equally satisfying ways of meeting important needs.

Defensive B—pathological. The defensive stage may be considered pathological if the person uses defense mechanisms to deny the continued existence of a partial barrier imposed by the disability. Diverse behavior may be displayed, depending on the defense mechanisms used. The person may try to conceal the disability; may

rationalize and say he does not want the things that are unattainable; may project negative feelings to others, claiming they cannot accept his disability although he has; and may try to convince others that he is well-adjusted. The existence of barriers imposed by the disability is denied.[7] A new compromise body image that can be accepted both consciously and unconsciously fails to develop. Psychotic reactions may result. Passive, dependent reactions may be manifested by a complete loss of motivation and a surrendering of all ambition. Psychological regression may become apparent. Pathological denial may be manifested by an inability to express negative feelings and a repression of anger.[13]

Under some additional stress the person may regress to an earlier stage and remain there permanently or may progress to adequate adjustment after a temporary regression.

Adjustment. If an adequate adjustment is attained, the person considers the disability as merely one of many personal characteristics. The disability is no longer considered a major barrier to be overcome. It is regarded as one of many assets or liabilities, and satisfying ways to meet personal needs and goals have been found.

It cannot be assumed that teaching the disabled person to do things will automatically lead to an adequate adjustment. Two other goals, held by many people, will need to be attained before adjustment is possible. The first goal lies in religion or personal philosophy. The person with religious beliefs must feel "right with God." All of the beliefs about the role of suffering in relation to God's influence on life must be worked through. The disability will be a barrier between the person and God as long as it is regarded as a punishment or the person believes that God surely will heal those who love Him. Second is the goal of achieving a feeling of personal adequacy. Because of the tendency in our society to relegate the disabled to an inferior status, the disabled person must be helped to discriminate between adequate and inferior on the basis of characteristics rather than on physique and productivity. The person must be helped to reach these more abstract goals before adjustment is attained.[7]

PSYCHOSOCIAL CONSIDERATIONS IN TREATMENT OF PHYSICAL DYSFUNCTION

In the treatment of physical dysfunction the client must be regarded as a whole person. The individual's capabilities, problems, interests, experiences, needs, fears, prejudices, beliefs, cultural influences, and reactions to the physical dysfunction are as important as the physical considerations in planning interaction strategies and the treatment program.[15]

The meaning of the disability to the client is the crucial factor in planning a sound approach in treatment and in aiding with the adjustment process. Therefore treatment directed to aid psychosocial adjustment must be based on individual reactions to the circumstances rather than on reactions and characteristics assumed to be similar among clients with the same physical disability or the same degree of severity of disability.[11]

Interpersonal relationships

The client will reflect attitudes of personnel and family. The psychological reactions and relationships between personnel and clients will affect the client's reaction to the disability and often the degree of participation in the rehabilitation program. The client must have someone who cares about him and someone who waits for him, or he may lose the will to live.[5] One or several of the rehabilitation workers dealing with the client may assume this role.

Becoming disabled alters a person's life situation not only in terms of functional performance but in social interactions with others as well. The newly disabled person knows that there has not been a change in selfhood because of the disability, yet that person may be assigned to an inferior status by the nondisabled and by professional "helpers." Customary behavior may stimulate responses very different from those that are usual or anticipated by the disabled individual. This may cause questioning of personal identity, appropriate roles, and expectations in performance ability. The early answers to such questions come from the rehabilitation personnel in everyday treatment situations. By their words and actions personnel may communicate answers to critical and perhaps unspoken questions of the disabled person.[6]

One of the problems in interpersonal relationships frequently encountered by disabled persons is the tendency of nondisabled persons to assess the limitations as more severe and restrictive than they actually are. Frequently when the nondisabled judge that the physical dysfunction precludes participation in a given activity or social situation, the disabled person knows that some level of participation is possible. The degree of difference between their assessments may make the difference between nonparticipation and nonacceptance. Since it is not possible for the nondisabled person to know the capabilities of the disabled person in a given situation, it is wise for the nondisabled to invite the participation of the disabled thus leaving him to determine whether or not performance is feasible. Even if participation appears patently impossible to the nondisabled, the invitation should still be made to avoid rejection and allow for the possibility of the disabled to participate in an alternative role from the ones most participants will be assuming. The disabled person may be willing to restructure the situation so that participa-

tion is possible. The changes devised to allow participation may be simple or complex, but should be left to the discretion of the disabled person and not structured by the preconceived notions of the nondisabled. The role of the nondisabled is to provide opportunities for participation in social interchange for the disabled.[9]

Interpersonal approach in treatment

The reactions of personnel can be positive or negative. Negative reactions will result in a negative response in the client. Such reactions increase the client's suffering and may result in negativistic behavior demonstrated by an apparent loss of motivation and uncooperative behavior.[5]

Behavior of personnel that connotes respect for the rights, capabilities, and ability of the disabled person to make judgments and be involved in the rehabilitation process communicates their belief in the disabled individual as a human being and a fully functioning adult. It is important for rehabilitation personnel to not automatically assign clients to an inferior status or treat them as dependent children. The communication of a belief in the capacities of the disabled is essential. An attitude of helping the disabled person to explore and discover possibilities in performance skills and social interchange is much more helpful than preconceived notions and conclusions about their capacities by the "experts." Involvement of the client on the rehabilitation team to the extent possible is a critical factor in communicating the belief that the disabled person can be a self-determining agent in the rehabilitation process.[6]

The focus of rehabilitation should be on helping the person to reformulate an approving self who wishes to continue with life despite important discontinuity with past identity. This means the development of a new self-image based on a sense of worth rather than on deficiency and self-contempt.

The goal of rehabilitation then is to promote ego integrity and feelings of self-worth. Early rehabilitation efforts should be directed toward shaping basic life goals, and later efforts should shift to the emotional, physical, and technical resources necessary for their accomplishment.

The job of rehabilitation workers is to help the disabled person feel that he, as a personality, still continues. Functional aid should be seen in the larger context of enhancing self-respect. Functional and physical progress can be ego builders and aid in the adjustment process. However, functional efforts in the early stages of rehabilitation should be strategies designed to help the client see that performance is possible and should serve as a promise for the future. Emphasis on functional achievements as ends in themselves for specific skill development can serve as a means of avoiding the affective implications of physical dysfunction that must be manifested and worked through.

Therefore the proper role of the rehabilitation worker is that of assistant to the client. Unfortunately most rehabilitation settings are founded on the medical model. The professionals are in the expert and authoritarian role while the clients are in a passive, dependent, and compliant role. Passivity and authoritarian direction are inappropriate for persons with chronic, permanent conditions. Their role is the principal investment, and the roles of personnel are secondary.

The client's self-enhancement is supported when rehabilitation workers abandon their sense of omnipotence and see themselves as assistants to the client as he goes about the job of reconstituting his life. The roles of the professional must shift from active authoritarian to a more passive mode of professional behavior. The role of the client must shift from passive recipient of services to active doer. The rehabilitation approach is more suitable than the medical model approach when treating physically disabled persons. Except for the period of acute illness or injury and the subsequent maintenance of good health the problems to be faced are social, emotional, functional, and vocational performance problems, for which the medical model is not suitable.[12]

Adverse or negative reactions of rehabilitation workers toward clients may stem from a variety of reasons. Personality incompatibility or prejudicial reactions to a particular age, sex, ethnic group, or physical dysfunction are some of the factors that can evoke a negative reaction. Awareness and admission of adverse reactions are the first steps in coping with them constructively. Some signs of adverse reactions to clients are (1) failure to keep appointments; (2) cutting treatment time short; (3) frequently arranging for the client to be treated by an aide, student, or other therapist; (4) unnatural and excessive politeness and service to the client; (5) a feeling of boredom when the client is present; (6) a tendency to ignore the client when others are present; (7) unrealistic optimism or pessimism about the client's prognosis or potential achievements; and (8) giving the client sketchy answers and inadequate instructions.[5]

To deal with adverse reactions to clients rehabilitation personnel who become aware of these reactions may undergo a self-analysis or analysis with the aid of peers or a psychological counselor to identify the underlying cause of the negative reaction, if it is not readily apparent. Discussion of such reactions with the client who evokes them is sometimes appropriate. If the reaction is caused by an asocial or inappropriate behavior that is within the client's capacity to change and if changed would aid his acceptance by others, discussion of the

feeling with the client may be helpful. Personnel may be able to change their reactions and reconstruct interaction with the client more positively through ongoing counseling with peers or a professional counselor. If these measures fail and the negative reactions cannot be dealt with and resolved, transferring the client to the care of another is essential to progress.

Pathological reactions in adjustment may be prevented if personnel can recognize the stage of adjustment that the client is experiencing and structure approaches and activities to accommodate the client's particular emotional needs at that point in the adjustment process. Clients should be encouraged to express their fears, anxieties, worries, and sense of loss. This must be done with tact and understanding. Personnel must expect that strong emotions exist in the client and must be prepared to invite the expression of these emotions and to cope with them. Personnel should not minimize the problems or enter into the client's denial. Attitudes of acceptance of the individual with the physical dysfunction will help his self-acceptance. A cheerful and optimistic attitude is useful, but the appropriate expression of irritation and anger by personnel may help the client realize that expressions of emotion are allowed and the acceptance of personnel will not be lost if such feelings are expressed.[5,13]

Early recognition of pathological reactions by personnel trained in personality development and the use of mental defense mechanisms is important. Personnel should observe for deep depression, suicidal tendencies, undue guilt or preoccupation with symptoms, bizarre behavior, confusion, paranoid symptoms, or schizophrenic behavior.[5]

Personnel should share their observations for reality testing and for referral of problems to the appropriate specialists with other members of the rehabilitation team. There should be a concerted effort of the team to deal with the normal adjustment process and minor problems. Assistance and special treatment by psychiatric or psychological specialists may be required to deal with pathological reactions. Evaluation and treatment of the client and counsel of personnel by these specialists may be helpful in dealing effectively with the client, coping with feelings toward the client, and helping the client progress toward a healthy adjustment. All professionals dealing with the client, then, need to be aware of his perception of self and of the immediate and extended interpersonal environment. The focus of rehabilitation should be on helping the client reconstruct the body image in accepting and approving terms.[12]

Geis[3] stresses self-definition and a sense of personal worth as critical factors in successful rehabilitation and suggests some methods for helping clients to value themselves positively. If the disabled person is to achieve successful adjustment and adaptation, he cannot continue to value himself in terms of a self-image that can never be.

The individual's definition of himself is the crucial factor, determining the degree of sense of worth and self-satisfaction that can be achieved. Things outside of the client do not satisfy him, rather, satisfaction is derived in terms of these things. The client determines which things will bring satisfaction in terms of his own definition and conception of self. If this is the case, what kind of self-definition must be achieved for success, and how can rehabilitation personnel help the client achieve a positive and worthwhile definition of self?

The goal of rehabilitation is to aid the client to change a self-defeating definition to one that is self-enhancing. When the client's standards for attractiveness, productivity, or achievement are fixed and he can only define self and measure his value in terms of these standards, then problems are encountered in the rehabilitation process and adjustment. Therapy involves helping the client to experience the fact that he does not have to achieve a certain standard of productivity to be worthwhile and that his need to do this is only a fixed belief. The client needs to be directed to satisfactions that are attainable and helped to value goals and self preferentially rather than by some absolute standard.

In treatment the traditional focus has been on helping the client develop better modes of "doing." An emphasis on doing only or becoming efficient at reaching performance goals may focus self-valuation on an extrinsic standard of productivity. What is needed is to add to treatment modalities techniques for helping the client to simply "be" and to value things in themselves. Geis[3] describes "being" as a spontaneous expressive activity that may be purposeless and nonstriving. It exists during such pursuits as fiestas, ballet, dancing, and leisure activities and witnessing theatrical performances, comic events, and sports events, where gratification is intrinsic and linked with the process rather than the goal or end result of the activity. In contrast, "doing" activity has its satisfaction linked with the effect or ultimate achievement of the end goal of the activity process. Before the onset of physical disability the client's self-definition and sense of personal worth, in most cases, have been based largely on "doing" behavior. With the onset of physical dysfunction there is a major loss of the self-satisfaction derived from "doing." This may evoke a reduced sense of self-worth, which can be improved by helping the client derive gratification, and increase value to self as a result, from "being" experiences. Treatment methods that emphasize the client's exploration, manipulation, personal interests and choices, enjoyment, delight, and play can facilitate self-satisfaction from "being."[3]

Group approaches

Besides the interpersonal interaction strategies to facilitate adjustment to physical dysfunction just cited, several group approaches have been proposed that can be applied in occupational therapy. Therapeutic communities, self-help groups, milieu therapy, and sensitivity training may be helpful ways to facilitate adjustment and the development of a positive self-image in the client.[12]

Kutner[8] states that "in the diagnostic work-up and medical treatment plan of the recently disabled patient, is is rather rare to include a listing of 'role disorders' accompanying the illness or injury. . . . They require not the cursory attention typically accorded them but specific and purposeful therapy." This statement has important implications for occupational therapy. The occupational therapist, concerned with the client's occupational performance in self-maintenance, work, play, and leisure roles, is the expert in role definition, role analysis, and role change. Indeed a list of "role disorders" should appear in the medical record contained in the occupational therapy reports. Kutner[8] suggests that milieu therapy may offer a solution for acquiring new roles, readapting old ones, and gaining the social and physical skills necessary to reach goals.

Milieu therapy is particularly appropriate for use by occupational therapists, since it uses environmental or residential settings as training ground for clients to practice social, interpersonal, and functional skills and to test their ability to deal with problems commonly encountered in the community. This approach to treatment has always been fundamental to occupational therapy practice.

The milieu therapy program engages the client in a variety of social encounters, both group and individual, and exposes the client to increasingly challenging problems. This same gradation can be applied to performance skills concomitantly. The experiences are structured to test social competence, judgment, problem-solving ability, and social responsibility.

The major therapeutic objective of milieu therapy is the maintenance of the achievements acquired in the rehabilitation program. It attempts to provide the client with the necessary social, psychological, and performance skills to overcome frustration, to deal effectively with new or risky social situations, to cope with rebuff or rejection, and to remain independent.

Most therapeutic efforts have been concentrated on physical restoration with the assumption that personal and social readjustment follow automatically when physical integrity is restored. When adjustment difficulties occur, it has been customary to call on social, psychological, and psychiatric services to deal with these special problems. In contrast, milieu therapy deals with the problems of adjustment to new or changed roles by structuring situations and environments to allow the client to adopt and test roles as part of the treatment process.[8]

The self-help group model is another approach to dealing with psychosocial adjustment to physical dysfunction. Jaques and Patterson[4] reviewed the growth and development of self-help groups in this country and describe their effectiveness in the aid and rehabilitation of their members. The self-help group is one that provides aid for each group member around specific problems or goals. Positive benefits to members of self-help groups include (1) gaining information and knowledge about the dysfunction or the problem, (2) learning coping skills from group members who are living successfully with the condition, (3) gaining motivation and support through communication with others who have similar experiences, (4) modeling the successful problem-solving behaviors of group members, (5) evaluating one's own progress, (6) belonging to and identifying with a group, and (7) finding self-help in a situation of mutual concern. The mutual aid or self-help group is an excellent means of maintaining rehabilitation gain and preventing deterioration of function. It provides modeling by members who are coping with stigma and problems of functioning and reintegrating life roles.

Certain operational assumptions are characteristic of the self-help approach. Individuals with shared problems come together. All group members maintain the status of peer relationships. Peers come together expecting to help themselves or one another. Behavior change is expected in each person at his own pace. Group members identify with the program, are committed to it, and practice its principles in daily life. There are regularly scheduled group meetings, but peers are available to one another as needed outside of group meetings. This allows for both individual and group modes of contact. The group process consists of acknowledging, revealing, and relating problems; receiving and giving feedback; and sharing hopes, experiences, encouragement, and criticism. Members are responsible for themselves and their behavior. Leadership develops and changes within the group on the basis of giving and receiving help. Status comes from giving and receiving help effectively.

Many persons who were not helped in professional relationships and experiences turned to and received aid in self-help groups, which arose to meet needs that professionals could not meet. The professional process and self-help group models can share experiences with one another under certain conditions. The professional must meet the conditions of common problems, peer relationship, and mutual aid and those professionals who cannot meet these conditions can only act as visitors or observers. A professional can act as a consultant or speaker to self-help groups if invited to do so by the group. However, professional therapeutic skills cannot be used as such inside the self-help group.[4]

The self-help group model or some modification of it has application in occupational therapy. It may have most potential for use in long-term rehabilitation programs, extended care facilities, or community day-care programs. Self-help groups could be initiated out of the common needs of the clients in the program. The focus on solving problems in functional performance can provide a safe area for sharing. Ultimately as group relationships are cemented and mutual support is achieved, group members may move freely to emotional and social concerns and problems of community reintegration. The occupational therapist and other concerned professionals could act as consultants, invited speakers, or group members if the necessary conditions outlined previously are met.

Summary

The occupational therapy program for clients with physical dysfunction must include objectives and methods designed to facilitate psychosocial adjustment. The treatment approaches include using therapeutic relationships, structuring a therapeutic environment, and using group and dyadic interpersonal experiences. Activities selected should aid the client in adjusting to the physical dysfunction and restructuring his life-style to achieve the maximum independence possible.

Occupational therapy uses methods that demand the action and involvement of the client in the rehabilitation process. In the initial stages of rehabilitation when depression and denial are present and ego strength is poor, formal teaching or discussion groups fail because the client cannot integrate verbal material that deals with psychological exploration. Therefore social, recreational, special interest, and activity groups can be used to facilitate participation in rehabilitation tasks.

The group process may include discussion of needs and feelings, mutual support, and learning skills for dealing with the health care agency, its personnel, and the community. In dealing with those with physical dysfunctions the therapist should plan and structure group experiences that enhance the development of social skills, allow opportunities to test interaction strategies, discover assets and new or modified roles, and practice problem-solving behavior.

The occupational therapist can facilitate a collaborative treatment program through the use of individual and group processes. The client's involvement in treatment planning is critical because the client who uses his skills in planning, sharing, playing, socializing, and making judgments is more likely to want to pursue daily living skills and other modalities for physical and functional improvements.

If the client is involved in this kind of programming, it will not be necessary to point out that all skills have not been lost and that there are still assets and capabilities that can be used. There is usually a concomitant and gradual increase in self-esteem and progress toward healthy adjustment and accommodation to the physical dysfunction.[14]

REVIEW QUESTIONS

1. List some of the life changes that occur with the onset of physical dysfunction.
2. Describe the physical and psychological suffering that may be caused by illness or injury.
3. What are some of the negative and positive secondary gains that may result from physical dysfunction?
4. How do body image and self-valuation affect the process of adjustment to physical dysfunction?
5. How does personality structure or adjustment pattern correlate with specific types of physical disabilities?
6. Describe two typical attitudes of the nondisabled toward the disabled.
7. Describe how rehabilitation workers may be demonstrating prejudice and reduced social status to their clients.
8. Define "stigma."
9. List and briefly describe the steps in the process of adjustment to physical dysfunction.
10. List the defense mechanisms that the disabled person may use to cope with physical dysfunction, and describe how they may be manifested.
11. What are the psychosocial factors that the therapist must consider in treatment planning?
12. How do the reactions of family, friends, and rehabilitation personnel affect treatment?
13. What is the role and helping pattern that rehabilitation workers should assume to facilitate the adjustment process?
14. List four signs of adverse reactions of personnel to clients.
15. Describe at least two ways adverse reactions of personnel to clients can be handled.
16. List signs of pathological adjustment to physical dysfunction.
17. What are some steps that should be taken if pathological reactions are recognized?
18. List three types of group approaches to treatment, and describe how each can aid in the psychosocial adjustment to physical dysfunction.

EXERCISE

This is an empathy experience that is designed to help the student experience some of the personal and interpersonal reactions outlined in this chapter.

1. Select a wheelchair, walker, crutches, arm sling, or training arm prosthesis, and use the device as you would if you were so disabled.
2. Use the device for a minimum of 2 hours to tolerance.
3. Perform all of your usual daily living activities, and appear in public, perhaps to shop, eat in a restaurant, or look for an apartment, during the experiential period.
4. During the experience take notes and write a brief report describing your personal responses to people and objects, your affect and attitudes while performing daily living skills, and while in public, reactions of others to you, your attitude toward dependency, if and how others offered assistance, and architectural barriers and how they foster dependency.

REFERENCES

1. English, R.W.: Correlates of stigma toward physically disabled persons. In Marinelli, R.P., and Dell Orto, A.E., editors: The psychological and social impact of physical disability, New York, 1977, Springer Publishing Co., Inc.
2. Garner, H.H.: Somatopsychic concepts. In Marinelli, R.P., and Dell Orto, A.E., editors: The psychological and social impact of physical disability, New York, 1977, Springer Publishing Co., Inc.
3. Geis, H.J.: The problem of personal worth in the physically disabled patient. In Marinelli, R.P., and Dell Orto, A.E., editors: The psychological and social impact of physical disability, New York, 1977, Springer Publishing Co., Inc.
4. Jaques, M.E., and Patterson, K.: The self help group model: a review. In Marinelli, R.P., and Dell Orto, A.E., editors: The psychological and social impact of physical disability, New York, 1977, Springer Publishing Co., Inc.
5. Jeffress, E.J.: Psychological implications of physical disability, Videotape no. ITV 86 A and 86 B, San Jose State University, Instructional Resources Center.
6. Kerr, N.: Staff expectations for disabled persons: helpful or harmful. In Marinelli, R.P., and Dell Orto, A.E., editors: The psychological and social impact of physical disability, New York, 1977, Springer Publishing Co., Inc.
7. Kerr, N.: Understanding the process of adjustment to disability. In Stubbins, J., editor: Social and psychological aspects of disability, Baltimore, 1977, University Park Press.
8. Kutner, B.: Milieu therapy. In Marinelli, R.P., and Dell Orto, A.E., editors: The psychological and social impact of physical disability, New York, 1977, Springer Publishing Co., Inc.
9. Ladieu-Leviton, G., Adler, D.L., and Dembo, T.: Studies in adjustment to visible injuries: social acceptance of the injured. In Marinelli, R.P., and Dell Orto, A.E., editors: The psychological and social impact of physical disability, New York, 1977, Springer Publishing Co., Inc.
10. Marinelli, R.P., and Dell Orto, A.E., editors: The psychological and social impact of physical disability, New York, 1977, Springer Publishing Co., Inc.
11. Shontz, F.: Physical disability and personality. In Marinelli, R.P., and Dell Orto, A.E., editors: The psychological and social impact of physical disability, New York, 1977, Springer Publishing Co., Inc.
12. Siller, J.: Psychological situation of the disabled with spinal cord injuries. In Stubbins, J., editor: Social and psychological aspects of disability, Baltimore, 1977, University Park Press.
13. Simon, J.I.: Emotional aspects of physical disability, Am. J. Occup. Ther. **15**:408-410, 1971.
14. Versluys, H.: Psychological adjustment to physical disability. In Trombly, C.A., and Scott, A.D.: Occupational therapy for physical dysfunction, Baltimore, 1977, The Williams & Wilkins Co.
15. Willard, H.S., and Spackman, C.S., editors: Occupational therapy, ed. 4, Philadelphia, 1971, J.B. Lippincott Co.

SUPPLEMENTARY READING

Fidler, G.S., and Fidler, J.W.: Doing and becoming: purposeful action and self actualization, Am. J. Occup. Ther. **32**:30, 1978.
Garrett, J.F., editor: Psychological aspects of physical disability, Rehabilitation Services Series No. 210, Washington, D.C., U.S. Government Printing Office.
Goffman, E.: Stigma, Englewood Cliffs, N.J., 1963, Prentice-Hall, Inc.
Heard, C.: Occupational role acquisition: a perspective on the chronically disabled, Am. J. Occup. Ther. **31**:243, 1977.
Mann, W., Godfrey, M.E., and Dowd, E.T.: The use of group coun-

seling in the rehabilitation of spinal cord injured patients, Am. J. Occup. Ther. **27**:73, 1973.

Moore, J.W.: The initial interview and interaction analysis, Am. J. Occup. Ther. **31**:29, 1977.

Neistadt, M., and Baker, M.F.: A program for sex counseling the physically disabled, Am. J. Occup. Ther. **32**:646, 1978.

Sidman, J.M.: Sexual functioning and the physically disabled adult, Am. J. Occup. Ther. **31**:81, 1977.

Tyler, N.B., and Kogan, K.L.: The reduction of stress between mothers and their handicapped children, Am. J. Occup. Ther. **31**:151, 1977.

Tyler, N.B., Kogan, K.L., and Turner, P.: Interpersonal components of therapy with young cerebral palsied, Am. J. Occup. Ther. **28**:395, 1974.

Vargo, J.W.: Some psychological effects of physical disability, Am. J. Occup. Ther. **32**:31, 1978.

Chapter 2

Occupational therapy evaluation of physical dysfunction

Evaluation of physical dysfunction is a process of gathering data and assessing performance and performance components, that is, motor, sensory integrative, cognitive, emotional, and psychological functions, that underlie adequate performance. Its purpose is to aid the occupational therapist in developing treatment objectives and treatment strategies based on the problems identified in the evaluation process. Results of an evaluation may indicate a specific direction for occupational therapy intervention or that occupational therapy is inappropriate or not feasible for the particular client or at a given time.

The evaluation process includes collecting data from the client, the medical record, other professionals, friends, and family members. The process continues with the administration of specific occupational therapy assessment tools and concludes with an analysis and summary of the results and the identification of problems and assets in the client's life situation. Treatment objectives and methods are then selected on the basis of this information. It is important that the client be involved, to the extent possible, throughout the evaluation and treatment planning processes.

As the treatment program progresses, periodic reevaluation is essential to assess the effectiveness of treatment and to modify it to suit current client needs. This may involve the deletion of unattainable goals, the modification of goals partially or completely achieved, and the addition of new goals as progress is made.

Evaluation also provides the therapist with a specific and concrete method of determining her own effectiveness as a planner and administrator of treatment. It provides her with specific information that can be communicated to other members of the rehabilitation team. Further, careful evaluation can enhance the development of occupational therapy. If evaluation data are collected systematically, they may be used for the development of more standardized evaluation instruments and may contribute to a better understanding of which evaluation and treatment techniques are suitable and effective in occupational therapy practice.

If the occupational therapist is to be an effective evaluator, she must be knowledgeable about the dysfunction, its causes, course, and prognosis; be familiar with a variety of evaluation methods, their uses, and proper administration; and be able to select evaluation methods that are suitable to the client and his dysfunction. This means that an understanding of all the possible dysfunctional performance and performance components and the applicable treatment principles is essential. In addition the therapist must approach the client with openness and without preconceived ideas about his limitations or personality. She must have good observation skills and be able to enlist the trust of the client in a short period of time.[28]

METHODS OF EVALUATION
Medical records

Data gathered from the medical record are an important part of the evaluation process. The medical record can provide information on the diagnosis, prognosis, current treatment regime, social data, psychological data, and other rehabilitation therapies. Daily notes from nurses and physicians can give information about current medications and the client's reactions and responses to the hospital, the treatment regime, and persons in the treatment facility.

Ideally the occupational therapist should have had the opportunity to study the medical record before she sees the client to begin specific evaluation. This is not always possible, however, and it may mean that the therapist has to begin the evaluation without benefit of the information gleaned from the medical record.

The information serves as a good basis for selecting methods of evaluation of and even approach to the patient. It suggests the problem areas and helps the therapist focus attention on the relevant factors in the situation.[28]

Interview

The initial interview is a valuable step in the evaluation process. It is a time when the occupational therapist gathers information on how the client perceives his roles, dysfunction, needs, and goals and a time when the client can learn about the role of the occupational therapist and occupational therapy in his rehabilitation program.[28] An important outcome of the initial interview is the beginning development of rapport and trust between therapist and client.

The initial interview should occur in an environment that is quiet and ensures privacy. A specified period of time, known to interviewer and client at the outset, should be set aside for the interview. The first few minutes of the interview may be devoted to getting acquainted and orienting the client to the occupational therapy area as well as the role and goals of occupational therapy in the treatment facility.

The therapist should have the interview planned by knowing what information is to be acquired and having some specific questions prepared. As the interview progresses, there should be an opportunity for the client to ask questions as well. The therapist must have good listening and observation skills to glean the greatest amount of information from the interview.

During the initial or opening phase of the interview, the therapist should explain her role, the purpose of the interview, and how the information is to be used. As the interview progresses, the therapist may seek the desired information by asking appropriate questions and guiding the responses and ensuing discussion so that they remain on relevant topics. The occupational therapist may wish to seek information about the client's family and friends, community and work roles, educational and work histories, leisure and social interests and activities, and the living situation to which he will return. Information about the way the client spends and manages time is important. This can be gleaned by using a tool such as the daily schedule described later in this chapter or the activity configuration described by Watanabe.[31]

The therapist should sense the client's attitude toward his dysfunction, implicitly or explicitly, during the interview. The client should have an opportunity to express what he sees as his primary problems and goals for rehabilitation. These may differ substantially from the therapist's judgment and must be given careful consideration when therapist and client reach the point of setting treatment objectives together.

The interview can be concluded with a summary of the major points covered, information gained, an estimate of problems and assets, and plans for further occupational therapy evaluation. The occupational therapist will probably need to take notes of or record the initial interview. The client should be advised of this in advance, understand the reasons why, know the uses to which the material will be put, and be allowed to view or listen to the record if he so desires.[28]

Observation

Some aspects of the evaluation of the client will be based on the occupational therapist's observation of the client during the interview and the evaluation procedures that follow. As treatment commences, the occupational therapist will be basing some of the reevaluation of the client on observations during treatment. The occupational therapist can gain much information by observing the client as he approaches or is approached. What is his posture, mode of ambulation, and gait pattern? How is he dressed? Is there obvious motor dysfunction? Are there apparent musculoskeletal deformities? What is the facial expression, tone of voice, and manner of speech? How are the hands held and used?

Besides these observations that can be made during the first few minutes of the initial contact with the client, occupational therapists use observation to evaluate performance of activities of daily living, vocational potential, and cognitive functions. Evaluation of these skills is usually carried out by observing the client perform them in real or simulated environments to determine the client's level of independence, speed, skill, need for special equipment, and feasibility for further training.

Formal evaluation procedure

Several formal modes of evaluation are used in occupational therapy. There are procedures with a systematic and widely accepted method of administration. Among these are the manual muscle test, joint range of motion measurement, hand function evaluations, coordination tests, motor evaluation of hemiplegia, and sensory evaluation. Standardized tests are also used by occupational therapists. Examples of some of these are the Jebsen-Taylor Test of Hand Function,[17] the Minnesota Rate of Manipulation Test, the Lincoln-Oseretsky Motor Development Scale, the Marianne Frostig Development Test of Visual Perception, and the Southern California Sensory Integration Tests. Hopkins and Smith[28] list these and several other standardized tests and their sources.

Motor evaluation
EVALUATION OF JOINT RANGE OF MOTION

Joint measurement is a primary evaluation procedure for those physical dysfunctions that could cause limitation of joint motion, for example, arthritis, fractures, burns, and hand trauma. Range of motion (ROM) is the arc of motion through which a joint passes. Passive ROM is the arc of motion through which the joint passes when moved by an outside force. Active ROM is the arc of motion through which the joint passes when moved by the muscles acting on the joint. The instrument used for measuring ROM is the goniometer.

The purposes for measuring ROM are to (1) determine limitations that interfere with function or may produce deformity, (2) determine additional range needed to increase functional capacity or reduce deformity, (3) keep a record of progression or regression, (4) measure progress objectively, (5) determine appropriate treatment goals, (6) select appropriate treatment modalities, positioning techniques, and other strategies to reduce limitations, and (7) determine the need for splints and assistive devices.

Principles of joint measurement

The evaluator should know the average normal ROM, how the joint moves, and how to position self, client, and joints for measurement. Before measuring, the evaluator should ask the client to move the part and observe the movement. The evaluator should move the part passively to see and feel how the joint moves.

Formal joint measurement is *not* necessary with every client. ROM may be quickly checked out by eye by using active ROM or by putting all joints through passive ROM. Normal ROM varies from one person to the next. Establish norms for each individual by measuring the uninvolved part if possible. If not possible use average ranges listed in the literature. Check records and interview the client for the presence of fused joints and other limitations due to old injuries. Do not try to force joints when resistance is met on passive ROM. Be aware that pain may limit ROM and crepitation may be heard on movement in some conditions.

General procedure—180° method of measurement

1. Have client comfortable and relaxed in appropriate position.
2. Explain and demonstrate to client what you are going to do, why, and how you expect him to cooperate.
3. Uncover joint to be measured.
4. Stabilize joints proximal to joint being measured.
5. Move part passively through available ROM to observe available ROM and get a sense of joint mobility.
6. At starting position place axis of goniometer over axis of joint. Place stationary bar on stationary bone and movable bar on moving bone. Avoid goniometer dial going off

semicircle by always facing curved side away from direction of motion.
7. Record number of degrees at starting position and remove goniometer. Do not attempt to hold goniometer in place while moving joint through ROM.
8. Evaluator should hold part securely above and below joint being measured and *gently* move joint through available ROM to determine full *passive* ROM. *Do not force joints.* Watch for signs of pain and discomfort. Unless otherwise indicated it is passive ROM that should be measured.
9. Reposition goniometer and record number of degrees at final position.
10. Remove goniometer and gently place part in resting position.

Recording results of measurements

The evaluator should record the number of degrees at the starting position and the number of degrees at the final position after the joint has passed through the maximum possible arc of passive motion. Normal ROM always starts at 0° and increases toward 180°. A limitation is indicated if the starting position is not 0°. For example:
1. Elbow.
    Normal: 0° to 140°
    Extension limitation: 15° to 140°
    Flexion limitation: 0° to 110°
2. Abnormal hyperextension of the elbow may be recorded by indicating the number of degrees of hyperextension *before* the 0° starting position.
    Normal: 0° to 140°
    Abnormal hyperextension: 20° to 0° to 140°
3. There are alternate methods of recording ROM. The evaluator is advised to learn and adopt the particular method required by the health care facility. One method is to record limitations in minus degrees of motion. For example, elbow extension limitation would be recorded as −15°/140°.

A sample of a form for recording ROM measurements is shown in Fig. 2-1.

Average normal ROM is listed in Table 1. It should be noted that movements of the shoulder (glenohumeral) joint are accompanied by scapula movement as outlined. Glenohumeral joint motion is highly dependent on scapula mobility, which gives the shoulder its flexibility and wide ranges of motion. Although it is not possible to measure scapula movement with the goniometer, the evaluator should assess scapula mobility before proceeding with shoulder joint measurements. If the scapula musculature is in a state of spasticity or contracture and the shoulder joint is moved into ranges of motion that require scapula mobility (for example, above 90° of flexion or abduction), joint damage can result.

When joint measurements may be performed in more than one position, for example, as in shoulder internal and external rotation, the evaluator should note on the record in which position the measurement was taken.

JOINT RANGE MEASUREMENTS

Patient's name_____ Chart no._____

Date of birth_____ Age_____ Sex_____

Diagnosis_____ Date of onset_____

Disability_____

3	LEFT 2	1	SHOULDER	1	RIGHT 2	3
			Flexion 0 to 160			
			Extension 0 to 60			
			Abduction 0 to 160			
			Internal rotation 0 to 80			
			External rotation 0 to 80			

			ELBOW AND FOREARM			
			Flexion 0 to 140			
			Supination 0 to 80			
			Pronation 0 to 80			

			WRIST			
			Flexion 0 to 75			
			Extension 0 to 70			
			Ulnar deviation 0 to 30			
			Radial deviation 0 to 20			

			THUMB			
			MP flexion 0 to 50			
			IP flexion 0 to 90			
			Abduction 0 to 50			

			FINGERS			
			MP flexion 0 to 90			
			MP hyperextension 0 to 45			
			PIP flexion 0 to 110			
			DIP flexion 0 to 80			
			Abduction 0 to 25			

			HIP			
			Flexion 0 to 120			
			Extension 0 to 30			
			Abduction 0 to 40			
			Adduction 0 to 35			
			Internal rotation 0 to 40			
			External rotation 0 to 40			

			KNEE			
			Flexion 0 to 135			

			ANKLE AND FOOT			
			Plantar flexion 0 to 45			
			Dorsiflexion 0 to 20			
			Inversion 0 to 35			
			Eversion 0 to 20			

Fig. 2-1. Form for recording joint ROM measurement.

Table 1. Average normal ROM

Joint	ROM	Associated girdle motion	Joint	ROM
Shoulder			**Elbow**	
Flexion	0° to 160°	Abduction, lateral tilt, slight elevation, slight upward rotation	Flexion	0° to 140°
			Extension	0°
Extension	0° to 60°	Depression, adduction, upward tilt	**Forearm**	
Abduction	0° to 160°	Upward rotation, elevation	Pronation	0° to 80°
Adduction	0°	Depression, adduction, downward rotation	Supination	0° to 80°
Horizontal abduction	0° to 40°	Adduction, reduction of lateral tilt	**Wrist**	
Horizontal adduction	0° to 130°	Abduction, lateral tilt	Flexion	0° to 75°
Internal rotation	0° to 80°	Abduction, lateral tilt	Extension	0° to 70°
External rotation	0° to 80°	Adduction, reduction of lateral tilt	Radial deviation (abduction)	0° to 20°
			Ulnar deviation (adduction)	0° to 30°
			Fingers*	
			MP flexion	0° to 90°
			MP hyperextension	0° to 45°
			PIP flexion	0° to 110°
			DIP flexion	0° to 80°
			Abduction	0° to 25°
			Thumb*	
			DIP flexion	0° to 90°
			MP flexion	0° to 50°
			Adduction, radial and palmar	0°
			Palmar abduction	0° to 50°
			Radial abduction	0° to 50°
			Opposition	
			Hip	
			Flexion	0° to 120° (bent knee)
			Extension	0° to 30°
			Abduction	0° to 40°
			Adduction	0° to 35°
			Internal rotation	0° to 40°
			External rotation	0° to 40°
			Knee	
			Flexion	0° to 135°
			Ankle and foot	
			Plantar flexion	0° to 40°
			Dorsiflexion	0° to 20°
			Inversion	0° to 35°
			Eversion	0° to 20°

*DIP—distal interphalangeal; MP—metacarpophalangeal; PIP—proximal interphalangeal.

Procedure for joint measurement
DIRECTIONS FOR JOINT MEASUREMENT—180° SYSTEM
Upper extremity[1,2,4]

Shoulder
  Flexion—0° to 160° (Fig. 2-2)
    POSITION OF THE SUBJECT: Seated or supine with humerus
      in external rotation.
    POSITION OF GONIOMETER: Axis is in center of humeral
      head just distal to acromion process on the lateral aspect
      of humerus. Stationary bar is parallel to trunk, and mov-
      able bar is parallel to humerus.

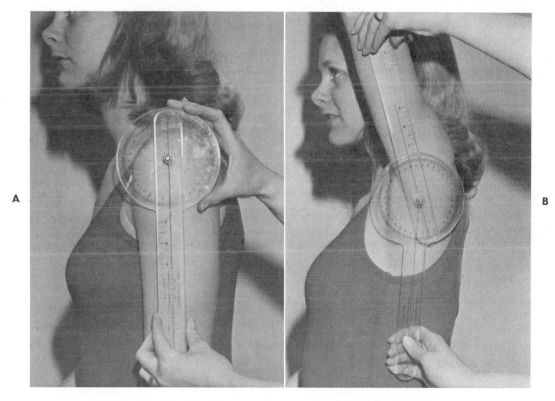

Fig. 2-2. Shoulder flexion. **A,** Starting position. **B,** Final position.

Extension—0° to 60° (Fig. 2-3)

   POSITION OF SUBJECT: Seated or prone with no obstruction
     behind humerus and humerus in internal rotation.

   POSITION OF GONIOMETER: Same as for flexion.

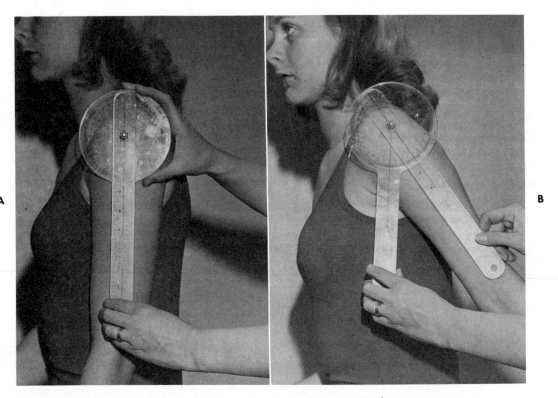

A   B

Fig. 2-3. Shoulder extension. **A**, Starting position. **B**, Final position.

Abduction—0° to 160° (Fig. 2-4)

POSITION OF SUBJECT: Seated or prone with humerus in external rotation. Measure on posterior surface.

POSITION OF GONIOMETER: Axis is approximately on acromion process on posterior surface of shoulder. Stationary bar is parallel to trunk, and movable bar is parallel to humerus.

Internal rotation—0° to 80° (Fig. 2-5)

POSITION OF SUBJECT: Seated with humerus adducted against trunk, elbow at 90°, and forearm at midposition and perpendicular to body.

ALTERNATE POSITION: (Fig. 2-6). Seated with humerus abducted to 90°, elbow flexed to 90°, and forearm parallel to floor.

POSITION OF GONIOMETER: Axis on olecranon process and stationary bar and movable bar parallel to forearm.

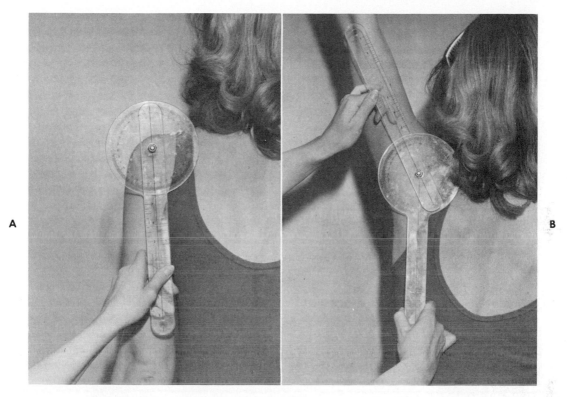

Fig. 2-4. Shoulder abduction. **A**, Starting position. **B**, Final position.

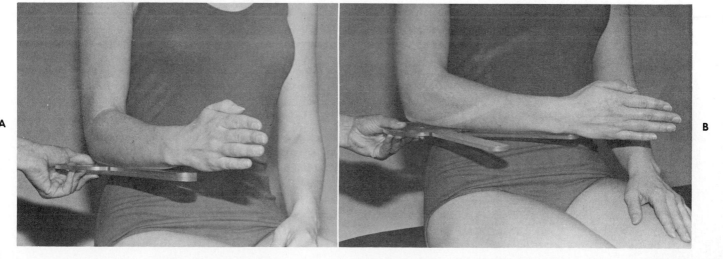

Fig. 2-5. Shoulder internal rotation. **A**, Starting position. **B**, Final position.

External rotation—0° to 80° (Fig. 2-7)
POSITION OF SUBJECT AND GONIOMETER: Same as for internal rotation.

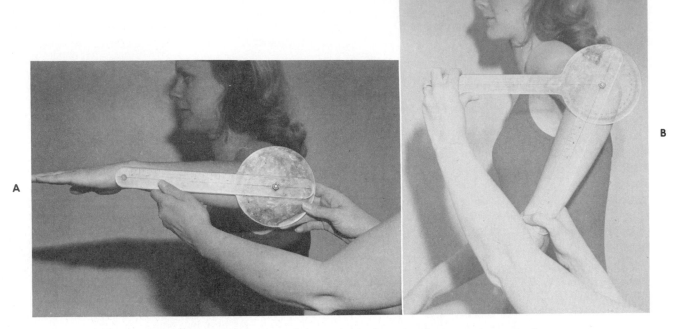

Fig. 2-6. Shoulder internal rotation, alternate method. **A,** Starting position. **B,** Final position.

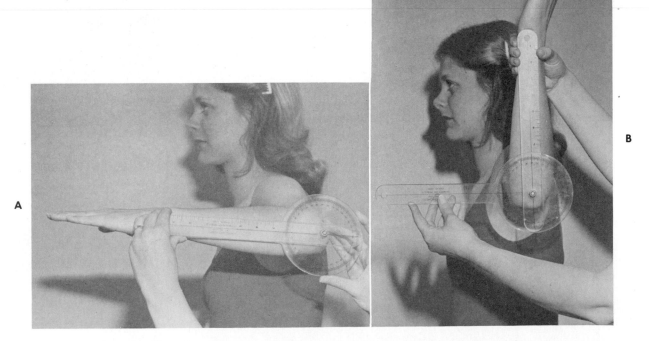

Fig. 2-7. Shoulder external rotation, alternate method. **A,** Starting position. **B,** Final position.

Elbow

Extension to *flexion*—0° to 140° (Fig. 2-8)

   POSITION OF SUBJECT: Standing, sitting, or supine with humerus adducted and externally rotated and forearm supinated.

   POSITION OF GONIOMETER: Axis is placed near lateral epicondyle of humerus approximately at base of elbow crease. Stationary bar is parallel to midline of humerus and movable bar is parallel to radius.

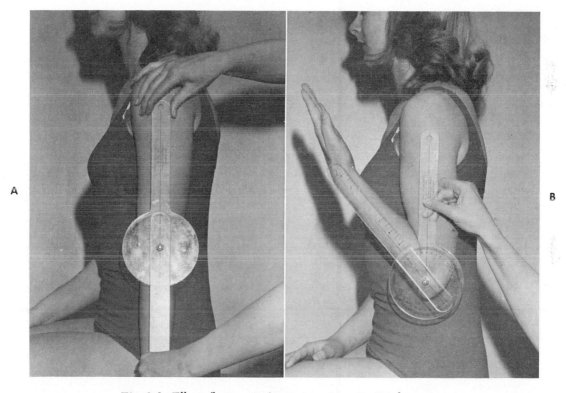

Fig. 2-8. Elbow flexion. **A,** Starting position. **B,** Final position.

Forearm

Supination—0° to 80° (Fig. 2-9)

POSITION OF SUBJECT: Seated or standing with humerus adducted, elbow at 90°, and forearm in midposition. Place pencil in hand so it is held by subject perpendicularly to floor.

POSITION OF GONIOMETER: Axis is at midpoint on the proximal phalanx of middle finger, and stationary bar is perpendicular to floor. Movable bar is parallel to pencil.

ALTERNATE METHOD: (Fig. 2-10). Subject is positioned same but without pencil in hand. Axis of goniometer is at ulnar border of volar aspect of wrist. Movable bar is resting against volar aspect of wrist, and stationary bar is perpendicular to floor.

Pronation—0° to 80° (Fig. 2-11)

POSITION OF SUBJECT AND GONIOMETER: Same as for supination.

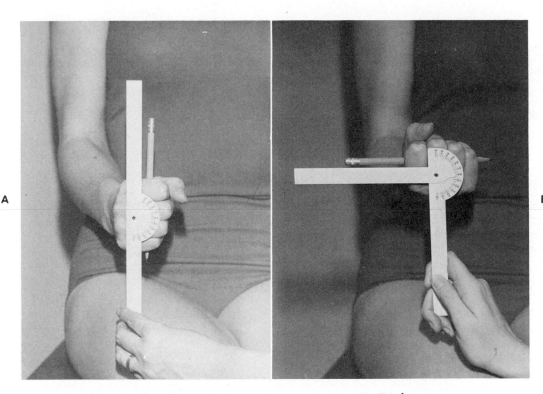

Fig. 2-9. Forearm supination. **A,** Starting position. **B,** Final position.

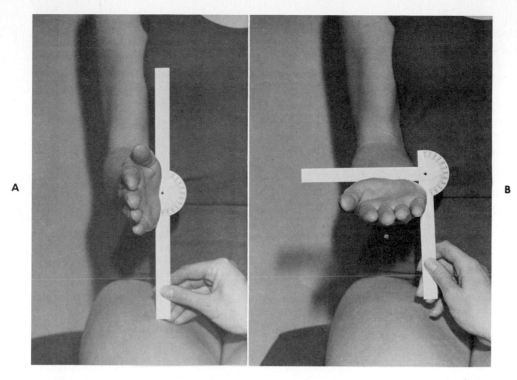

Fig. 2-10. Supination, alternate method. **A,** Starting position. **B,** Final position.

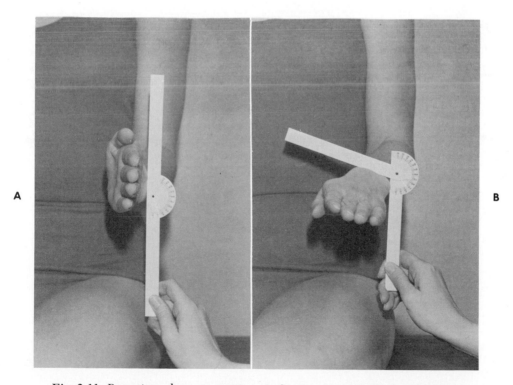

Fig. 2-11. Pronation, alternate position. **A,** Starting position. **B,** Final position.

Wrist

Flexion—0° to 75° (Fig. 2-12)

POSITION OF SUBJECT: Seated with forearm in midposition and hand and forearm resting on table on ulnar border.

POSITION OF GONIOMETER: Axis is on lateral aspect of wrist just distal to radial styloid in anatomical snuff box. Stationary bar is parallel to radius, and movable bar is parallel to metacarpal of index finger.

Extension—0° to 70° (Fig. 2-13)

POSITION OF SUBJECT AND GONIOMETER: Same as for wrist flexion.

Ulnar deviation—0° to 30° (Fig. 2-14)

POSITION OF SUBJECT: Seated with forearm pronated and palm of hand resting flat on table surface.

POSITION OF GONIOMETER: Axis is on dorsum of wrist at base of third metacarpal. Stationary bar is parallel to center of pronated forearm, and movable bar is parallel to third metacarpal.

Radial deviation—0° to 20° (Fig. 2-15)

POSITION OF SUBJECT AND GONIOMETER: Same as for ulnar deviation.

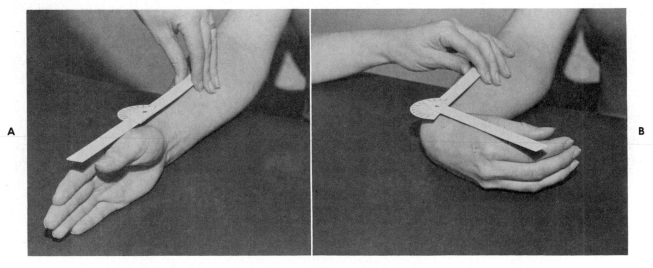

A   B

Fig. 2-12. Wrist flexion. **A,** Starting position. **B,** Final position.

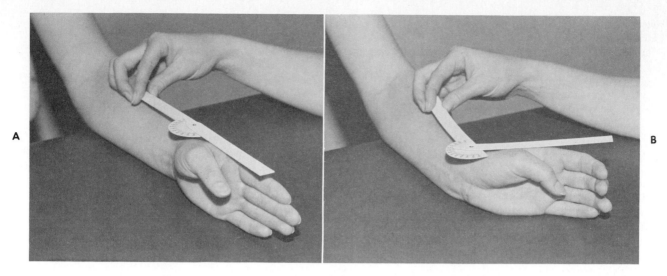

Fig. 2-13. Wrist extension. **A,** Starting position. **B,** Final position.

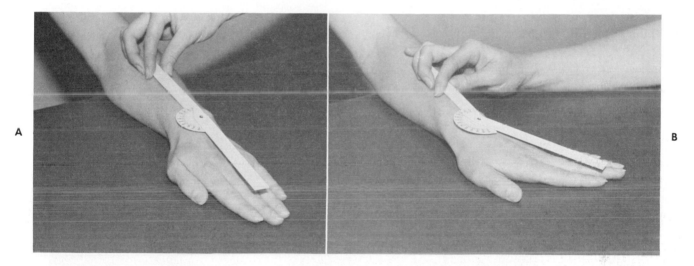

Fig. 2-14. Wrist ulnar deviation. **A,** Starting position. **B,** Final position.

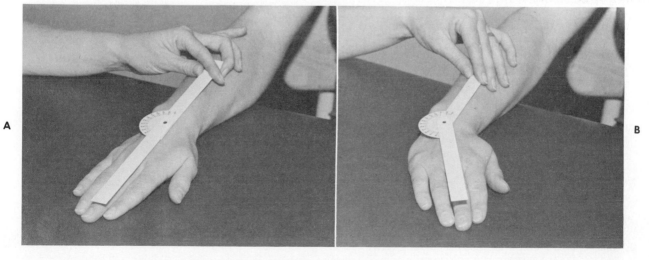

Fig. 2-15. Wrist radial deviation. **A,** Starting position. **B,** Final position.

Fingers

Metacarpophalangeal (MP) flexion—0° to 90° (Fig. 2-16)

POSITION OF SUBJECT: Seated with forearm in midposition, wrist at 0° neutral, and forearm and hand supported on firm surface on ulnar border.

POSITION OF GONIOMETER: Axis is centered on top of middle of MP joint. Stationary bar is on top of metacarpal, and movable bar is on top of proximal phalanx.

MP hyperextension—0° to 45° (Fig. 2-17)

POSITION OF SUBJECT: Seated with forearm in midposition, wrist at 0° neutral, and forearm and hand supported on a firm surface on ulnar border.

POSITION OF GONIOMETER: Axis is over lateral aspect of MP joint of index finger. Stationary bar is parallel to metacarpal, and movable bar is parallel to proximal phalanx. Fifth finger MP joint may be measured similarly. ROM of third and fourth fingers can be estimated by comparison.

MP abduction—0° to 25° (Fig. 2-18)

POSITION OF SUBJECT: Seated with forearm pronated and hand palm down, resting on firm surface. Fingers straight.

POSITION OF GONIOMETER: Axis is centered over MP joint being measured. Stationary bar is over corresponding metacarpal, and movable bar is over corresponding proximal phalanx.

Proximal interphalangeal (PIP) flexion—0° to 110° (Fig. 2-19)

POSITION OF SUBJECT: Seated with forearm in midposition, wrist at 0° neutral, and forearm and hand supported on a firm surface on ulnar border.

POSITION OF GONIOMETER: Axis is centered on dorsal surface of PIP joint being measured. Stationary bar is placed over proximal phalanx, and movable bar is over distal phalanx.

Distal interphalangeal (DIP) flexion—0° to 80° (Fig. 2-20)

POSITION OF SUBJECT: Seated with forearm in midposition, wrist at 0° neutral, and forearm and hand supported on the ulnar border on a firm surface.

POSITION OF GONIOMETER: Axis is on dorsal surface of DIP joint. Stationary bar is over middle phalanx, and movable bar is over distal phalanx.

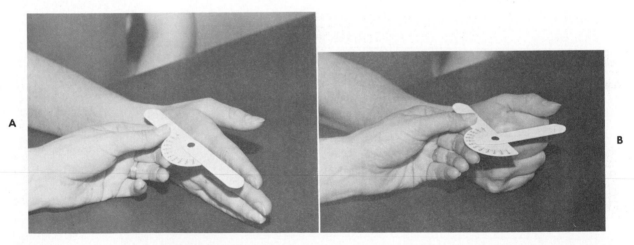

Fig. 2-16. MP flexion. **A,** Starting position. **B,** Final position.

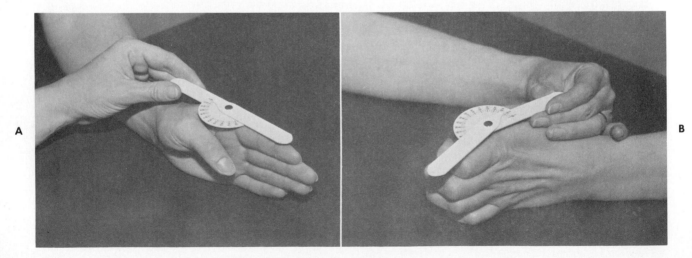

Fig. 2-17. MP hyperextension. **A,** Starting position. **B,** Final position.

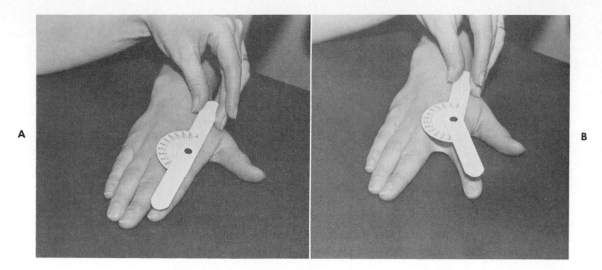

Fig. 2-18. MP abduction. **A,** Starting position. **B,** Final position.

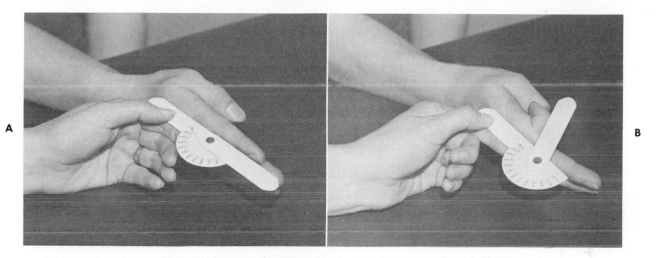

Fig. 2-19. PIP flexion. **A,** Starting position. **B,** Final position.

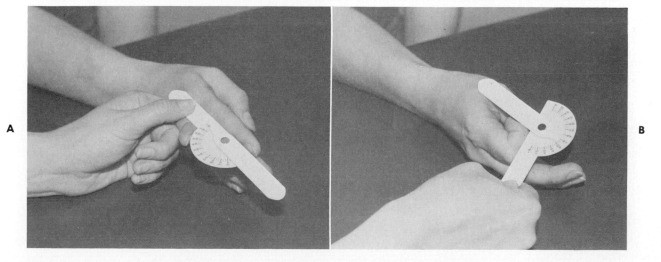

Fig. 2-20. DIP flexion. **A,** Starting position. **B,** Final position.

Thumb

MP flexion—0° to 50° (Fig. 2-21)

POSITION OF SUBJECT: Same as described for PIP and DIP finger flexion, but forearm is in partial supination.

POSITION OF GONIOMETER: Axis is on dorsal surface of MP joint. Stationary bar is over thumb metacarpal, and movable bar is over proximal phalanx.

Interphalangeal (IP) flexion—0° to 90° (Fig. 2-22)

POSITION OF SUBJECT: Same as described for PIP and DIP finger flexion.

POSITION OF GONIOMETER: Axis is on dorsal surface of IP joint. Stationary bar is over proximal phalanx, and movable bar is over distal phalanx.

Radial abduction (carpometacarpal [CMC] extension)—0° to 50° (Fig. 2-23)

POSITION OF SUBJECT: Seated with forearm pronated and hand palm down, resting flat on firm surface.

POSITION OF GONIOMETER: Axis is over CMC joint at base of thumb metacarpal. Stationary bar is parallel to radius, and movable bar is parallel to thumb metacarpal.

Palmar abduction—0° to 50° (Fig. 2-24)

POSITION OF SUBJECT: Seated with forearm at 0° midposition, wrist at 0°, and forearm and hand resting on ulnar border.

POSITION OF GONIOMETER: Axis is over CMC joint at base of thumb metacarpal. Stationary bar is over radius, and movable bar is over thumb metacarpal.

OPPOSITION (Fig. 2-25): Deficits in opposition may be recorded by measuring distance between pad of the thumb and pad of fifth finger with a centimeter ruler.

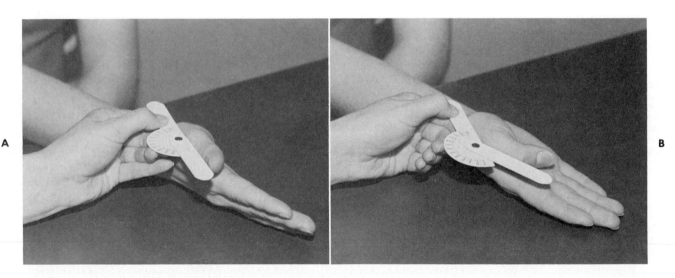

Fig. 2-21. Thumb MP flexion. **A,** Starting position. **B,** Final position.

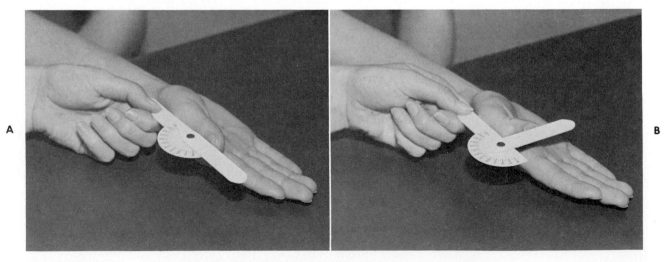

Fig. 2-22. Thumb IP flexion. **A,** Starting position. **B,** Final position.

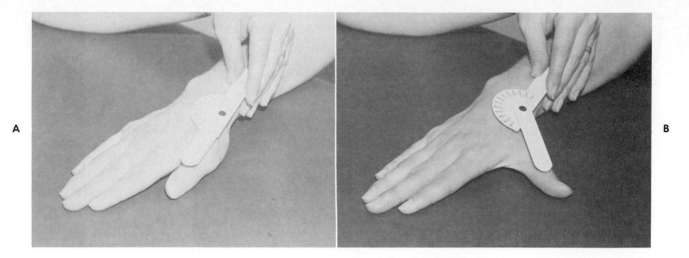

Fig. 2-23. Radial abduction. **A,** Starting position. **B,** Final position.

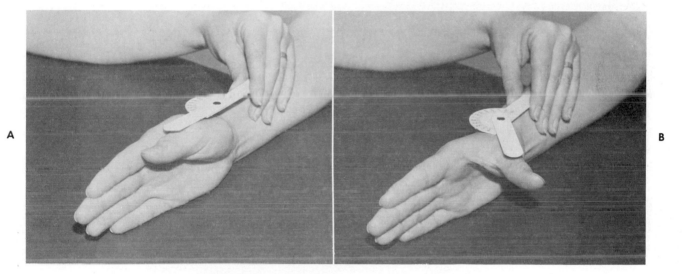

Fig. 2-24. Palmar abduction. **A,** Starting position. **B,** Final position.

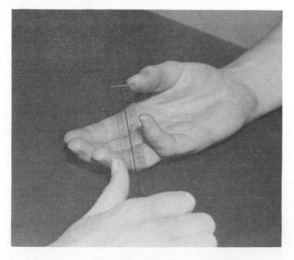

Fig. 2-25. Thumb opposition to fifth finger.

Lower extremity[14,29]

Hip

    Flexion—0° to 120° (Fig. 2-26)

        POSITION OF SUBJECT: Supine lying with hip and knee in extension.

        POSITION OF GONIOMETER: Axis is on lateral aspect of hip over greater trochanter of femur. Stationary bar is at middle of lateral aspect of lower trunk, and movable bar is parallel to long axis of femur on lateral aspect of thigh.

    Extension (hyperextension)—0° to 30° (Fig. 2-27)

        POSITION OF SUBJECT: Prone lying with hip and knee at 0° neutral extension.

        POSITION OF GONIOMETER: Same as for hip flexion.

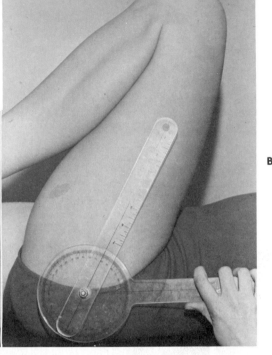

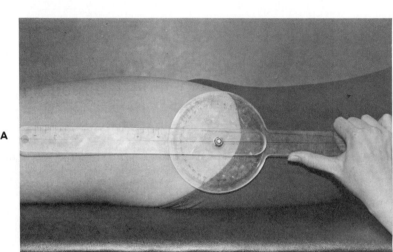

Fig. 2-26. Hip flexion. **A,** Starting position. **B,** Final position.

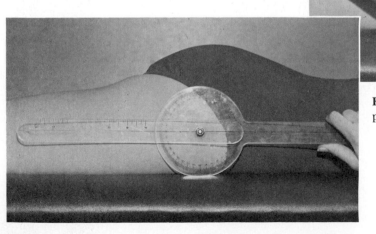

Fig. 2-27. Hip extension. **A,** Starting position. **B,** Final position.

Abduction—0° to 40° (Fig. 2-28)

POSITION OF SUBJECT: Supine lying with legs extended.

POSITION OF GONIOMETER: Axis is placed on anterior superior iliac spine. Stationary bar is placed on a line between two anterior superior iliac spines and movable bar is parallel to longitudinal axis of femur over anterior aspect of thigh. Note that starting position is at 90° for this measurement, and recording of measurement should be adjusted to accommodate to this exception to usual positioning of goniometer by subtracting 90° from total number of degrees obtained in arc of joint motion.

Adduction—0° to 35° (Fig. 2-29)

POSITION OF SUBJECT AND GONIOMETER: Same as for hip abduction.

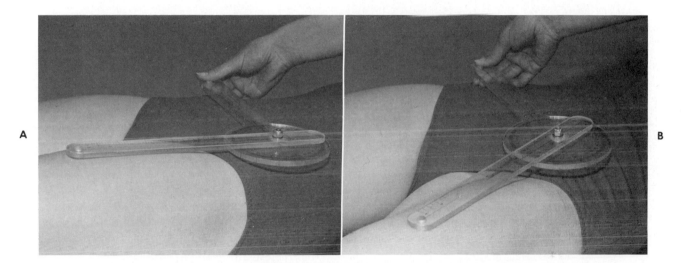

Fig. 2-28. Hip abduction. **A,** Starting position. **B,** Final position.

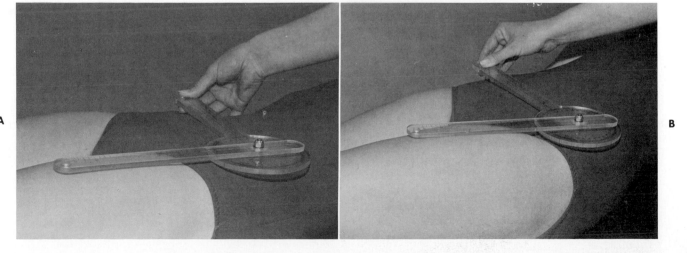

Fig. 2-29. Hip adduction. **A,** Starting position. **B,** Final position.

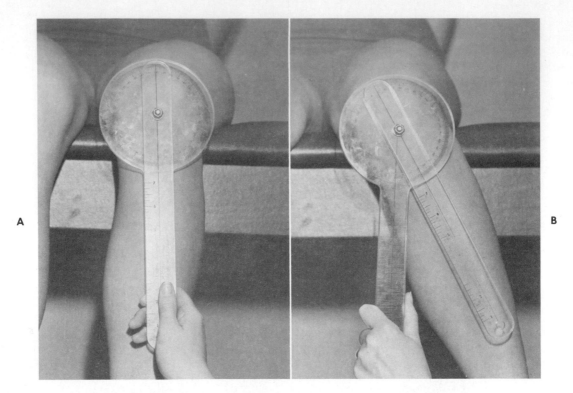

Fig. 2-30. Hip internal rotation. **A,** Starting position. **B,** Final position.

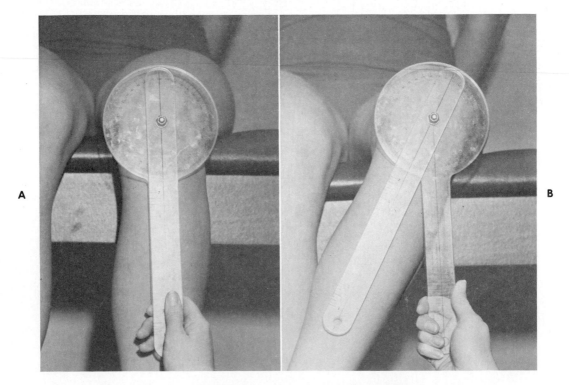

Fig. 2-31. Hip external rotation. **A,** Starting position. **B,** Final position.

Internal rotation—0° to 40° (Fig. 2-30)

POSITION OF SUBJECT: Seated or supine with hip and knee flexed to 90°.

POSITION OF GONIOMETER: Axis is on center of patella of knee. Stationary and movable bars are parallel to longitudinal axis of tibia on anterior aspect of lower leg. Stationary bar remains in this position, perpendicular to floor, while movable bar follows tibia as hip is rotated.

External rotation—0° to 40° (Fig. 2-31)

POSITION OF SUBJECT AND GONIOMETER: Same as for internal rotation.

Knee

Extension-flexion—0° to 135° (Fig. 2-32)

POSITION OF SUBJECT: Prone lying with legs extended.

POSITION OF GONIOMETER: Axis is centered on lateral aspect of knee joint at tibial condyle. Stationary bar is on lateral aspect of thigh to parallel longitudinal axis of femur. Movable bar is parallel to longitudinal axis of tibia on lateral aspect of leg.

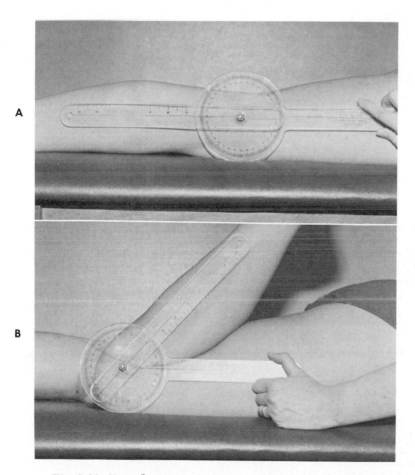

Fig. 2-32. Knee flexion. **A,** Starting position. **B,** Final position.

Ankle

Dorsiflexion—0° to 20° (Fig. 2-33)

POSITION OF SUBJECT: Supine lying or seated with knee flexed. Ankle is at 90° neutral position.

POSITION OF GONIOMETER: Axis is placed approximately 1 inch below medial melleolus. Stationary bar is parallel to midline of lower leg and movable bar parallel with first metatarsal. Note that measurement begins at 90° so that this must be subtracted when recording joint measurement.

Plantar flexion—0° to 45° (Fig. 2-34)

POSITION OF SUBJECT AND GONIOMETER: Same as for dorsiflexion.

Inversion—0° to 35° (Fig. 2-35)

POSITION OF SUBJECT: Sitting or supine with knee flexed and ankle in 90° neutral position.

POSITION OF GONIOMETER: Axis is placed at lateral border of foot near heel. Stationary bar is parallel to longitudinal axis of tibia on lateral aspect of leg. Movable bar is parallel to plantar surface of heel.

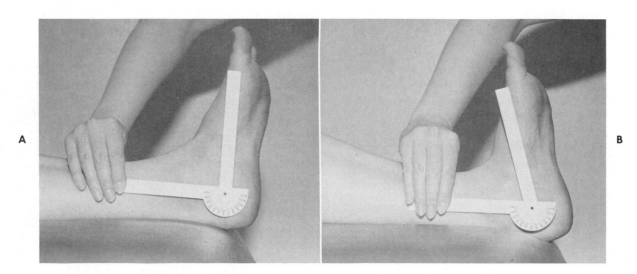

Fig. 2-33. Ankle dorsiflexion. **A,** Starting position. **B,** Final position.

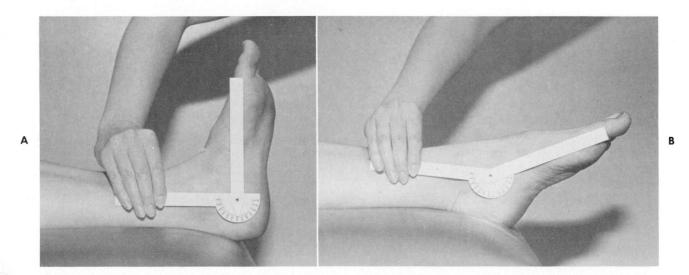

Fig. 2-34. Ankle plantar flexion. **A,** Starting position. **B,** Final position.

Eversion—0° to 20° (Fig. 2-36)

POSITION OF SUBJECT: Same as for inversion.

POSITION OF GONIOMETER: Axis is on medial border of foot just proximal to metatarsal-phalangeal joint. Stationary bar is parallel to longitudinal aspect of tibia on medial aspect of lower leg. Movable bar is parallel to plantar surface of sole. Note that measurements for inversion and eversion both begin at 90°. Therefore this amount must be subtracted from total when recording measurement.

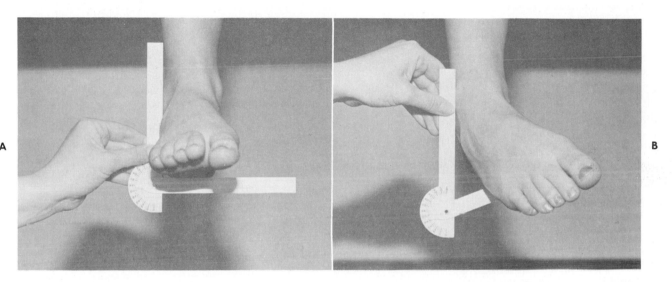

Fig. 2-35. Inversion. **A,** Starting position. **B,** Final position.

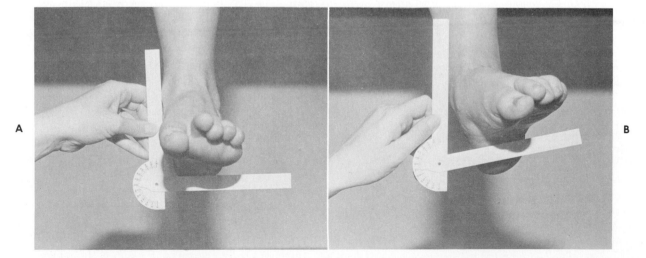

Fig. 2-36. Eversion. **A,** Starting position. **B,** Final position.

EVALUATION OF MUSCLE STRENGTH

The reader is referred to one of the following resources for instructions on specific manual muscle testing procedures:

Daniels, Lucille, and Worthingham, Catherine: Muscle testing: technique of manual examination, Philadelphia, 1980, W. B. Saunders Co.

Kendall, Henry O., Kendall, Florence P., and Wadsworth, Gladys E.: Muscles, testing, and function, Baltimore, 1971, The Williams & Wilkins Co.

Trombly, Catherine A., and Scott, Anna D.: Occupational therapy for physical dysfunction, Baltimore, 1977, The Williams & Wilkins Co.

The manual muscle test is a means of measuring the maximum contraction of muscles or muscle groups. It is used to determine amounts of muscle power and to record gains and losses in muscle power. The criteria used to measure strength are the amount of ROM through which the joint passes and the amount of resistance against which the muscle can contract.

Candidates for the muscle test are persons with lower motor neuron dysfunctions (LMN), orthopedic dysfunctions, and primary muscle diseases.

The manual muscle test cannot measure muscle endurance, that is, the number of times the muscle can contract at its maximum level, muscle coordination, or motor performance capabilities of the client. The manual muscle test cannot be used accurately with clients who have spasticity due to upper motor neuron (UMN) disorders. The reasons are that in these disorders muscles are often hypertonic, muscle tone and ability to perform movements are influenced by primitive reflexes and position of the head and body in space, and movements tend to occur in gross synergistic patterns that make it impossible for the client to isolate joint motions, which is demanded in the manual muscle testing procedures.[6,9,19] Methods for measuring motor performance of persons with UMN lesions will be reviewed later in this chapter.

Validity of the manual muscle test depends on careful observation of movement, careful and accurate palpation, correct positioning, consistency of procedure, and experience of the examiner.

General principles of manual muscle testing

Gravity factors influencing muscle function. A gravity-assisted movement is toward the floor and is never used in the testing procedure. The gravity-eliminated position and movement are parallel to the floor and are used with trace, poor, and poor plus grades. Movements against gravity are away from the floor or toward the ceiling and are used with grades fair, good, and normal. Movements against gravity and resistance are performed away from the floor with added manual or mechanical resistance and are used with fair plus (F+) to normal (N) grades.

Muscle grades. In manual muscle testing muscles are graded according to the following criteria:

Number grade	Word/letter grade	Definition
0	Zero (0)	No muscle contraction can be seen or felt.
1	Trace (T)	Contraction can be felt, but there is no motion.
2−	Poor minus (P−)	Part moves through an incomplete ROM with gravity eliminated.
2	Poor (P)	Part moves through a complete ROM with gravity eliminated.
2+	Poor plus (P+)	Part moves through incomplete ROM (less than 50%) against gravity or through complete ROM with gravity eliminated against slight resistance.
3−	Fair minus (F−)	Part moves through an incomplete ROM (more than 50%) against gravity.
3	Fair (F)	Part moves through complete ROM against gravity.
3+	Fair plus (F+)	Part moves through a complete ROM against gravity and slight resistance.
4	Good	Part moves through a complete ROM against gravity and moderate resistance.
5	Normal	Part moves through complete ROM against gravity and full resistance.

Procedure for muscle testing. Muscle testing should be performed according to a standard procedure to ensure accuracy and consistency of the examiner. First, the client should be *positioned* for the specific muscle test to be performed. If the examiner has some idea of the amount of available muscle strength, she can position the client for the estimated grade, that is, gravity-eliminated or against-gravity position. If the muscle power cannot be estimated, the client can be positioned for fair (F), then repositioned for lower muscle grade if necessary. The second step in the procedure is to *stabilize* the part proximal to the part being tested to isolate the muscle group and eliminate substitutions. Third, the examiner *observes* the movement after asking the client to move the part through the available ROM. During this visual observation the examiner *palpates* muscle fibers or tendons to see if the muscle being tested is contracting. After the client has moved the part through his available ROM, the examiner *resists* the motion while the client holds the part at the end of the joint excursion. Finally, the examiner *grades* the muscle strength according to the preceding definitions of muscle grades.

MUSCLE EXAMINATION

Patient's name_____ Chart no._____

Date of birth_____ Name of institution_____

Date of onset_____ Attending physician _____MD

Diagnosis:

LEFT							RIGHT		
				Examiner's initials					
				Date					
			NECK	Flexors	Sternocleidomastoid				
				Extensor group					
			TRUNK	Flexors					
				Rt. ext. obl. / Lt. int. obl. } Rotators { Lt. ext. obl. / Rt. int. obl.					
				Extensors	{ Thoracic group / Lumbar group				
				Pelvic elev.	Quadratus lumb.				
			HIP	Flexors	Iliopsoas				
				Extensors	Gluteus maximus				
				Abductors	Gluteus medius				
				Adductor group					
				External rotator group					
				Internal rotator group					
				Sartorius					
				Tensor fasciae latae					
			KNEE	Flexors	{ Biceps femoris / Inner hamstrings				
				Extensors	Quadriceps				
			ANKLE	Plantar flexors	{ Gastrocnemius / Soleus				
			FOOT	Invertors	{ Tibialis anterior / Tibialis posterior				
				Evertors	{ Peroneus brevis / Peroneus longus				
			TOES	MP flexors	Lumbricales				
				IP flexors (first)	Flex. digit. br.				
				IP flexors (second)	Flex. digit. l.				
				MP extensors	{ Ext. digit. l. / Ext. digit. br.				
			HALLUX	MP flexor	Flex. hall. br.				
				IP flexor	Flex. hall. l.				
				MP extensor	Ext. hall. br.				
				IP extensor	Ext. hall. l.				

Measurements:

Cannot walk   Date   Speech

Stands   Date   Swallowing

Walks unaided   Date   Diaphragm

Walks with apparatus   Date   Intercostals

KEY

5	N	Normal	Complete range of motion against gravity with full resistance.
4	G	Good*	Complete range of motion against gravity with some resistance.
3	F	Fair*	Complete range of motion against gravity.
2	P	Poor*	Complete range of motion with gravity eliminated.
1	T	Trace	Evidence of slight contractility. No joint motion.
0	0	Zero	No evidence of contractility.
	S or SS		Spasm or severe spasm.
	C or CC		Contracture or severe contracture.

*Muscle spasm or contracture may limit range of motion. A question mark should be placed after the grading of a movement that is incomplete from this cause.

Fig. 2-37. Muscle examination. (Adapted with the express permission and authority of the March of Dimes Birth Defects Foundation.)

Continued.

LEFT							RIGHT			
				Examiner's initials						
				Date						
				SCAPULA Abductor	Serratus anterior					
				Elevator	Upper trapezius					
				Depressor	Lower trapezius					
				Adductors	Middle trapezius					
					Rhomboids					
				SHOULDER Flexor	Anterior deltoid					
				Extensors	Latissimus dorsi					
					Teres major					
				Abductor	Middle deltoid					
				Horiz. abd.	Posterior deltoid					
				Horiz. add.	Pectoralis major					
				External rotator group						
				Internal rotator group						
				ELBOW Flexors	Biceps brachii					
					Brachioradialis					
				Extensor	Triceps					
				FOREARM Supinator group						
				Pronator group						
				WRIST Flexors	Flex. carpi rad.					
					Flex. carpi uln.					
				Extensors	Ext. carpi rad. l. & br.					
					Ext. carpi uln.					
				FINGERS MP flexors	Lumbricales					
				IP flexors (first)	Flex. digit. sub.					
				IP flexors (second)	Flex. digit. prof.					
				MP extensor	Ext. digit. com.					
				Adductors	Palmar interossei					
				Abductors	Dorsal interossei					
				Abductor digiti quinti						
				Opponens digiti quinti						
				THUMB MP flexor	Flex. poll. br.					
				IP flexor	Flex. poll. l.					
				MP extensor	Ext. poll. br.					
				IP extensor	Ext. poll. l.					
				Abductors	Abd. poll. br.					
					Abd. poll. l.					
				Adductor pollicis						
				Opponens pollicis						
				FACE:						

Additional data:

Fig. 2-37, cont'd. Muscle examination.

To perform manual muscle testing accurately the examiner should have a good working knowledge of muscles and their functions, the position of muscles, direction of muscle fibers, and their angle of pull on the joints. She should know the joints and their motions and the innervation of the muscles, be familiar with muscle testing procedures and know how to observe for and rule out substitutions during the test, and be able to palpate muscles accurately and estimate normal strength for each individual client. Fig. 2-37 is a sample of a form for recording muscle grades after specific manual muscle testing.

Functional muscle testing

It is not always necessary to perform a specific manual muscle test on a client referred for occupational therapy services. In some health care facilities the specific muscle testing is the responsibility of the physical therapy service. The occupational therapist may wish, then, to perform a quick functional muscle test to get a "feel" for the strength and motion capabilities of the client. In dysfunctions where muscle weakness is not a primary or significant symptom, it may not be important to perform discrete muscle testing, but a general estimate of strength is desirable and adequate to plan treatment and measure progress. In still other instances a quick functional muscle test may be performed to identify areas of significant weakness that deserve more discrete testing. Thus the functional muscle test may serve as a screening tool.

The functional muscle test should be performed while the client is comfortably seated in a sturdy chair or wheelchair.

In all of the tests the subject is allowed to complete the test motion before the examiner applies resistance. The resistance is applied at the end of the range of motion while the subject maintains the position and resists the force applied by the examiner. The therapist may make modifications in positioning to suit individual needs. As in the manual muscle test, the examiner should stabilize proximal parts and attempt to rule out substitutions. A functional muscle test of the upper extremities is outlined here. It is assumed that the reader is familiar with joint motions, their prime movers, and muscle grades before performing this test.

Functional muscle test

Scapular elevation (upper trapezius and levator scapula): Subject elevates shoulders, and examiner pushes down on shoulders into depression.

Scapular abduction (serratus anterior): With subject's arms positioned in 90° of elbow and shoulder flexion, examiner pushes at shoulder into scapular adduction.

Scapular adduction (middle trapezius and rhomboids): Subject extends shoulder and flexes elbow fully, producing scapular adduction. Examiner pushes at shoulder joint into scapular abduction.

Scapular depression (lower trapezius, latissimus dorsi): Subject extends arm down at side of body as if reaching to floor. Examiner attempts to push arm up at a point just proximal to elbow joint. Muscles act to stabilize scapula and prevent elevation.

Shoulder flexion (anterior deltoid and coracobrachialis): With subject's shoulder flexed to 90° and elbow flexed or extended, examiner pushes down on arm proximal to elbow into extension.

Shoulder extension (latissimus dorsi and teres major): Subject moves shoulder into full extension. Examiner pushes from behind at a point proximal to elbow into flexion.

Shoulder abduction (middle deltoid and supraspinatus): Subject abducts shoulder to 90° with elbow flexed or extended. Examiner pushes down on arm just proximal to elbow into adduction.

Shoulder horizontal adduction (pectoralis major, anterior deltoid): Subject crosses arms in front of chest. Examiner reaches from behind and attempts to pull arms back into horizontal abduction at a point just proximal to elbow.

Shoulder horizontal abduction (posterior deltoid, teres minor, infraspinatus): Subject moves arms from full horizontal adduction as just described to full horizontal abduction. Examiner pushes forward on arms just proximal to elbow into horizontal adduction.

Shoulder external rotation (infraspinatus and teres minor): Subject holds arm in 90° of shoulder abduction and 90° of elbow flexion, then externally rotates shoulder through available ROM. Examiner supports or stabilizes upper arm proximal to elbow and pushes from behind at dorsal aspect of wrist into internal rotation.

Shoulder internal rotation (subscapularis, teres major, latissimus dorsi, pectoralis major): Subject begins with arm as described for external rotation but performs internal rotation. Examiner supports or stabilizes upper arm as before and pulls up into external rotation at volar aspect of wrist.

Elbow flexion (biceps, brachialis): With forearm supinated and shoulder externally rotated subject flexes elbow from full extension. Examiner sits opposite subject and stabilizes upper arm against trunk while attempting to pull forearm into extension at volar aspect of wrist.

Elbow extension (triceps): With subject's upper arm supported in 90° of abduction (gravity-eliminated position) or 160° shoulder flexion (against-gravity position), he extends elbow from full flexion. Examiner pushes forearm into flexion at dorsal aspect of wrist.

Forearm supination (biceps, supinator): Upper arm is stabilized against trunk by subject or examiner. Elbow is flexed to 90°, and forearm is in full pronation. Subject supinates forearm. Examiner grasps distal forearm and attempts to rotate it into pronation.

Forearm pronation (pronator teres, pronator quadratus): Subject is positioned as described for forearm supination except forearm is in full supination. Subject pronates forearm. Examiner grasps distal forearm and attempts to rotate it into supination.

Wrist flexion (flexor carpi radialis, flexor carpi ulnaris, palmar-

is longus): Subject's forearm is supported on its dorsal surface on a tabletop or armrest. He moves hand up from tabletop, using wrist flexion. Examiner is seated next to or opposite subject and pushes on palm of hand, giving equal pressure on radial and ulnar sides into wrist extension or down toward tabletop.

Wrist extension (extensor carpi radialis longus and brevis, extensor carpi ulnaris): Subject's forearm is supported on a tabletop or armrest, resting on its volar surface. Hand is lifted from tabletop, using wrist extension. Examiner sits next to or opposite subject and pushes on dorsal aspect of palm, giving equal pressure at radial and ulnar sides into wrist flexion or down toward tabletop.

Finger MP flexion and IP extension (lumbricales and interossei): With forearm and hand supported on tabletop on dorsal surface, examiner stabilizes palm and subject flexes MP joints while maintaining extension of IP joints. Examiner pushes into extension with index finger across proximal phalanges or pushes on tip of each finger into IP flexion and MP extension.

Finger IP flexion (flexors digitorum profundus and sublimis): Subject is positioned as described for MP flexion. He flexes IP joints while maintaining extension of MP joints. Examiner attempts to pull fingers back into extension by hooking tips of her fingers with those of subject.

Finger MP extension (IP joints flexed) (extensor digitorum communis, extensor indicis proprius, extensor digiti minimi): Subject's forearm and hand are supported on a table surface resting on ulnar border. Wrist is stabilized by examiner in 0° neutral position. Subject moves MP joints from flexion to full extension (hyperextension) while keeping IP joints flexed. Examiner pushes fingers at PIP joints simultaneously into flexion.

Finger abduction (dorsal interossei, abductor digiti minimi): Subject's forearm is resting on volar surface on a table. Examiner may stabilize wrist in slight extension so that hand is raised slightly off supporting surface. Subject abducts fingers. Examiner attempts to push fingers into adduction two at a time. First, index finger and middle fingers are pushed together, then, ring finger and middle fingers, and finally, little finger and ring fingers. To give resistance examiner may use same two fingers on her own hand as are being tested to equalize force being given. Since these muscles are very small, they are easily overcome in normal hand if palmar prehension force of examiner is used to give resistance.

Finger adduction (palmar interossei): Subject is positioned as described for finger abduction. He adducts fingers tightly. Examiner attempts to pull fingers apart one at a time. First, index finger is pulled away from middle finger, then, ring finger is pulled away from middle finger, and finally, little finger is pulled away from the ring finger. In normal hand adducted finger "snaps" back into adducted position when examiner pulls it into abduction and lets go quickly. An alternate method would be for examiner to place her index finger between two of subject's fingers and have him adduct against it, thus estimating amount of force or pressure that subject is exerting.

Thumb MP and IP flexion (flexor pollicis brevis and flexor pollicis longus): Subject's forearm should be supported on a firm surface, with elbow flexed at 90° and forearm in 45° supination. Thumb is flexed across palm. Examiner should pull on tip of thumb into extension.

Thumb MP and IP extension (extensor pollicis brevis, and extensor pollicis longus): Subject is positioned same as for thumb MP and IP flexion. He extends thumb away from palm. Examiner pushes on tip of thumb into flexion.

Thumb palmar abduction (abductor pollicis longus and abductor pollicis brevis): Subject is positioned as described for thumb flexion and extension. He is asked to abduct thumb away from palm in a plane perpendicular to palm. Subject resists movement at metacarpal head into adduction.

Thumb adduction (adductor pollicis): Subject is positioned as for all other thumb movements. Thumb is adducted to palm. Examiner attempts to pull thumb into abduction at metacarpal head or proximal phalanx.

Opposition of thumb to fifth finger (opponens pollicis, opponens digiti minimi): Subject is positioned with elbow flexed to 90° and dorsal surface of forearm and hand resting on a tabletop or armrest. He opposes thumb to fifth finger, making pad-to-pad contact. Examiner attempts to pull fingers apart, applying force at metacarpal heads of both fingers.

Motor evaluation of hemiplegic patient

For the reasons stated earlier in the discussion on muscle testing, it is not appropriate for the manual muscle test to be used to measure motor function of hemiplegics. Brunnstrom[9] in *Movement Therapy in Hemiplegia* described an evaluation procedure that assesses muscle tone, stage of recovery, movement patterns, motor speed, and prehension patterns of the upper extremity. Landen and Amizich[19] described a functional muscle examination that assesses functional movement patterns that can be performed in a position of function, that is, standing or sitting. These two tests are summarized here. The reader is referred to the original sources for more detail.

Brunnstrom's hemiplegia evaluation[9]. The evaluation is based on the recovery stages after the onset of hemiplegia (Chapter 4). The test requires the client to perform motor acts that are graduated in complexity and require increasingly finer neuromuscular control. Thus the degree of recovery of the central nervous system can be evaluated.

Progress through the recovery stages is gradual, and signs of two stages may be apparent at any given time in the client's recovery. Since it is not possible to establish an absolute demarcation between one recovery stage and the next, the client may be classified as stages 2 and 3 or 3 and 4, for example. This indicates that he is progressing from one stage to the next. The upper extremity evaluation portion of the Hemiplegia Classification and Progress Record is presented in Fig. 2-38. The reader should refer to this while reading the directions for test administration, which have been summarized from *Movement Therapy in Hemiplegia.*

HEMIPLEGIA—CLASSIFICATION AND PROGRESS RECORD

Upper limb-test sitting

Name_____ Age_____ Date of onset_____ Side affected_____

Date

_____ Passive motion sense: Shoulder_____ Elbow_____

_____ Pronation-supination _____Wrist flexion-extension _____

_____ 1.   NO MOVEMENT INITIATED OR ELICITED _____

_____ 2.   SYNERGIES OR COMPONENTS FIRST APPEARING. Spasticity developing_____

_____   Flexor synergy_____

_____   Extensor synergy_____

_____ 3.   SYNERGIES OR COMPONENTS INITIATED VOLUNTARILY. Spasticity marked_____

	FLEXOR SYNERGY	ACTIVE JOINT RANGE		REMARKS
_____	Shoulder girdle Elevation_____			
_____	Retraction_____			
_____	Shoulder joint Hyperextension_____			
	Abduction_____			
	External rotation_____			
_____	Elbow Flexion_____			
_____	Forearm Supination_____			
	EXTENSOR SYNERGY			
_____	Shoulder Pectoralis major_____			
_____	Elbow Extension_____			
_____	Forearm Pronation_____			
_____ 4.	MOVEMENTS Hand to sacral			
	DEVIATING region____			
_____	FROM BASIC Raise arm forward-			
	SYNERGIES. horizontally____			
_____	Spasticity Pronate-supinate			
	decreasing elbow at 90°			
_____ 5.	RELATIVE Raise arm sideways-			
	INDEPENDENCE horizontally____			
_____	OF BASIC Raise arm			
	SYNERGIES. over head____			
_____	Spasticity Pronate-supinate			
	waning elbow extended___			
_____ 6.	MOVEMENT COORDINATION NEAR			
	NORMAL. Spasticity minimal_____			

Fig. 2-38. Hemiplegia classification and progress record. (From Brunnstrom, S.: Movement therapy in hemiplegia, New York, 1970, Harper & Row, Publishers, Inc.)

Continued.

HEMIPLEGIA—CLASSIFICATION AND PROGRESS RECORD

Upper limb-test sitting—cont'd

Name_____

Date_____

SPEED TESTS for Classes 4, 5, 6   Strokes per 5 seconds

Hand from	Normal			
lap to chin	Affected			
Hand from lap	Normal			
to opposite knee	Affected			

_____ Passive motion sense, digits_____

_____ Fingertip recognition_____

_____ Wrist stabilization for grasp   1. Elbow extended_____
                                          2. Elbow flexed_____

_____ Wrist flexion and extension   1. Elbow extended_____
_____ Fist closed   2. Elbow flexed_____

_____ Wrist circumduction _____

DIGITS

_____ Mass grasp_____ Dynamometer test   Normal_____lb.
                                                        Affected____lb.

_____ Mass extension_____

_____ Hook grasp (handbag, 2 lb.)_____

_____ Lateral prehension (card)_____

_____ Palmar prehension (pencil)_____

_____ Cylindrical grasp (small jar)_____

_____ Spherical grasp (ball) _____Catch_____ Throw_____

_____ Indiv. thumb movements hands in lap   1. Vertical movements_____
_____ Ulnar side down   2. Horizontal movements_____

_____ Individual finger movements_____

_____ Button and unbutton shirt   Using both hands_____
                                           Using affected hand only_____
_____ Other skilled activities_____

Fig. 2-38, cont'd. Hemiplegia classification and progress record.

Gross sensory testing. The sensory evaluation precedes the motor evaluation and includes assessment of passive motion sense and touch localization in the hand. Tests of passive motion sense of the shoulder, elbow, forearm, wrist, and fingers are carried out by procedures similar to those described in Section 2 of this chapter. Results are recorded on the first and second pages of the form (shown in Fig. 2-38, *A* and *B*).

Fingertip recognition is evaluated by asking the subject to localize touch stimuli to specific fingers. The subject is seated with forearms pronated and resting on a pillow in his lap. The test is given with the vision occluded after a rehearsal in full view. The palmar surface of the fingertips is lightly touched with a pencil eraser in a random sequence. The subject must indicate which finger is being touched. Results are recorded on the second page of the form (in Fig. 2-38, *B*).

Motor tests, upper extremity.[9] The subject is classified in stage 1 when no voluntary movement of the affected arm can be initiated. The examiner should move the limb passively through the synergy patterns (Chapter 13) and assess the degree of resistance to passive movement. The subject should be asked to attempt movement during these maneuvers. During recovery stage 1 the limb will be predominantly flaccid and will feel heavy, there will be little or no resistance to passive movement, and the subject will be unable to initiate or effect any movement voluntarily. At this time the subject is likely to be confined to bed and be too weak for extensive evaluation.

During recovery stage 2 spasticity begins to increase, and the limb synergies or some of their components may be evoked on voluntary effort or as associated reactions. The flexor synergy usually appears first.[9] The examiner may again move the limb passively, alternating between flexor and extensor synergy patterns. She should ask the subject to "help" in the movements. Thus it is possible to assess degree of spasticity and whether the subject's voluntary efforts are evoking any movement responses.

During recovery stage 3 spasticity is increased and may be marked. The limb synergies or some of their components are performed voluntarily. The subject may remain at this stage for a long period of time. Severely involved hemiplegics may never progress beyond it. The pectoralis major, pronators, and wrist and finger flexors may be very spastic, causing limited performance of their antagonists.

The subject is seated, and the complete flexor synergy is demonstrated by the examiner. The subject is asked to perform the movement pattern with the unaffected side to ascertain that he understands the directions. He is then asked to perform the movement pattern with the affected side after a command such as "Touch your ear" or "Touch your mouth," which gives purpose and direction to the effort.

A similar procedure is used to evaluate performance of the extensor synergy. The subject is asked to reach forward and downward to touch the examiner's hand, which is held between the subject's knees.

The responses may be influenced by the predominant spasticity seen in components of each of the synergies. For instance, the very spastic pectoralis major and elbow flexors may predominate during the subject's efforts and result in the subject reaching across the thorax to touch the opposite shoulder.

The status of the synergies is recorded on the evaluation form in terms of the active joint range achieved for each motion in the pattern. The joint ranges are estimated and recorded as 0, 1/4, 1/2, 3/4, or full range.

When the subject has reached recovery stage 4, there is a decrease in spasticity, and he is capable of performing gross movement combinations that deviate from the limb synergies. Brunnstrom chose three movements to represent stage 4. These are (1) placing the hand behind the body to touch the sacral region, (2) raising the arm forward to 90° of shoulder flexion with elbow extended, and (3) pronating and supinating the forearm with the elbow flexed to 90° and stabilized close to the side of the body. The subject performs all of the movements while seated, and as in all test items, no facilitation is allowed. During the test for pronation-supination, bilateral performance is allowed so that the examiner can make a comparison of the two sides.

Further decrease of spasticity and ability to perform more complex combinations of movement characterize recovery stage 5. The subject is relatively free of the influence of the limb synergies and performs the stage 4 movements with greater ease. Three movements chosen to represent stage 5 are (1) raising the arm to 90° of shoulder abduction with the elbow extended and forearm pronated, (2) raising the arm forward, as in stage 4, but above 90° of shoulder flexion, and (3) pronating and supinating the forearm with the elbow extended. The third movement is performed with the arm in the forward or side horizontal position and is not isolated from shoulder internal and external rotation.

Individuals who progress to recovery stage 6 will be able to perform isolated joint motions and demonstrate coordination that is comparable or nearly comparable to that of the unaffected side. On close observation the trained observer may detect some awkwardness of movement, and there may be some incoordination when rapid movement is attempted. The subject may be evaluated while performing a variety of daily living tasks, provided that recovery of hand function has kept pace with recovery of arm function.

The tests of motor speed on the second page of the evaluation form (Fig. 2-38, *B*) may be used to assess spasticity during any recovery stage, provided the subject has enough range of active motion to perform the necessary movement. The tests are especially useful in stages 4, 5, and 6. The normal side is tested first for comparison, then, the affected side is tested. The two movements that are tested are (1) hand to chin and (2) hand to opposite knee. The subject is seated in a sturdy chair without armrests. His trunk should be stabilized against the back of the chair, and the head should be erect. The hand is closed, but not tightly, and rests in the lap. For the hand-to-chin test the forearm is at 0° neutral between pronation and supination. The examiner asks the client to bring the hand from lap to chin as rapidly as possible, first with the unaffected side, and then with the affected side and records the number of full back-and-forth movements accomplished in 5 seconds. If speed is slow due to marked spasticity, half movements may be counted. The same procedure is followed for the hand-to-opposite knee test, except that the forearm is positioned in full pronation on the lap. The hand is moved from the lap to the opposite knee, using full range of elbow extension. These two tests measure the spasticity of elbow flexors and extensors.

Wrist stabilization, which is automatic during normal grasp, is often lacking after a stroke. Therefore it is important to evaluate wrist stabilization during fist closure. This is done with the elbow both flexed and extended. During the recovery stages when the synergies are dominant, the wrist will tend to flex when the elbow flexes. The subject is asked to make a fist while the elbow is extended across the front of the body. He is then asked to make a fist while the elbow is flexed at the side of the body. Whether the wrist remains stabilized in the neutral position or extends slightly is observed. This test is followed by a request for wrist flexion and extension with the fist closed. The subject holds an object such as a wide (1¾ inches) dowel in the hand and extends and flexes the wrist. This is done in the elbow-extended and elbow-flexed positions as on the previous test.

Circumduction of the wrist indicates significant recovery to the advanced stages. When evaluating the ability to perform this movement, the examiner should stabilize the forearm in pronation. The upper arm should be stabilized against the trunk.

Mass grasp is tested with a dynamometer, which measures pounds of pressure of grasp strength. The normal side is tested first, then the affected side is tested, and the results are recorded for comparison. Mass extension is evaluated by asking the subject to release and actively extend the fingers to the degree possible. Whether active extension was accomplished and the approximate amount of range achieved should be noted on the form. Active release to full range of extension is very difficult for many persons with cerebrovascular accident (CVA).

All types of prehension are evaluated in order of their difficulty. Everyday tasks that require the particular prehension pattern should be used. Hook grasp may be assessed by asking the subject to hold a handbag. Holding a card demands lateral prehension. Palmar prehension is required for grasping a pencil. Cylindrical grasp may be assessed by asking the subject to hold a small, narrow jar. Grasping a ball requires spherical grasp. The subject's ability to catch and throw the ball may be observed. These are difficult activities for hemiplegics, since they require rapid grasp and release, coordination of the entire limb, and time-space judgment. In all of the prehension tests the normal side should be observed first for purposes of comparison.

Individual thumb movements are evaluated with the subject's hand resting in the lap, ulnar side down. The normal side is observed first, then the affected side is observed. The subject is asked to move the thumb up and down (flexion-extension) and side to side (adduction-abduction).

Individual finger movements are evaluated by asking the subject to tap the index and middle fingers on the tabletop or on a pillow held in the lap. Isolated control of MP flexion and extension is observed and noted on the evaluation form.

Fine, coordinated use of the affected hand/arm and of both hands together usually is indicative of advanced recovery. Subjects who have succeeded well at the prehension tests may be asked to button and unbutton a shirt, first using both hands, then using the affected hand only. Other skilled activities, such as writing, threading a needle, removing a small bottle cap, and picking up and placing ¼-inch mosaic tiles, may be used to further test skilled hand use.

• • •

The reader is referred to the original source for a description of the evaluation of trunk balance and ambulation.

Functional muscle examination.[19] Landen and Amizich finalized the Functional Muscle Examination and Gait Analysis in 1962. This test was devised to meet the need for an evaluation more suitable than the manual muscle test to assess motor function after UMN lesions. Since the optimal goal of rehabilitation is "voluntary muscle control in a position of function, sitting or standing," it seemed wise to these researchers to evaluate their subjects in these positions. Some of the advantages of the Functional Muscle Examination are that it is not time-consuming, is easily administered, can be understood by other professionals, and aids the therapist in treatment planning and provides a record of progression or regression. This test may be particularly useful in assessing potential for functional use of the affected upper extremity in activities of daily living.

FUNCTIONAL MUSCLE EXAMINATION FOR UPPER MOTOR NEURON LESIONS

SCALE:

0 – Patient unable to perform activity   N – Normal strength endurance coord.
1 – Partial performance only   S – Spasticity
2 – Performance possible not practical   C – Contracture
3 – Adequate for daily use   T – Tremor

LEFT				Examiner / Date		Examiner / Date		RIGHT		
				A. Neck (sitting)						
				Flex from complete extension						
				Extend from complete flexion						
				Turn to side						
				B. Upper extremities (sitting)						
				Reach up						
				Bring hand to mouth						
				Reach out straightening elbow						
				Hand behind back						
				Pronate-supinate						
				Grasp and hold (medium and large objects)						
				Pinch (oppose thumb to index finger)						
				Straighten fingers with wrist neutral						
				C. Dexterity						
				Button garments (small-medium-large)						
				Write						
				D. Lower extremities						
				Lift heel to opposite knee (sitting)						
				Stand from sitting position						
				Extend from flexion with heelstrike (standing)						
				Stand on toes alternately						
				Stand on heels alternately						
				Sidestep to right						
				Sidestep to left						
				Balance on one leg						
				Step up (maximum in inches)						
				E. Trunk						
				Sit from lying position						
				Bend to side and return						
				Rotate trunk and return						
				Bend forward at hips and return						
				Hike hip						

Name (last, first, MI)	Grade	SN	Branch	Ward

Test requested by:

Diagnosis:

Comments on reverse side   Army—Ft. Mason, Calif.

Fig. 2-39. Functional muscle examination for UMN lesions. (Reprinted from PHYSICAL THERAPY 43(1):39, 1963 with permission of the American Physical Therapy Association.)

The form for recording the scores on the Functional Muscle Examination is found in Fig. 2-39. Landen and Amizich set up the following rules for administering the test*:

1. Since this is basically a test of muscle strength, endurance, and co-ordination, the patient is tested without any adaptive or supportive equipment that he might normally use. The only exception is a corset or other form of trunk support, if necessary, to maintain the erect position for testing the extremities.
2. All sitting tests should be performed in a straight chair without arms.
3. All standing tests should be done in the parallel bars using one hand on the bars for balance.
4. Grades of three (3) and normal (N) are recorded in black, all others in red.
5. Neck motions may be limited, primarily in older people, by arthritis or other conditions not involved in the patient's immediate problem. If the range of motion is not adequate for his daily use, then a grade of one (1) should be given and this explained in the comments.
6. We use the same standard of testing the upper extremities regardless of hand dominance.
7. *Reach-up* and *reach-out* are tests of the shoulder and elbow. Mild resistance by the tester may be necessary to determine a grade of normal (N). Hand function is covered by other test activities and should not influence the grading of the shoulder and elbow.
8. *Hand behind back* is tested here for extension and internal rotation of the shoulder with elbow flexion and forearm pronation, as a motion basic to dressing activities.
9. *Pronation* and *supination* are tested with the arms adducted and the elbows flexed to 90°.
10. *To grasp and hold medium and large objects*, a 3-inch roll of tape might be used for a medium object and a 32-ounce bottle (half full) for a large object.
11. *Pinch*, in this instance, means opposition of the thumb and index finger. A piece of paper held between the pads of the thumb and index finger as the tester tries to pull the paper away is a good way to determine grades of two (2), three (3), and normal (N).
12. In testing *buttoning garments* the patient should be given the best grade possible for any size button and the size should be indicated by circling small, medium, or large. A small button would usually be ¼ inch to ⅜ inch in diameter; a medium button ⅝ inch to ⅞ inch, and a large button anything over 1 inch. Since this is usually a bimanual activity, grade as such. If one hand is less dextrous than the other, grade accordingly.
13. *Write* indicates handedness. If the patient can sign his name but not write more than that, this usually would be considered possible, not practical, and a grade of two (2) is given. If his normal occupation requires much writing, this should be noted in the comments if the grade is less than normal (N).
14. *Lift heel to opposite knee* is a test of hip flexion, abduction, and external rotation with knee flexion. These motions, together or in part, may be important to the patient in such things as dressing, transfer activities, and ambulation.
15. *Stand from sitting position* is a test of combined strength (such as quadriceps, gluteus maximus, and trunk) not individual muscle ability. Use grades of (2), (3), or (N) to indicate method used to accomplish activity.
16. *Extend from flexion with heelstrike* is the motion performed during the second stage of the swing phase of walking and is tested here to determine the ability to dorsiflex while the knee is extending.
17. *Sidestep to right and left* tests abduction and adduction of the legs as the patient steps to one side and then the other.
18. *Balance on one leg* is tested standing still. Balance in ambulation will be tested in the Gait Analysis Test.
19. In *stepping-up* the patient should be allowed to keep one hand on a rail for balance just as he does in the parallel bars for the other standing tests. The maximum height he can climb, without pushing with his arm, should be recorded.
20. *Sit from lying position* is not a test of abdominal strength as such, but rather of the patient's ability to do this with any combination of muscle actions. How he does it will be reflected in a grade of three (3) or normal (N) and may be explained under comments if necessary.
21. In *bending motions of the trunk*, the hands should be allowed to reach toward the floor as the patient attempts to perform the activity. If his balance is poor, the activity might be graded a two (2) from the standpoint of safety.
22. *Hiking* the hip reflects the strength of the stance leg as well as the muscles which elevate the pelvis, lateral abdominals or latissimus, on the side being tested. This is done by asking the patient to stand on one leg and hike the opposite hip, keeping the hip and knee extended.

The reader is referred to the original source for the Gait Analysis portion of the test.

HAND EVALUATION

LORRAINE PEDRETTI, M.S., O.T.R., and MARY KASCH, O.T.R.

The purposes of hand evaluation are to identify (1) functional limitations, (2) substitution patterns that are being used to perform daily activities, and (3) deformities or positions and use patterns that are likely to enhance the development of deformities. The identification and measurement of causes of deformity, substitution patterns, and performance limitations may assist with diagnosis.

Arm and hand function are mutually dependent and have an intimate relationship in effective function.[10] Some upper extremity movements are more valuable for

---

*Reprinted from PHYSICAL THERAPY 43:43-44, 1963 with the permission of the American Physical Therapy Association.

□ Mary Kasch, Director of hand therapy, Hand Surgery Associates, Sacramento, Calif.

function than others. Finger performance is limited without wrist stability. Skilled hand performance depends on wrist stability, mobility, and ability to make fine adjustments in position. It also depends on arm and shoulder stability and mobility for fixing or positioning the hand for functioning. Functions of the thumb are of greater importance than those of any one finger. A hand with a mobile thumb and one or two fingers is more functional than a hand with no thumb and four fingers. Shoulder, elbow, and wrist function are less valuable when hand function is limited.

Evaluation of hand function

Physical evaluation. The effect of the dysfunction on anatomical structures is the first consideration in evaluating hand function. The joints must be assessed for their mobility, ROM, deforming tendencies, and existing deformities. The ligaments must be evaluated for laxity or contracture and their ability to maintain joint stability. Tendons must be examined for integrity, contracture, or overstretching; muscles are tested for strength and function. The degree of mobility, elasticity, adherence, and trophic changes in the skin should be observed. The vascular system is assessed by observing the skin color and temperature of the hand and evaluating for presence of edema. The latter may be done by measuring hand volume.

Hand volume is measured to assess the presence of extra or intracellular edema. It is generally used to determine the effect of treatment and activities. By measuring volume at different times of the day the effects of rest versus activity may be measured as well as the effects of splinting or treatment designed to reduce edema.

A volumeter may be made using the instructions of Brand and Wood[9] or it may be purchased.[12] The equipment must be well-calibrated and always placed in the same position on the same table. The patient must sit in the same position each time, and place the hand in the volumeter in the same manner. The evaluation is performed as follows:

1. A plastic volumeter is filled and allowed to empty into a 500 ml graduated cylinder until the water reaches spout level. The cylinder is then emptied and dried thoroughly.
2. The patient is instructed to immerse the hand in the plastic volumeter, being careful to keep the hand supinated.
3. The hand is lowered until it rests gently between the middle and ring fingers on the dowel rod. It is important that the hand does not press onto the rod.
4. The hand remains still until no more water drips into the cylinder.

5. The hand is removed, the cylinder is placed on a level surface, and a reading is made.

Nerve function is evaluated by assessing active motion and sensation. Sensation may be evaluated for light touch, superficial pain, temperature, and position sense, using methods described later in this chapter. In addition some special tests may be applied to the hand to determine its sensibility. These are tests for vibration, moving touch, constant touch, and two-point discrimination (2 PD).

Vibration is tested first with a 30 cps tuning fork. The fork should be at room temperature. The patient faces the therapist with his hand resting lightly in the therapist's hand so that feedback will not come from the table. As with other sensibility tests, the uninvolved hand is tested first for reference. After the patient understands what is being asked, the therapist starts the tuning fork and rests it lightly on the proximal palm. It is moved distally until the patient is no longer able to identify the vibration. It should be stressed that the patient must distinguish between pressure and vibration. After the patient has recovered the ability to detect moving touch and constant touch to the tip of the finger, vibration of 256 cps may be tested. Testing is performed in the same manner.[13]

Moving touch is tested using the eraser end of a pencil. The eraser is placed in an area of normal sensibility and, pressing lightly, is moved to the distal fingertip. The patient notes when the perception of the stimulus changes. Light and heavy stimuli may be applied and noted.[10]

Constant touch is tested by pressing with the eraser end of a pencil, first in an area with normal sensibility and then moving distally. The patient responds when the stimulus is altered again; light and heavy stimuli may be applied.[16]

Originally described by Weber in the nineteenth century the test for 2 PD is used to assess the functional level of sensation. Moberg[23] refers to the ability to see with the hand for complex function as *tactile gnosis*. Most examiners today continue to feel that the 2 PD test has a high positive correlation with sensory function or tactile gnosis.

The test is performed as follows[21]:
1. The patient's vision is occluded.
2. An area of normal sensation is tested as a reference, using a blunt caliper or bent paper clip.
3. The calipers are set 10 mm apart and are randomly applied longitudinally in line with the digital nerves, with one or two points touching. The skin should not be blanched by the caliper. The distance is decreased until the patient no longer feels two distinct points, and that distance is measured. From 3 to 4 seconds should be allowed between

applications, and the patient should have four out of five correct responses.[16] Because this test indicates sensory function, it is usually administered at the tips of the fingers. It may be used proximally to test nerve regeneration. Normal two-point discrimination at the fingertip is 6 mm or less.[7]

Functional evaluation. Evaluation of hand function or performance is important because the physical evaluation does not measure the client's ingenuity and ability to compensate for loss of strength, ROM, sensation, or presence of deformities.[10] The effect of the hand dysfunction on the use of the hand in activities of daily living should be observed by the occupational therapist. In addition some type of a standardized performance evaluation, such as the Jebsen-Taylor Test of Hand Function[17] or the Carroll Quantitative Test of Upper Extremity Function,[10] should be administered.

The Jebsen-Taylor Test of Hand Function[17] was developed to provide objective measurements of standardized tasks with norms for client comparison. It is a short test that is easy to administer, is inexpensive, and is put together by the person administering the test. The test consists of seven subtests, including (1) writing a short sentence, (2) turning over 3 × 5-inch cards, (3) picking up small objects and placing them in a container, (4) stacking checkers, (5) eating (simulated), (6) moving empty large cans, and (7) moving weighted large cans. Norms are provided for dominant and nondominant hands for each subtest and also are divided by sex and age. Instructions for fabricating the test, as well as specific instructions for administering the test, are provided by the authors.[17] This has been found to be a good test for overall hand function.

The Quantitative Test of Upper Extremity Function described by Carroll[10] was designed to measure ability to perform general arm and hand activities used in daily living. It is based on the assumption that complex upper extremity movements used to perform ordinary activities of daily living can be reduced to specific patterns of grasp and prehension of the hand, supination and pronation of the forearm, flexion and extension of the elbow, and elevation of the arm.

The test consists of six parts, including (1) grasping and lifting four blocks of graduated sizes to assess grasp; (2) grasping and lifting two pipes of graduated sizes from a peg to test cylindrical grip; (3) grasping and placing a ball to test spherical grasp; (4) picking up and placing four marbles of graduated sizes to test fingertip prehension or pinch; (5) putting a small washer over a nail and putting an iron on a shelf to test placing; and (6) pouring water from pitcher to glass and glass to glass, placing hand on top of head, behind head, and to mouth, and writing the name to assess pronation, supination, and elevation of the arm. The test uses simple, inexpensive,

and easily acquired materials. Details of materials and their arrangement, test procedures, and scoring can be found in the original source. Melvin[22] lists a variety of additional hand function evaluations.

The physical evaluation should precede the functional evaluation because awareness of physical dysfunction can result in a critical analysis of functional impairment and an understanding of why the client functions as he does.[22]

Observation.[33] The occupational therapist should observe the appearance of the hand and arm. The position of the hand and arm at rest and the carrying posture can yield valuable information about the dysfunction. How the client "treats" the disease or injury should be observed. Is it overprotected and carefully guarded or ignored? The skin condition of the hand and arm should be noted. Are there lacerations, sutures, or evidence of recent surgery? Is the skin dry or moist? Are there scales or crusts? Does the hand appear swollen? Does the hand have an odor? Is the skin normally mobile? Palmar skin is less mobile than dorsal skin normally. Are there contractures of the web spaces? The therapist should observe the relationship between hand and arm function as the client moves about and performs test items or tasks. If the client has difficulty assuming the functional position, the therapist may assist by stabilizing the client's wrist and placing the thumb in opposition. This is done by grasping the client's hand with the middle and little fingers over the dorsum of the wrist and hand, the thumb over the dorsum of the thenar area, and the index and middle fingers placed in the thumb web space between the index finger and thumb. With this assistance the therapist can observe the client's ability to perform palmar prehension, opposition to all fingers, and spherical and cylindrical grasp.

The therapist should ask the client to perform some simple bilateral activities of daily living, such as buttoning a button, putting on a shirt, opening a jar, and threading a needle, and observe the amount of spontaneous movement and use of the affected hand and arm. Is it relatively or completely static or slightly to completely dynamic when required for function?

Clinical tests for specific dysfunction

Peripheral neuropathy. Several quick clinical observations to detect dysfunction of peripheral nerves are available, based on the sensory and motor function of the individual nerve.

The ulnar nerve may be tested by asking the client to make a cone with the fingers or abduct and adduct the fingers. The radial nerve may be tested by asking the client to extend the wrist and fingers. Median nerve function is tested by asking the client to oppose the thumb to the fingers and flex the fingers.[11] The median nerve may be affected by carpal tunnel compression in conditions such as rheumatoid arthritis. Early signs of median nerve compression are sensory in nature and may be tested in two ways. First, to elicit Tinel's sign of median nerve compression, the examiner taps over the volar aspect of the wrist at the base of the thumb metacarpal. A positive response of paresthesias along the median distribution in the thumb is indicative of compression. Phalen's test involves complete passive flexion or extension of the wrist to elicit the same response described for Tinel's sign. The complete passive flexion or extension increases the nerve compression and results in the abnormal sensory response.

It is important to test for median nerve compression periodically in clients with rheumatoid arthritis involving the wrist, since synovial proliferation under the transverse carpal ligament can cause compression on the median nerve. It is important to correct this problem before it progresses to include motor dysfunction of the muscles innervated, which are so critical to hand function.

Deformities of rheumatoid arthritis.[20,22] Involvement of the wrist and finger joints in this disease can result in mild to severe hand dysfunction and deformity. A few of the more common deformities and their tests are described here. The reader is referred to *Rheumatic Disease: Occupational Therapy and Rehabilitation* by Jeanne L. Melvin* for a comprehensive discussion of rheumatoid arthritis, its deformities, and treatment.

To test for tightness (contracture) or adherence of the extensor digitorum communis (EDC) tendon, position the wrist at neutral. Then passively flex the MP, PIP, and DIP joints fully. If full flexion is not possible, this indicates shortening or adherence of the EDC tendon. This test is a preliminary step for the tests for all types of swan-neck deformity.

Swan-neck deformity (Chapter 9) results in hyperextension of the PIP joint and incomplete extension or slight flexion of the DIP joint. There are three causes of swan-neck deformity, and it is important for the therapist and physician to know the underlying cause if appropriate treatment is to be instituted.

The type I swan-neck deformity is due to intrinsic muscle tightness. To test for this type the test for extrinsic muscle tightness is applied first to prove that the extensor tendons do not have adhesions. Then the MP joint is passively moved into hyperextension, and the PIP joint is flexed. Resistance to PIP flexion indicates intrinsic tightness. The PIP joint will not flex fully in this position if the intrinsic muscles are shortened. The reason for this is that the lumbricales act to extend the IP

joints during MP flexion. By hyperextending MP and flexing PIP joints these muscles are fully stretched. If they have become shortened, there will be insufficient elasticity or length to achieve the test position. Intrinsic muscles become weak, scarred, and shortened when they are invaded by pannus during the rheumatoid disease process.

The type II swan-neck deformity is due to rupture of the lateral slips of the extensor tendons. To test for this type the test for extrinsic tightness is applied first to prove that there is no adherence of the extensor tendon. Then the MP joint is moved into hyperextension, and the PIP joint is flexed to prove that there is no intrinsic tightness. Then the client should extend the finger actively. If there is a type II swan-neck deformity, the DIP joint will drop into flexion because ruptured lateral slips of the EDC cannot function to extend the joint. The middle slip of the EDC, acting on the PIP joint, pulls too hard and hyperextends the joint when active extension is attempted, resulting in the swan-neck appearance. This type of swan-neck deformity is due to tendon ruptures resulting from inflammatory infiltration of pannus and attrition from bony spurs.[20]

Rupture of the flexor digitorum sublimis (FDS) tendon causes the type III swan-neck deformity. To test for this the test for extrinsic tightness is applied as before. The MP joint is moved into hyperextension, and the PIP joint is flexed to rule out intrinsic tightness. The client is then asked to flex the finger into the palm actively. If the FDS tendon is ruptured, it will not be possible to flex the PIP joint. Then tendon rupture is due to synovitis of the PIP joint with infiltration of the FDS tendon, causing its rupture, or to bony spurs producing tendon erosion.[20,22]

Another common deformity of the fingers in rheumatoid arthritis is the boutonnière deformity (Chapter 9). This appears as flexion at the PIP joint and hyperextension at the DIP joint. There are two types. Type I boutonnière deformity is due to rupture of the central slip of the EDC tendon. To test for this type the client should actively extend the finger. Loss of active PIP extension is indicative of the rupture. The deformity is described as mild if the loss is 5° to 10°, as moderate if the loss is 10° to 30°, and as severe if 30° or more is lost.[22] The central slip of the extensor tendon is ruptured due to inflammatory infiltration or bony spurs. Therefore it cannot function to extend the PIP joint on which it acts. The lateral slips slide volarly below the normal angle of pull and act to flex the PIP joint and hyperextend the DIP joint, resulting in the typical boutonnière appearance.[20]

The type II boutonnière deformity is due to a nodule or thickening of the FDS tendon at the entrance to the flexor tunnel (tendon sheath). This is caused by a rheu-

*Melvin, J.L.: Rheumatic disease: occupational therapy and rehabilitation, Philadelphia, 1977, F.A. Davis Co.

matoid nodule on the FDS tendon that blocks or makes difficult the slipping of the tendon through its sheath, preventing full extension of the PIP joint.[20] To test for this type of deformity, the examiner should ask the client to fully flex the PIP joint and then to extend the joint and should observe for an inconsistency in the degree of active extension with repetitive motion or a frank inability to extend the finger once it is fully flexed. The examiner may palpate a click or crepitation at the point where the nodule is pulled through the sheath. The palpation point is in the palm distal to the palmar creases at the base of the involved finger. The deformity is described as mild if there is inconsistent, painless triggering during active motion; as moderate if there is constant triggering during active motion or if it is intermittent but painful; and as severe if it prevents full active motion and is severely painful.[22]

Ulnar drift at the MP joints is another common deformity of rheumatoid arthritis. The therapist may test for the deformity by measuring the degrees of excess mediolateral motion at the MP joints during active extension. This measurement should be compared with the normal ROM. The severity of the ulnar drift is described as follows:

Severity	Index finger	Fingers 3 to 5
Mild	20° to 30°	0° to 10°
Moderate	30° to 50°	10° to 30°
Severe	50° or more	30° or more[22]

MP subluxation is also seen in the rheumatoid hand. It is the volar subluxation of the proximal phalanx on the metacarpal head. The therapist can test for this deformity by palpating over the dorsum of the joint when it is at the 0° neutral position. If there is subluxation, a "step" can be felt between the metacarpal and the first phalanx. The deformity is described as mild if the step is palpable, but full extension is possible; as moderate if the step is visible, palpable, and there is a slight limitation of extension; and as severe if there is gross malalignment and definite limitation of ROM.[22]

Subluxation of the wrist is a volar slippage of the carpal bones on the radius. It is caused by weakness of the supporting ligaments caused by chronic synovitis. To test for wrist subluxation the therapist should palpate from the distal radius to the carpals on the dorsal side of the forearm. If there is subluxation, there will be a step. It may be merely palpable if mild, visible if moderate, and grossly malaligned if severe.[22]

Dorsal burn of the hand. Dorsal skin is normally loose, mobile, and elastic to allow for grasp and prehension, which require stretching and mobility of the dorsal skin. If skin contracture develops due to burn injury, the metacarpal transverse arch is flattened, the MP joints

are pulled into extension, and the IP joints are pulled into flexion. This is the clawhand or intrinsic minus position. The burned hand may slip into this nonfunctional state by first being allowed to rest in the position of ease. Edema may mask the deformity and make the hand appear to be in a functional position when, in fact, the claw is hiding in the swelling.

If not prevented with appropriate positioning, splinting in the antideformity position, and exercising, the deformity can progress to a severe clawhand with permanent contracture of the dorsal skin of the hand, overstretching of the lumbricales, and permanent contracture of the MP collateral ligaments. This precludes any flexion at the MP joints and severely limits hand function. The therapist cannot wait to observe or test for the development of the deformity but must act to prevent it with splinting, positioning, and bandaging from the first day of the burn injury.[25,30]

EVALUATION OF REFLEXES AND REACTIONS

Following central nervous system (CNS) injury or disease the nervous system may revert to an earlier level of development. Primitive reflexes may reappear, and equilibrium and protective reactions may be disturbed, limiting voluntary motor function and performance.

It is important to evaluate reflexes and reactions in adults with CNS disease to measure the level of CNS function; establish a baseline for recovery; inhibit or use the reflex activity as appropriate with the selected treatment approach; and determine the kind of positioning, motion, and sensory stimuli that could facilitate more mature motor responses.

Fiorentino[15] has designed methods for testing the reflexes and reactions in children with CNS dysfunction. Many of these are appropriate for use with adults. Bobath[6] describes methods of evaluating muscle tone, abnormal motor patterns, voluntary movement, balance, and protective reactions of adults with hemiplegia. The reader is referred to these sources for a more detailed discussion of reflex maturation and evaluation.

Summary of reflexes and reactions

Spinal level. Reflexes mediated at the spinal level are the flexor withdrawal, extensor thrust, and crossed extension. These are normally present in the first 2 months of life.[15]

Brain stem level. Reflexes mediated at the brain stem level are static, postural reflexes that cause a change in muscle tone throughout the body. The changed tone is in response to a change of the position of the head in space or in relation to the body. The reflexes included are the asymmetrical tonic neck reflex (ATNR), symmetrical tonic neck reflex (STNR), and tonic labyrinthine reflex (TLR). Associated reactions and the positive and negative supporting reactions are also mediated at the brain stem level. These reflexes and reactions are present in the first 4 to 6 months of life.[15]

Midbrain level. Righting reactions are integrated at the midbrain level. They interact with one another to effect the normal head-to-body relationship in space and to each other. The righting reactions begin developing after birth and reach maximum effect at 10 to 12 months of age. As cortical control of voluntary movement increases, they are gradually inhibited and disappear by the end of the fifth year of life. Their effect on motor performance is to enable rolling over, sitting up, and assuming the quadrupedal position. Reactions included are the neck righting, body righting acting on the body, and labyrinthine righting and optical righting acting on the head.[15]

Cortical level. Cortical level reactions are the result of the efficient interaction of the cerebral cortex, basal ganglia, and cerebellum. The maturation of equilibrium reactions results in the ability to deal with bipedal motor skills. Equilibrium reactions occur when muscle tone is normalized and enable the adaptation to changes in the body's center of gravity. They begin to develop at 6 months of age and continue throughout life. Equilibrium and righting reactions that act to recover balance and maintain the normal position of the head in space should be possible in the prone, supine, quadrupedal, sitting, kneel-standing, squatting, and standing positions.[15]

Innate primary reactions.[29] Innate primary reactions are primitive movements present at birth that involve total patterns of flexion and extension. These include primary standing, reflex stepping, placing reactions of the upper and lower limbs, grasp reflex, sucking reflex, and rooting reflex. Primary standing is present from birth to 6 or 8 months of age.[29] Reflex stepping is normal in the first 4 to 8 weeks of life.[5] The placing reactions of the lower limbs are present in the first month of life and those of the upper limbs are present for the first 6 months of life. The grasp, sucking, and rooting reflexes are present for the first 3 to 4 months of life.[29]

Automatic movement reactions. Automatic movement reactions are produced by changes of the position of the head in space. Included are the Moro reflex, Landau reflex, and protective extensor thrust. The Moro reflex is normal from 0 to 4 months of age. The Landau reflex is normally present from 6 months to 2½ years of age. The protective extensor thrust begins in the arms at about 6 months of age and is present throughout life.[15]

Evaluation techniques

The following are methods for evaluation of some of the reflexes and reactions just described. The methods may have to be adapted to accommodate to the size and physical abilities of the client being evaluated.

Spinal level

Extensor thrust[15]
POSITION: Supine lying, head in midposition, one leg extended and the other flexed
STIMULUS: Stimulation to sole of foot of flexed leg
NEGATIVE RESPONSE: Controlled maintenance of leg in flexion
POSITIVE RESPONSE: Uncontrolled extension of stimulated leg
NORMAL: Positive reaction up to 2 months of age

Flexor withdrawal[15]
POSITION: Supine lying, head in midposition, legs extended
STIMULUS: Stimulation to sole of foot
NEGATIVE RESPONSE: Maintained extension or voluntary withdrawal of stimulated leg
POSITIVE RESPONSE: Uncontrolled flexion of stimulated leg
NORMAL: Positive response is present from birth to 2 months of age

Brain stem level

Asymmetrical tonic neck reflex (ATNR)[5,15]
POSITION: Supine lying
STIMULUS: Rotation of head to either side
NEGATIVE RESPONSE: No reaction in limbs
POSITIVE RESPONSE: Extension of arm and leg on jaw side, flexion of arm and leg on skull side; response is more pronounced in arms
NORMAL: Positive response is present up to 6 months of age; never obligatory

Symmetrical tonic neck reflex (STNR)[5,15,29]
POSITION: Quadruped
STIMULUS 1: Forward flexion of head
NEGATIVE RESPONSE: No change in muscle tone or position of limbs
POSITIVE RESPONSE: Increased flexor tone in arms and increased extensor tone in legs or flexion of arms and extension of legs
STIMULUS 2: Extension of head
NEGATIVE RESPONSE: No change in muscle tone or position of limbs
POSITIVE RESPONSE: Increased extensor tone in arms and increased flexor tone in legs or extension of arms and flexion of legs
NORMAL: Same as for ATNR

Tonic labyrinthine reflex (TLR)[5,15]
POSITION: Supine lying, head in midposition, limbs extended
STIMULUS 1: Supine position is stimulus
NEGATIVE RESPONSE: No increase in extensor tone of limbs when moved passively
POSITIVE RESPONSE: Increased overall extensor tone of neck, arms, and legs
POSITION: Prone lying, head in midposition, limbs extended
STIMULUS 2: Prone position is stimulus
NEGATIVE RESPONSE: No increase of flexor tone in neck, trunk, arms, or legs
POSITIVE RESPONSE: Increased overall flexor tone; inability to extend neck, back, or limbs, or adduct scapulae

NORMAL: Positive response is present in first 4 months of life, disappears by fifth month

Positive supporting reaction[5,15]

POSITION: Standing, or holding subject in standing

STIMULUS: Pressure of soles against supporting surface; bounce subject several times on soles of feet

NEGATIVE RESPONSE: No increase in tone; legs flex voluntarily

POSITIVE RESPONSE: Legs develop supporting tone, become rigid, and support body weight for a short period

NORMAL: Positive reaction may occur normally from 3 to 8 months of age

Negative supporting reaction[5,15]

POSITION: Lift subject to standing

STIMULUS: Weight bearing

NEGATIVE RESPONSE: Loosening or relaxation of extension, progressing from proximal to distal musculature, which allows flexion for reciprocation

POSITIVE RESPONSE: Persistence of the positive supporting reaction; no release of extensor tone

NORMAL: Positive response should not persist beyond 8 months of age

Midbrain level

Neck righting[5,29]

POSITION: Supine lying, head in midposition, limbs extended

STIMULUS: Rotation of head to one side, actively or passively

NEGATIVE RESPONSE: Body does not rotate and follow rotation of head

POSITIVE RESPONSE: Body follows by turning in one piece, like a log, following in direction of head

NORMAL: Positive reaction is present from 0 to 6 months of age; negative reaction should not persist beyond 1 month of age

Body righting reaction acting on the body[15,29]

POSITION: Supine lying, head in midposition, limbs extended

STIMULUS: Active or passive rotation of head

NEGATIVE RESPONSE: Body rotates in one piece, with a neck righting response

POSITIVE RESPONSE: Segmental rotation of trunk, first shoulders, then pelvis

NORMAL: Negative response—0 to 6 months of age
Positive response—6 to 18 months of age

Labyrinthine righting reaction acting on the head[5,15,29]

POSITION: Prone, supine, or vertical positions in space; subject's vision is occluded

STIMULUS: Prone or supine positions are test stimuli or in vertical position body is tilted laterally

NEGATIVE RESPONSE: Head does not raise or right itself to normal face-vertical position

POSITIVE RESPONSE: Head tends to seek vertical position in space regardless of position of body and independent of vision

NORMAL: Positive response is present from 2 to 6 months of age throughout life

Optical righting reaction[15]

POSITION: Prone, supine, or vertical positions in space, with eyes open

Stimuli and responses are same as for labyrinthine righting reaction acting on head, described earlier

Cortical level

Equilibrium reaction[5,15,29]

POSITION: Supine or prone lying, quadruped, kneel-standing, sitting, or standing

STIMULUS: Tipping or rocking subject or supporting surface, depending on position, sufficiently to disturb balance

NEGATIVE RESPONSES: Failure to make automatic movements to right head and body; no protective reactions

POSITIVE RESPONSES: Automatic movements to maintain balance, right head and body; protective reactions

NORMAL: Positive reactions in prone and supine begin at about 6 months of age; in quadruped position positive responses begin at about 8 months of age; in sitting at 10 to 12 months of age; in kneel-standing at about 15 months of age; and in standing from 15 to 18 months; these reactions remain throughout life

Innate primary reactions[29]

Reflex stepping[5,29]

POSITION: Supported in upright position, with some weight bearing on feet

STIMULUS: Lean subject forward; contact and pressure of soles on supporting surface

RESPONSE: Rhythmic alternate stepping

NORMAL: First 4 to 8 weeks of life

Grasp reflex or tonic palmar reflex[26,29]

STIMULUS: Contact of object or pressure to palm of hand from ulnar side

RESPONSE: Flexing of fingers, grasping of stimulus object

NORMAL: Present at birth, diminishing by 4 or 5 months of age

Rooting reflex[5,29]

STIMULUS: Touching or stroking outward on corner of lips or on cheeks

RESPONSE: Tongue, lip, and head move to follow stimulus

NORMAL: From birth to 3 or 4 months of age

Sucking reflex[5,27]

STIMULUS: Stimulation to lips, gums, or front of tongue

RESPONSE: Sucking, swallowing motions

NORMAL: Present at birth, diminishing by 4 months of age[27]

Automatic movement reactions

Moro reflex[5,15,29]

POSITION: Semireclining or supine lying

STIMULUS: Striking pillow beside head or dropping head backward

NEGATIVE RESPONSE: Minimal or absent movement of limbs

POSITIVE RESPONSE: Extension (or flexion) and abduction of arms and spreading of fingers

NORMAL: First 4 to 6 months of age

Landau reflex[15,29]

POSITION: Prone, suspended in space, supported under chest

STIMULUS: Passive or active neck extension

NEGATIVE RESPONSE: Spine and legs remain flexed

POSITIVE RESPONSE: Back and legs extend

NORMAL: Positive response begins about 4 to 6 months of age and disappears by 2 years of age[15,27]

Protective extension or parachute reactions[5,15]

POSITION: Suspended in prone position with arms extended overhead

STIMULUS: Move head suddenly toward the floor, holding subject at pelvis; for adults, where this position is not feasible, a sudden displacement of erect trunk will evoke protective extension, in the direction of the trunk movement, by arm or leg

NEGATIVE RESPONSE: Arms do not extend to protect head

POSITIVE RESPONSE: Protective extension of appropriate limb to protect head and attempt to recover balance

NORMAL: Begins in arms at about 6 months of age; develops first with forward responses, progresses to sideward, and then backward responses; is present throughout life

SECTION TWO
Sensory-perceptual-cognitive evaluation

All persons with peripheral nervous system or CNS disease or damage should be tested for sensory and perceptual dysfunction. For those with peripheral neuropathy, tests of light touch, superficial pain, pressure, thermal sensitivity, position and motion sense (proprioception), and stereognosis should be applied. For those with CNS dysfunction, additional tests of visual perception should be applied. Examples of diagnoses that require

sensory testing are thermal injuries (burns), peripheral nerve injuries and diseases, spinal cord injuries and diseases, brain injuries and diseases, and fractures and arthritis, when there is peripheral nerve involvement or to help determine if there is peripheral nerve involvement.

The purposes of performing sensory-perceptual evaluation are to determine the need for teaching precautions against injury or compensatory techniques such as visual guidance for movement and for initiating a program of sensory reeducation. Sensory loss may affect the client's use of splints and braces, since he may be unaware of pressure points during use. Sensory loss may also affect controlled use of a dynamic splint, since the client's sensory feedback is faulty.

For these reasons the occupational therapist can use results of the sensory-perceptual evaluation to select appropriate treatment objectives and methods. In addition in some diagnoses sensory status and progress may provide valuable information that can indicate prognosis for recovery.[3]

TESTS FOR SENSATION

The following tests are nonstandardized evaluation tools designed to test the sensation of adults with central or peripheral nervous system dysfunction. It is important for the examiner to orient the subject to the test procedures and the rationale for administering the tests. The examiner should be sure the subject understands

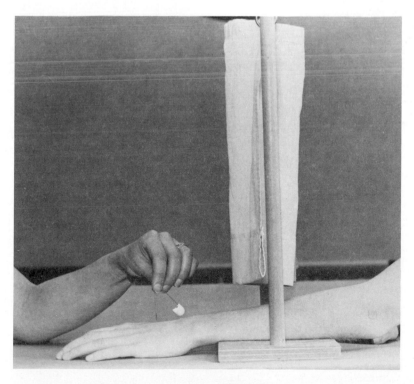

Fig. 2-40. Test for superficial pain sensitivity.

FORM FOR RECORDING SCORES ON
TESTS OF SENSATION

Department of Occupational Therapy

Name_____ Age_____ Sex_____

Diagnosis_____ Disability_____

Date_____

TEST FOR SUPERFICIAL PAIN	LEFT	RIGHT
Use a large safety pin and touch random locations with sharp and dull ends on anterior and posterior surfaces. Indicate on diagram: 　Intact:　　+ 　Impaired:　− 　Absent:　　0	Anterior Posterior	Anterior Posterior

TEST FOR LIGHT TOUCH SENSITIVITY	LEFT	RIGHT
Use a cotton swab and touch random locations on anterior and posterior surfaces. Indicate on diagram: 　Intact:　　+ 　Impaired:　− 　Absent:　　0	Anterior Posterior	Anterior Posterior

Fig. 2-41. Form for recording scores on test of sensation.

how he is to respond. His vision can be occluded by shielding parts to be tested from view. The subject should not be blindfolded nor asked to keep his eyes closed.

A blindfold can be a source of sensory distraction and can be very anxiety provoking to subjects with sensory, perceptual, and balance disturbances. It is difficult for many individuals with CNS dysfunction to maintain eye closure because of apraxia and motor impersistence, in addition to the reasons just stated. Therefore to occlude vision it is preferable to use a folder or small screen under which the subject can place his hands and forearms.

Test for superficial pain[3]

PURPOSE: To make a gross evaluation of superficial pain sensitivity.

LIMITATIONS: Persons with receptive aphasia cannot be validly tested.

MATERIALS: A small curtain between two uprights or a manila folder to occlude subject's vision. A large safety pin or sharpened pencil.

CONDITIONS: A nondistracting environment where subject (S) is seated at a narrow table. Affected hand and forearm should rest comfortably on table. Examiner (E) sits opposite S on other side of table.

METHOD: S's hand and forearm are hidden from his view by placing them between uprights and under curtain or by E holding a manila folder over them. Affected hand and forearm are touched lightly at random locations, using sharp and dull stimuli in random order (Fig. 2-40). A few trial stimuli should be conducted with S watching to be sure that he un-

derstands test and knows how to respond. Test may be conducted entirely on an unaffected area first to establish a standard and determine that instructions are understood. If spasticity is a problem, E may support hand on dorsal surface and hold thumb in radial abduction and extension to secure relaxation for palmar testing. Each stimulus should be applied with same degree of pressure.

NOTES: Calloused or toughened areas (for example, palms) may be normally less sensitive than other areas. If S is fearful of a safety pin, a pencil or broken swab stick may be used.

RESPONSES: S should be asked to say "sharp" or "dull" in response to each stimulus. If aphasic or dysarthric E should ask S to indicate his response by pointing to appropriate side of an open safety pin in S's view.

SCORING: E marks a plus at stimulus point on scoring chart for a correct response, a minus for an incorrect or unduly delayed response, and a zero for no response. Space for recording results of evaluation is presented in Fig. 2-41.

Test for light touch sensitivity[32]

PURPOSE: To determine S's ability to recognize and localize light touch stimuli.

LIMITATIONS: Patients with receptive aphasia cannot be validly tested.

MATERIALS: A small curtain between two uprights or a manila folder to occlude vision. A cotton swab.

CONDITIONS: A nondistracting environment where S is seated at a narrow table. Affected hand and forearm rest comfortably on table. E sits opposite subject.

METHOD: S's hand and forearm are hidden from his view by placing it under curtain or by E holding manila folder over them. Hand and forearm are touched lightly with a cotton

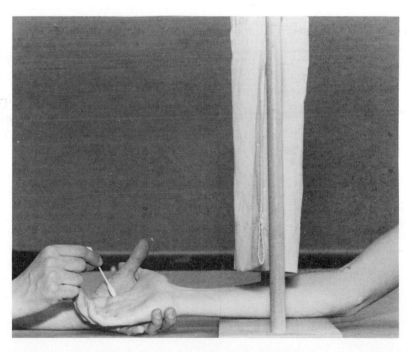

Fig. 2-42. Test of light touch sensitivity.

swab at random locations. A few trial stimuli should be administered while S is watching to be sure he understands procedure and how to respond. Test may be administered on an uninvolved area first to establish a standard. If spasticity is a problem, E may support hand on dorsal surface and hold thumb in radial abduction and extension to secure relaxation of fingers for palmar testing (Fig. 2-42).

RESPONSES: After each stimulus, E asks S if he was touched (recognition). S responds by nodding or saying "yes" or "no." Curtain or folder is removed after each stimulus, and S is asked to point to place where he was touched, using unaffected hand if possible. If this cannot be done, S is asked to describe location, and E should select locations that are easy to name (for example, over PIP joint).

SCORING: On scoring chart E marks a plus for ability to recognize and localize touch stimuli, a minus for ability to recognize only, and a zero for inability to recognize or localize a stimulus. Fig. 2-41 includes space for recording scores on test for touch sensitivity.

STANDARDS: Deviation of 1½ to 3 cm is normal, depending on area of hand or arm touched. Responses should be more accurate on hand than on forearm.

Test for pressure sensitivity

Pressure sensitivity may be tested in exactly the same manner as described for light touch, except that the E should press hard enough with the cotton swab to dent and blanch the skin. If light touch sensitivity is severely impaired or absent, pressure sensitivity may be intact and may provide important sensory feedback to compensate and enhance function.

Test for thermal sensitivity

PURPOSE: To determine S's ability to discriminate between extremes of hot and cold and to detect variations in temperature at four levels.

LIMITATIONS: Persons with receptive aphasia cannot be validly tested.

MATERIALS: Four test tubes (¾-inch diameter) with stoppers.

CONDITIONS: A nondistracting environment where the S is seated comfortably at a table with both hands and forearm resting on table.

METHOD:

Subtest I: Two test tubes are used, one filled with very cold water and one with very hot water. Ice water may be used for cold and hottest tap water tolerable to normal touch used for hot. Stoppers are placed in tubes. E touches sides of test tubes to skin surfaces to be tested in random order and at random locations, being sure to cover test area thoroughly (Fig. 2-43).

Subtest II: Four test tubes are used, one filled with very cold water, one with tepid water, one with warm water, and one with hot water. E should color code stoppers as follows: yellow—hot, green—warm, orange—tepid; and red—cold. Place stoppers in test tubes. E asks S to touch or hold test tubes with affected hand(s) in random order. If S is unable to hold tubes, E may touch each one to S's palm and fingertips.

Subtest III: Using same four test tubes as in subtest II filled with water of like temperature, S is asked to hold each one

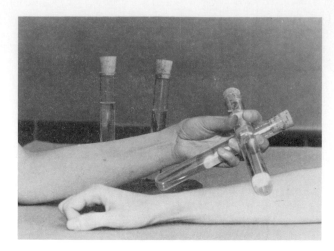

Fig. 2-43. Test of thermal sensitivity.

with both hands simultaneously. If S is unable to hold tube with affected hand, E may hold tube to palmar surface of fingers of that hand while S touches tube with fingers of unaffected hand. S is asked to compare feeling of heat or cold in both hands, that is, does temperature feel same or different to affected and unaffected hands.

RESPONSES:

Subtest I: S responds "hot" or "cold" in response to each stimulus. If S is aphasic, E should work out an alternate nonverbal response before beginning tests.

Subtest II: S is asked to arrange test tubes on table from hottest to coldest in order from left to right. E checks correctness of order by color-coded stoppers and/or feeling tubes herself.

Subtest III: S is asked to tell whether sensation of warmth or cold is same to both hands or whether a given temperature is warmer or cooler to one hand or the other. This is an entirely subjective estimate and cognitive status of S may influence response.

SCORING (Fig. 2-44):

Subtest I: E marks a plus on form if temperature is correctly identified, and marks a zero if S cannot tell hot from cold. Subtests II and III are not administered if S cannot succeed at subtest I.

Subtest II: E marks appropriate blanks on form with a check and the appropriate letter to indicate S's responses

Subtest III: E marks appropriate blanks on form with a check to indicate S's responses.

STANDARD: Normal adults should be able to complete all items on this test successfully.

TESTS OF PERCEPTION

Test for proprioception[32]

PURPOSE: To evaluate S's senses of motion and position.

MATERIALS: Curtain on uprights shown on test for light touch sensitivity (Fig. 2-42) or a manila folder. For testing elbow and shoulder, if space and equipment permit, a curtained screen high and wide enough to conceal subject's arm when he holds it overhead or out in front of him when in a seated

TEST FOR THERMAL SENSITIVITY

SUBTEST I.

Test site (fill in location tested)   Score (+, 0)

Dates			

Use diagram to record scores on test of arms

LEFT   RIGHT

Anterior   Anterior

Posterior   Posterior

SUBTEST II.

	Date	Date	Date
Arrange test tubes in correct order			
Arrange test tubes in wrong order			

Indicate arrangement of test tubes by filling in spaces below with
H for hot, W for warm, T for tepid, and C for cold.

Date:

SUBTEST III.

	Date	Date	Date
Temperature feels the same to both hands			
Temperature feels different to each hand			
All feel warmer to affected hand			
All feel cooler to affected hand			
All feel warmer to unaffected hand			
All feel cooler to unaffected hand			
Hottest is intolerably hot to affected hand			
Coldest is intolerably cold to affected hand			

Fig. 2-44. Form for recording scores on test of thermal sensitivity.

position. Curtain on screen should be full, continuous and attached at top only. If such a screen is not available, a blindfold may be used that is as small and comfortable as possible.

CONDITIONS: Test should be conducted in privacy in a non-distracting environment. When fingers and wrist are being tested, S should be seated at a table with screen in front of him in a position to accommodate affected hand and forearm comfortably. E should sit opposite S on other side of screen in a position comfortable to accommodate S's hand for conducting test. When elbow and shoulder are being tested, S should be seated and curtain screen placed at his affected side. Curtain should be draped over his shoulder in such a

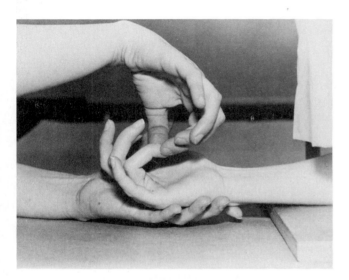

Fig. 2-45. Position sense test of fingers.

manner that he is unable to see his affected arm. If screen is not available, blindfold should be used.

RESPONSES: To determine appreciation of direction of movement S should be instructed to respond "up" (away from floor) and "down" (toward floor) or "out" (away from body) and "in" (toward body) as soon as he perceives direction of movement. Aphasic subjects may respond by pointing in appropiate direction. If there is one unaffected extremity, as in hemiplegia, subject should be asked to imitate with unaffected extremity final position in which part rests after examiner has ceased movement to determine appreciation of position.

METHOD:

Test of fingers: Test positions are index finger flexion, middle finger extension, thumb extension, and little finger flexion. These should be presented in random order. No range should be carried to such an extreme as to elicit pain or a stretch reflex. S's hand and forearm should be placed under curtain, resting on dorsal surface. When testing a right hand, E should support S's hand in his left palm and hold thumb out of way with his left thumb if necessary. This position should induce relaxation of fingers if S has flexor spasticity. With his right hand E should grasp finger to be tested on each side at distal phalanx to avoid giving pressure cues with her thumb and index finger. Finger being tested should be separated from others and should be kept from touching palm to avoid cues from contact. Position of E's hands is reversed when testing a left hand (Fig. 2-45).

Test of wrist: Test positions are wrist flexion and extension. The ranges should not be carried to such an extreme as to elicit tendon action or a stretch reflex. E's and S's hands are positioned as for testing fingers. However, E makes a somewhat firmer grasp at sides of S's hand, reducing contact between her palm and back of S's hand.

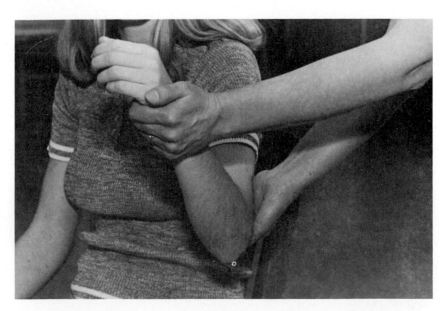

Fig. 2-46. Position and motion sense test of elbow and shoulder.

FORM FOR RECORDING TESTS OF PERCEPTION

Department of Occupational Therapy

Name _____ Age _____ Sex _____ Onset _____

Diagnosis/disability_____

Date_____

TEST OF PROPRIOCEPTION

	Index finger flexion	Middle finger extension	Thumb extension	Little finger flexion	Wrist flexion	Wrist extension	Elbow extension	Shoulder flexion	Shoulder internal rotation	Shoulder flexion-abduction
Appreciation of direction of movement										
Appreciation of position										
Remarks:										

TEST OF STEREOGNOSIS

COMMON OBJECTS	+, -, 0	DESCRIPTION
Pencil		
Fountain pen		
Sunglasses		
Key		
Nail		
Safety pin		
Teaspoon		
Quarter		
Leather coin purse		
Remarks:		

Fig. 2-47. Form for recording scores on tests of perception.

Test of elbow and shoulder: Starting position for all motions is with S's arm at his side, shoulder supported in 20° to 30° of abduction, elbow supported at 90° of flexion, and wrist stabilized at neutral. Test positions are elbow extension, shoulder flexion, shoulder internal rotation, and shoulder flexion-abduction (halfway between 90° of flexion and 90° of abduction). Test position should be presented in random order. Ranges should not be carried to such an extreme as to elicit a stretch reflex or cause pain, if there is joint tightness. S should be seated away from table. Curtained screen should be arranged at S's test side as described or blindfold put in place. E should stand at S's test side and guide limb passively through test positions. When testing a right arm E's right hand should be placed along ulnar border of S's hand and wrist, stabilizing wrist at neutral. E's left hand should be placed on dorsal surface of upper arm just proximal to elbow. Position is reversed when testing left arm. E may carry out all test positions for elbow and shoulder without changing position of her hands (Fig. 2-46).

SCORING (Fig. 2-47):

Appreciation of direction of movement: E records plus if direction is correctly perceived or zero if direction is not perceived.

Appreciation of position: E records plus if correct response is given, minus if response is nearly correct, and zero if response is obviously incorrect or no response is given.

Remarks: E comments on S's reactions, unusual statements, and observations, as well as individual variations in test procedure adapted for specific dysfunctions, on the recording form.

Test for stereognosis[32]

PURPOSE: To evaluate S's ability to perceive tactile properties and identity of common objects.

MATERIALS: Uprights with curtain described in test for light touch. Pencil, fountain pen, sunglasses, key, nail, large safety pin, metal teaspoon, quarter and small leather coin purse.

CONDITIONS: Test should be conducted in privacy in a nondistracting environment. S should be seated at a table with curtain in front of him in a position that accommodates affected hand and forearm comfortably. E should sit opposite S. If S is unable to manipulate test objects because of motor weakness, E should assist S to manipulate them in as near normal a manner as possible.

METHOD: S's hand is under curtain, resting on dorsal surface on table. Objects are presented in random order. Manipulation of objects is allowed and encouraged. Manipulation of objects may be assisted by E if S's hand is partially or completely paralyzed.

RESPONSES: S should be asked to name object or describe its properties if he cannot name it. Aphasic patients may view a duplicate set of test objects after each trial and point to a choice.

SCORING: E marks plus if object is identified quickly and correctly and minus if there is a long delay before identification of object or if S can only describe properties (for example, size, texture, material, shape) of object. E marks a zero if S cannot identify object or its properties (Fig. 2-47).

Test for body scheme[32]

PURPOSE: To evaluate S's ability to recognize and name individual fingers on himself and E, identify body parts, differentiate between right and left, visualize body scheme, and recognize presence of disability.

MATERIALS: A lap board may be used for testing finger identification if S is in a wheelchair. Otherwise S may be seated at a table for finger identification test.

CONDITIONS: Test should be conducted in privacy in a nondistracting environment. S should be seated away from table so he has a good view of himself. E should sit on S's side at such an angle that S can see him clearly. If subject is hemiplegic, E should sit on unaffected side.

RESPONSES:

Finger identification: Names of fingers are to be clarified before test. They should be called thumb, index, middle, ring, and little fingers. S should be instructed to lift or point to appropriate finger as E names them.

Identification of body parts: S should be instructed to point to or raise appropriate parts of body as E names them. Correct part on either side of body is acceptable for full score.

Concept of right and left: S is to point to or raise appropriate parts of body as they are named. Part and side specified are essential for full score.

Visualization of body scheme and recognition of illness: S is to respond "yes" or "no" to a series of questions regarding body orientation and presence of illness. Aphasic subjects may nod "yes" or "no" in response.

METHOD:

Finger identification: On himself S should be asked to identify thumb, ring, little, and index fingers, as E names them. On E S should be asked to identify thumb, index, ring, and little fingers.

Identification of body parts: E should name hand, ear, cheek, knee, shoulder, and mouth, and S should point to or raise appropriate part.

Concept of right and left: E should name right hand, left knee, right foot, left elbow, left ear, right shoulder, left thumb, and right middle finger. S should lift or point to appropriate part and side.

Visualization of body scheme and recognition of illness: S should be instructed to respond with "yes" or "no" to following questions:

Are your feet at the tops of your legs?
Is your hand below your elbow?
Is your knee above your hip?
Are your (E names affected parts) weak, paralyzed?
Are your eyes above your nose?
Do you have one chin?
Are you now in perfect health?
Is your (right, left) leg as strong as (right, left)?
Is your mouth larger than your hand?

Questions may be modified to suit individual cases. Correct answers to questions regarding recognition of illness may vary from case to case.

SCORING (Fig. 2-48):

Finger identification: E records plus if correct identification

TEST OF BODY SCHEME

FINGER IDENTIFICATION	+, 0	LOCATION NAMED, IF INCORRECT
Self: Thumb		
Ring		
Little		
Index		
Examiner: Thumb		
Index		
Ring		
Little		

IDENTIFICATION OF BODY PARTS	+, 0	LOCATION NAMED, IF INCORRECT
Hand		
Ear		
Cheek		
Knee		
Shoulder		
Mouth		

CONCEPT OF RIGHT AND LEFT	+, -, 0	LOCATION NAMED, IF INCORRECT
Right hand		
Left knee		
Right foot		
Left elbow		
Left ear		
Right shoulder		
Left thumb		
Right middle finger		

VISUALIZATION OF BODY SCHEME/ RECOGNITION OF ILLNESS	+, 0	SUBJECT'S COMMENTS
Feet at top of legs?		
Hand below elbow?		
Knee above hip?		
Are your____ weak, paralyzed?		
Arm and leg weak?		
Eyes above nose?		
One chin?		
Perfect health now?		
Right limbs as strong as left?		

Remarks:

Fig. 2-48. Form for recording scores on test of body scheme.

is made and zero for incorrect identification. E also indicates incorrect locations named in response.

Identification of body parts: E records plus for correct identification and zero for incorrect identification.

Concept of right and left: E records plus for correct part and side, minus for correct part and wrong side or incorrect part and correct side, and zero for both incorrect part and side. E also specifies location of S's incorrect responses.

Visualization of body scheme and recognition of illness: E records plus for correct answers and zero for incorrect answers. E also records responses and comments S makes to questions.

DISCUSSION: Body scheme perception may also be evaluated by asking the subject to draw a picture of a man or woman, as appropriate, or assemble a human figure puzzle. These two tasks require several other perceptual and cognitive functions besides body scheme awareness. The examiner should be aware of this if the subject fails at these tasks. To validate responses on any of the methods the subject may be tested in all three ways.

Test of motor planning (praxis)

Praxis is the ability to plan and copy demonstrated acts or carry out movements commonly associated with tools and implements (for example, comb or typewriter) or action words (for example, stir or kick). This skill is critical to success in rehabilitation programs, since much of the training in activities of daily living (ADL), exercises, activities, and work-related tasks involves carrying out demonstrated and verbal instructions, using tools and implements, and learning new movement patterns to perform old familiar tasks. The purpose of testing praxis is to determine the subject's capacity to plan and carry out the motor skills essential to progress.

The tests described are for quick clinical evaluation.

Subtest I: Ability to copy demonstrated acts

PROCEDURE: Examiner (E) sits or stands opposite subject (S). E performs random movements with arms and or legs (for example, strikes poses) and asks S to mimic or copy movements. Initially E should first use symmetrical postures, then asymmetrical, and then postures involving crossing midline. If S has one or more paralyzed limbs, E should not use mirror counterpart of that limb on self in demonstrations.

RESPONSES: Responses should be a mirror image of E's postures. Same procedure may be followed, using hand postures to evaluate fine motor planning, except that E sits next to S on unaffected side (if S is hemiplegic).

EVALUATION: Observe for speed and accuracy of responses.

Intact: S responds quickly and accurately to at least 90% of stimuli.

Impaired: S's responses are delayed or are less than 90% accurate.

Absent: S does not respond accurately to most of stimuli.

Subtest II. Ability to perform movements associated with action words or tools (ideomotor praxis)

PROCEDURE: E hands S an implement used in daily life, (for example, comb, toothbrush) and asks S to show her what to do with it or how to use it.

RESPONSES: S should actually perform or pantomime movements associated with implement.

EVALUATION: Any confusion or delays can be interpreted as some impairment. Inappropriate use of implement or complete inability to use it correctly can be interpreted as a significant dysfunction in praxis.

PROCEDURE: E asks S to pantomime movements that go with action verbs. Suggested test items are stir, rub, brush, comb, beat eggs, and typewrite.

RESPONSES AND EVALUATION: S should be able to carry these

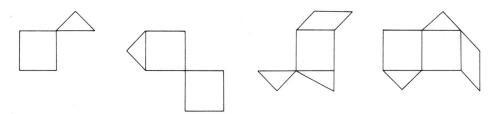

Fig. 2-49. Simple block designs may be used to assess form perception and spatial relationships.

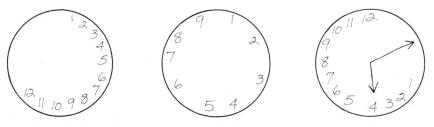

Fig. 2-50. Examples of responses that may be indicative of impaired perception of spatial relationships.

out quickly and accurately. Hesitation and delayed responses may be interpreted as impairment. Inaccurate or no response may be interpreted as a significant impairment of praxis.

Tests of visual form and space perception

Tests of visual form and space perception require constructional praxis. The second requires visual memory and number sequencing. Therefore poor performance could be partially or entirely due to dysfunctions in these skills and not to visual form and space perception impairment. It is wise to test for praxis and visual memory before administering these tests. Also, performance on both tests could be affected by homonymous hemianopsia and neglect of the affected side.

Test of form perception and spatial relationships

MATERIALS: One set of parquetry blocks, pencil, and paper.
PROCEDURE: E sits next to S on unaffected side. E selects five pairs of blocks from set for self and for S (four squares, four triangles, two diamonds). E arranges block designs, first using two, then three, four, and five blocks and asks S to duplicate pattern *after* each set is presented. S may not construct patterns at same time that E is performing (Fig. 2-49).
EVALUATION: Evaluation of performance is based on E's experience and judgment. If form and space perception are intact, S will have no difficulty with this task and may be presented with increasingly complex visual spatial patterns in same manner or may be challenged to copy block designs from paper patterns. Signs of dysfunction may be noted in (1) confusion between forms (for example, diamond and triangle), (2) reversals and inversions of patterns, (3) difficulty positioning block in relation to others (for example, uses a trial and error approach to setting a block down in pattern), (4) placing correct form in wrong position, and (5) omitting a form from pattern. If response is incorrect, E asks whether it looks same as model. If response is "no," E challenges S to attempt to correct it. Often S cannot make corrections but perceives pattern accurately.

Test of spatial relationships

MATERIALS: 8½ × 11-inch piece of plain paper and a pencil.
PROCEDURE: E draws a large circle on paper for S. E asks S to draw a clock face in circle, first arranging numbers, then placing hands at a designated hour.
EVALUATION: Again evaluation is based on E's experience and judgment. Signs of dysfunction may be noted in (1) tendency to space numbers incorrectly (for example, all squeezed together or spread out so they do not fit on clock face) and (2) tendency to be unable to place hands in correct positional relationships (Fig. 2-50).

Test for homonymous hemianopsia (visual field defect)

PROCEDURE: S is seated and asked to fix gaze on an object directly in front of him (6 to 10 feet away). "Object" can be a volunteer or assistant who can observe that S maintains eye fixation. E stands at S's side and holds a pencil or small flashlight. E gradually moves flashlight into S's peripheral visual field and asks S to say "now" or hold up his hand

as soon as he sees flashlight. Flashlight should be held 10 to 15 inches from S's head. This should be repeated four to six times to determine accuracy of response (Fig. 2-51).
EVALUATION: Moving flashlight should be perceived at approximately 180° point on an imaginary circle around S's head at sides of eye. Responses may be recorded on a graph (Fig. 2-52).

COGNITIVE EVALUATION

Cognitive functions may be disturbed by head injury, stroke (CVA), or other diseases involving the brain. Following disease or injury impairments in functions such as judgment, memory, reasoning, problem solving, ab-

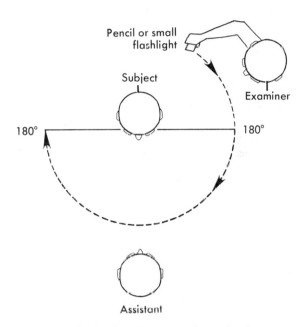

Fig. 2-51. Method of evaluating subject for homonymous hemianopsia (visual field defect).

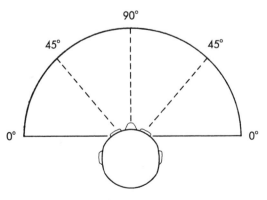

Fig. 2-52. Graph for recording visual field defect. On semicircle shade in number of degrees of estimated visual field defect.

stract thinking, concentration, sequencing, reading, computation, and generalization of learning may be evident.

The occupational therapist should observe for deficits in these functions throughout her interaction with the client during evaluation and treatment procedures. She should note apparent problems, and describe in evaluation and progress reports behaviors that support her judgment.

Cognitive dysfunctions and behaviors for observation are described in Chapters 13 and 14.

SECTION THREE
Performance evaluation

The performance evaluation focuses on the client's abilities and limitations in performing activities of self-maintenance, work, and play-leisure. It is a primary purpose of occupational therapy to facilitate skill in performance of these essential tasks of living. It is important to help the client to create a balance in the quantity of activity in each of these three performance areas, which is healthy for him in terms of personality, skills, limitations, needs, values, and life-style.

For the therapist to assay the client's performance profile, the evaluation could begin with the charting of a daily or weekly schedule.

THE DAILY SCHEDULE

The therapist should interview the client to get a detailed account of his activities for a typical day (or week) in his life prior to the onset of physical dysfunction and at present after the onset of dysfunction. Information that should be elicited is outlined as follows:

Rising hour
Morning activities with hours
    Hygiene
    Dressing
    Breakfast
    Work-leisure-home management
    Child care
    Luncheon
Afternoon activities with hours
    Work-leisure-home management
    Child care
    Rest
    Social activities
    Dinner
Evening activities with hours
    Leisure-social activities
    Preparation for retiring
Bedtime

Amount of time spent on each activity should be recorded carefully. During the interview the therapist should be careful not to allow the client to gloss over or omit any of the daily activities by cuing him with appropriate questions.

The therapist might ask "What time did you get up?" "What was the first thing that you did?" "When did you eat lunch?" "Who fixed it for you?" The review of the former daily schedule may evoke many recollections of family, friends, and social, community, vocational, and leisure activities about which the client may share information freely. At times this digression from the schedule itself is desirable to elicit a well-rounded picture of the client in his roles and relationships, as well as some ideas of his needs, values, and personal goals. In other instances tangential conversation should be limited or discouraged to focus the client's attention on the specific daily schedule.

If memory or communication disorders make the construction of the daily schedule impossible in the manner described, friends or family members may be consulted to get an approximation of the client's activities pattern that may be helpful for goal setting and activity selection.

A second daily schedule of present activities pattern in the treatment facility or at home, if the client is an outpatient, is then constructed. It is important during this interview to ask the client who helps him with each activity, and how much assistance he believes he needs and receives. A discussion and comparative analysis of these two schedules between therapist and client should yield valuable information about the client's needs, values, satisfaction-dissatisfaction with the activities pattern, primary and secondary goals for change, interests, motivation, interpersonal relationships, and fears. On the basis of this information and the activity analysis it becomes possible to set priorities for treatment objectives according to the client's needs and values rather than the therapist's priorities. Activities that will be meaningful to the client as an individual and in his particular social group, and may be appropriate for use in the intervention plan, begin to emerge. Their potential for facilitation of change may be presented, and selection of therapeutic modalities to meet objectives that have been agreed on can be made.

ACTIVITIES OF DAILY LIVING (ADL) EVALUATION

Procedures for conducting the ADL evaluation are discussed in Chapter 4. The emphasis there is on evaluation of self-care tasks. Fig. 2-53 is a suggested form for recording results of self-care performance evaluation. There are a wide variety of such forms, although they are all somewhat similar. Many treatment facilities have

Text continued on p. 73.

```
                    OCCUPATIONAL THERAPY DEPARTMENT

                  ACTIVITIES OF DAILY LIVING EVALUATION


Name_____Age_____Diagnosis_____ Dom._____

Mode of ambulation_____ Disability_____

     Grading key:    I = Independent          D = Dependent
                   MiA = Minimal assistance   NA = Not applicable
                   MoA = Moderate assistance    0 = Not evaluated
                   MaA = Maximal assistance

TRANSFERS AND AMBULATION
```

	Date	Independent	Assisted	Dependent
Tub or shower				
Toilet				
Wheelchair				
Bed and chair				
Ambulation				
Wheelchair management				
Car				

```
BALANCE FOR FUNCTION

          Adequate  Inadequate
Sitting  _____|_____
Standing _____|_____
Walking  _____|_____

SUMMARY OF EVALUATION RESULTS

Date_____
Intact  Impaired                                        REMARKS
                    SENSORY STATUS
_____|_____    Touch          _____
_____|_____    Pain           _____
_____|_____    Temperature    _____
_____|_____    Position sense _____
_____|_____    Olfaction      _____
_____|_____    Stereognosis   _____
_____|_____    Visual fields (hemianopsia)_____

                    PERCEPTUAL/CONCEPTUAL TESTS
_____|_____    Follow directions_____
_____|_____    Visual spatial (form)_____
_____|_____    Visual spatial (block design)_____
_____|_____    Make change _____
_____|_____    Geometric figures (copy)_____
_____|_____       Square, circle, triangle, diamond _____
_____|_____    Praxis _____

                    FUNCTIONAL RANGE OF MOTION
_____|_____    Comb hair—two hands _____
_____|_____    Feed self _____
_____|_____    Button collar button _____
_____|_____    Tie apron behind back_____
_____|_____    Button back buttons _____
_____|_____    Button cuffs _____
_____|_____    Zip side zipper _____
_____|_____    Tie shoes_____
_____|_____    Stoop _____
_____|_____    Reach shelf _____
```

Fig. 2-53. ADL evaluation. (Adapted from Activities of Daily Living, evaluation form OT 461-1, Hartford, Conn., Sept. 1963, The Hartford Easter Seal Rehabilitation Center.)

Continued.

ADL SKILLS

EATING | Date | | | | | | REMARKS

Butter bread
Cut meat
Eat with spoon
Eat with fork
Drink with straw
Drink with glass
Drink with cup
Pour from pitcher

UNDRESS | Date | | | | | | REMARKS

Pants or shorts
Girdle or garter belt
Brassiere
Slip or undershirt
Dress
Skirt
Blouse or shirt
Slacks or trousers
Bandana or necktie
Stockings
Nightclothes
Hair net
Housecoat or bathrobe
Jacket
Belt and/or suspenders
Hat
Coat
Sweater
Mittens or gloves
Glasses
Brace
Shoes
Socks
Overshoes

DRESS | Date | | | | | | REMARKS

Pants or shorts
Girdle or garter belt
Brassiere
Slip or undershirt
Dress
Skirt
Blouse or shirt
Slacks or trousers
Bandana or necktie
Stockings
Nightclothes
Hair net
Housecoat or bathrobe
Jacket
Belt and/or suspenders
Hat
Coat
Sweater
Mittens or gloves
Glasses
Brace
Shoes
Socks
Overshoes

Fig. 2-53, cont'd. ADL evaluation.

FASTENINGS

Date						REMARKS
	Grade					
Button						
Snap						
Zipper						
Hook and eye						
Garters						
Lace						
Untie shoes						
Velcro						

HYGIENE

Date						REMARKS
	Grade					
Blow nose						
Wash face, hands						
Wash extremities, back						
Brush teeth or dentures						
Brush or comb hair						
Set hair						
Shave or put on makeup						
Clean fingernails						
Trim fingernails, toenails						
Apply deodorant						
Shampoo hair						
Use toilet paper						
Use tampon or sanitary napkin						

COMMUNICATION

Date						REMARKS
	Grade					
Verbal						
Read						
Hold book						
Turn page						
Write						
Use telephone						
Type						

HAND ACTIVITIES

Date						REMARKS
	Grade					
Handle money						
Handle mail						
Use of scissors						
Open cans, bottles, jars						
Tie package						
Sew (baste)						
Sew button, hook and eye						
Polish shoes						
Sharpen pencil						
Seal and open letter						
Open box						

Fig. 2-53, cont'd. ADL evaluation.

Continued.

COMBINED PERFORMANCE
    ACTIVITIES

Date	Grade				REMARKS
Open-close refrigerator					
Open-close door					
Remove and replace object					
Carry objects during locomotion					
Pick up object from floor					
Remove, replace light bulb					
Plug in cord					

OPERATE

Date	Grade				REMARKS
Light switches					
Doorbell					
Door locks and handles					
Faucets					
Raise-lower window shades					
Raise-lower venetian blinds					
Raise-lower window					
Open and close drawer					
Hang up garment					

Fig. 2-53, cont'd. ADL evaluation.

OCCUPATIONAL THERAPY DEPARTMENT

ACTIVITIES OF HOME MANAGEMENT

Name_____ Date_____

Address_____

Age_____ Weight_____ Height_____ Role in family_____

Diagnosis_____ Disability_____

Mode of ambulation_____

Limitations or contraindications for activity____ _____

DESCRIPTION OF HOME

    1. Private house _____
        No. of rooms _____
        No. of floors _____
        Stairs _____
        Elevators _____

    2. Apartment house _____
        No. of rooms _____
        No. of floors _____
        Stairs _____
        Elevators _____

    3. Diagram of home layout (attach to completed form)

Will patient be required to perform the following activities? If not, who will perform?

Meal preparation _____ _____
Baking _____ _____
Serving _____ _____
Wash dishes _____ _____
Marketing _____ _____
Child care
  (under 4 years) _____ _____
Washing _____ _____
Hanging clothes _____ _____
Ironing _____ _____
Cleaning _____ _____
Sewing _____ _____
Hobbies or
  special interest _____ _____

Does patient really like housework? Yes_____ No_____

Fig. 2-54. Activities of home management. (Adapted from Occupational Therapy Department, University Hospital, Ohio State University, Columbus, Ohio.)

Continued.

```
                    ACTIVITIES OF HOME MANAGEMENT

   Sitting position:    Chair_____ Stool_____ Wheelchair_____
   Standing position:   Braces_____ Crutches_____ Canes_____
   Handedness: Dominant hand_____Two hands_____One hand only_____ Assistive_____

      Grading key:   I = Independent              MaA = Maximal assistance
                   MiA = Minimal assistance         D = Dependent
                   MoA = Moderate assistance         O = Not evaluated
```

CLEANING ACTIVITIES	Date					REMARKS
	Grade					
Pick up object from floor						
Wipe up spills						
Make bed (daily)						
Use dust mop						
Shake dust mop						
Dust low surfaces						
Dust high surfaces						
Mop kitchen floor						
Sweep with broom						
Use dust pan and broom						
Use vacuum cleaner						
Use vacuum cleaner attachments						
Carry light cleaner tools						
Use carpet sweeper						
Clean bathtub						
Change sheets on bed						
Carry pail of water						

MEAL PREPARATION	Date					REMARKS
	Grade					
Turn off water						
Turn off gas or electric range						
Light gas with match						
Pour hot water from pan to cup						
Open packaged goods						
Carry pan from sink to range						
Use can opener						
Handle milk bottle						
Dispose of garbage						
Remove things from refrigerator						
Bend to low cupboards						
Reach to high cupboards						
Peel vegetables						
Cut up vegetables						
Handle sharp tools safely						
Break eggs						
Stir against resistance						
Measure flour						
Use eggbeater						
Use electric mixer						
Remove batter to pan						
Open oven door						
Carry pan to oven and put in						
Remove hot pan from oven to table						
Roll cookie dough or piecrust						

Fig. 2-54, cont'd. Activities of home management.

ACTIVITIES OF HOME MANAGEMENT—cont'd

MEAL SERVICE | Date | Grade | | | | | REMARKS

Set table for four
Carry four glasses of water to table
Carry hot casserole to table
Clear table
Scrape and stack dishes
Wash dishes (light soil)
Wipe silver
Wash pots and pans
Wipe up range and work areas
Wring out dishcloth

LAUNDRY | Date | Grade | | | | | REMARKS

Wash lingerie (by hand)
Wring out, squeeze dry
Hang on rack to dry
Sprinkle clothes
Iron blouse or slip
Fold blouse or slip
Use washing machine

SEWING | Date | Grade | | | | | REMARKS

Thread needle and make knot
Sew on buttons
Mend rips
Darn socks
Use sewing machine
Crochet
Knit
Embroider
Cut with shears

HEAVY HOUSEHOLD ACTIVITIES
WHO WILL DO THESE? | Date | Grade | | | | | REMARKS

Wash household laundry
Hang clothes
Clean range
Clean refrigerator
Wax floors
Marketing
Turn mattresses
Wash windows
Put up curtains

Fig. 2-54, cont'd. Activities of home management.

Continued.

WORK HEIGHTS   SITTING/STANDING

Best height for   Wheelchair_____ Chair_____ Stool_____

   Ironing   _____

   Mixing   _____

   Dish washing   _____

   General work   _____

Maximum depth of counter area (normal reach) _____

Maximum useful height above work surface   _____

Maximum useful height without counter surface_____

Maximum reach below counter area   _____

Best height for chair   _____

Best height for stool with back support   _____

SUGGESTIONS FOR HOME MODIFICATION

_____

_____

_____

_____

_____

_____

_____

_____

_____

_____

_____

_____

Fig. 2-54, cont'd. Activities of home management.

developed their own forms. The practitioner must learn and use the system of recording used in the particular treatment facility.

Home management tasks are evaluated similarly to self-care tasks. The client should first be interviewed to elicit a description of the home and former and present home management responsibilities. Those tasks that the client will need to perform when returning home, as well as those that he would like to perform, should be ascertained during the interview. If there are communication disorders, aid of friends or family members may be enlisted to get the information needed. The client may also be questioned about his ability to perform each task on the activities list. However, the evaluation is much more meaningful if this is followed by a performance evaluation in the ADL kitchen or apartment of the treatment facility or in the client's home if possible.

The initial tasks should be simple one- or two-step procedures that are not hazardous, such as wiping a dish, sponging off the table, or turning the water on and off. As the evaluation progresses, tasks graded in complexity and involving safety precautions should be performed, such as making a sandwich and a cup of coffee and vacuuming the carpet. It is assumed here that the therapist has already evaluated motor, sensory, perceptual, and cognitive skills. Consequently she should select tasks and exercise safety precautions in keeping with the client's capabilities and limitations.

Traditionally, home management skills were thought to apply primarily to women clients. However, they are appropriate for men and sometimes for children and adolescents as well. In our modern society men are more often living independently or sharing home management responsibilities with the partner. In some homes it will be necessary for a role reversal to occur after onset of a physical disability, and the woman partner may seek employment outside the home for the first time, while the disabled man remains at home. If he will be there alone, at the very least he needs to be able to prepare a simple meal, employ safety precautions, and get emergency aid if needed. The occupational therapist can evaluate potential for remaining at home alone through the activities of home management evaluation. Fig. 2-54 is a suggested form for recording results of the home management evaluation.

HOME EVALUATION

When the discharge from the treatment facility is anticipated, a home evaluation should be carried out. The purpose of the home evaluation is to facilitate the client's maximum independence in his living environment. Ideally it should be performed by the physical and occupational therapists together on a visit to the client's home with the client and family members or housemates present. Budgetary and time factors may not allow two professional workers to go to the client's home, however. Therefore either the physical or occupational therapist should be able to perform the evaluation.

Before the visit the client and a family member should be interviewed to determine the client's and family's expectations and the roles the client will assume in the home and community. The cultural or family values regarding a disabled member may influence role expectations and whether or not independence will be encouraged. Willingness and financial ability to make modifications in the home can also be determined.[29]

Sufficient time should be scheduled for the home visit so that the client can demonstrate the required transfer and mobility skills. The therapist may also wish to ask the client to demonstrate selected self-care and home management tasks, which were learned at the treatment facility, in his home environment. The client should use the ambulation aids and any assistive devices that he is accustomed to during the evaluation. The therapist should bring a measuring device to determine, for example, width of doorways, height of stairs, and height of bed.

The therapist can begin by explaining the purposes and procedure of the home evaluation to the client and others present, if not done prior to the visit. She can proceed to take the required measurements while surveying the general arrangement of rooms, furniture, and appliances. It may be helpful to sketch the size and arrangement of rooms for later reference and attach these to the home visit checklist (Fig. 2-55). Once this is completed, the client is involved in demonstrating his mobility and transfer skills as designated on the form and in demonstrating performance of essential self-care and home management tasks. The client's ability to use the entrance to the home and transfer to and from an automobile, if to be used, should be included in the home evaluation.

During the performance evaluation the therapist should be observing for safety factors, ease of mobility and performance, and limitations imposed by the environment. If the client requires assistance for transfers and other activities, the caretaker should be instructed in the methods that are appropriate.

At the end of the evaluation the therapist can make a list of problems. Additional safety equipment, assistive devices, home rearrangement, or alteration may be necessary to solve these. The most frequently needed changes are installation of a ramp or railings at the entrance to the home; removal of scatter rugs, extra furniture, and bric-a-brac; removal of door sills; addition of safety grab bars around the toilet and bathtub; rearrangement of furniture to accommodate a wheelchair;

HOME VISIT CHECKLIST

Name_____ Therapist_____

Address_____ Date_____

Diagnosis_____ Disability_____

Type of home   Apartment_____ Floor, if apt._____

                Private home_____ No. of rooms_____ No. of floors_____

ENTRANCE TO HOME
1. Elevator_____ Stairs_____
2. Number of stairs_____
3. Height of stairs_____
4. Is there a handrail?_____Left_____Right_____(facing house)
5. Are there other entrances that can be used? Describe_____
    _____
    _____
6. Is construction of a ramp feasible?_____
7. Is addition of a handrail feasible?_____
    Comments_____
    _____
    _____

BEDROOM
1. Width of doorway_____
2. Is there a doorsill?_____
3. Height of bed_____
4. Is bed suitable for attachment of side rails?_____ trapeze bar?_____
5. Can furniture be arranged more conveniently?_____
6. Can patient reach closets?_____ bureaus?_____
7. Is there room for a wheelchair to maneuver?_____
8. Is there room for additional furniture (e.g., commode seat)?_____

BATHROOM
1. Width of doorway_____
2. Is there a doorsill?_____
3. Type of bathtub: roll rim_____ square rim_____wide square rim_____
4. Can wheelchair get close to sink?_____ toilet?_____bathtub?_____
5. Is tub enclosed by shower curtain?_____ sliding doors?_____
6. Is there a separate shower stall?_____
7. Is bathroom on same floor as bedroom?_____ living room?_____ kitchen?_____
8. Is it feasible to install handrails on bathtub?_____ walls?_____ toilet?____
9. Additional comments_____
    _____
    _____
    _____
    _____

Fig. 2-55. Home visit checklist. (Adapted from The Hartford Easter Seal Rehabilitation Center, 1964, Hartford, Conn.)

KITCHEN
1. Width of doors_____
2. Is there a doorsill?_____
3. Is there room for movement of wheelchair?_____
4. Are cupboards within reach?_____
5. Can patient use kitchen utilities (e.g., range, sink, refrigerator)?_____
6. Is rearrangement of furniture feasible?_____
7. Additional comments_____
    _____
    _____
    _____

OTHER ROOMS
1. Width of doors_____
2. Are there doorsills?_____
3. Are light switches in easy reach?_____
4. Would furniture rearrangement be feasible?_____
5. Is telephone conveniently located?_____
6. If needed, is there suitable space for installation of parallel bars?_____

FUNCTIONAL ACTIVITIES OF PATIENT
1. Can patient enter and leave home independently?_____
    If not, what assistance is needed?_____
2. Can the patient move about the home freely?_____
    If not, comment on limitations. _____
    _____
    _____
3. Which transfer activities is patient unable to perform independently?_____
    Bed to wheelchair_____
    Chair to bed _____
    Toilet_____
    Bathtub_____
    Shower_____
    Automobile_____
4. Self-care activities: Comment on performance and limitations imposed by home
    environment, if any._____
    _____
    _____
5. Home management activities_____
    _____
    _____

PROBLEM LIST
_____
_____
_____
_____

RECOMMENDATIONS FOR HOME MODIFICATION/SPECIAL EQUIPMENT
_____
_____
_____
_____
_____
_____
_____

Fig. 2-55, cont'd. Home visit checklist.

rearrangement of kitchen storage; and lowering of the clothes rod in the closet.[29]

When the home evaluation is completed, the therapist should write a report summarizing the information on the form and describing the client's performance in the home. The report should conclude with a summary of the problems the client is encountering and recommendations for their solution that would facilitate independence. Any equipment or alterations that are recommended should be specific in terms of size, building specifications, costs, and sources.

These recommendations are carefully reviewed with the client and his family. This is done with tact and diplomacy in a way that gives them options and freedom to refuse or consider alternative possibilities. Family finances may be a limiting factor in carrying out needed changes. The social worker may be involved in working out funding for needed equipment and alterations, and the client should be made aware of this service when cost is discussed.[29]

The therapist should include her recommendations regarding the feasibility of the client's discharge to the home environment or his remaining in or managing the home alone, if these apply.

If a home visit is not possible, much of the information can be gained by interviewing the client and family member following a trial home visit. The family member or caretaker may be instructed to complete the home visit checklist and provide photographs or sketches of the rooms and their arrangements. Problems encountered by the client during the trial home visit should be discussed and the necessary recommendations for their solution made, as described earlier.[29]

PREVOCATIONAL AND VOCATIONAL EVALUATION

Prevocational and vocational evaluation and training programs are specialized areas in occupational therapy. The ultimate goal of such programs is to estimate the client's vocational potential, measure basic skills necessary for work, and aid in setting appropriate vocational goals.

The occupational therapist is an appropriate evaluator of prevocational and vocational potential because of her personal skills and professional knowledge. She is interested in working with people; has the ability to perceive, observe, and analyze performance and performance problems; has knowledge of dysfunctions; possesses teaching and motivating skills; can perform activity and task analyses; and knows or has the ability to learn a wide variety of work-related tasks and skills.[18]

Prevocational evaluation, usually performed by the occupational therapist, includes evaluation of physical assets and limitations; ADL performance, including transfer and transportation skills; perceptual and cognitive functions; and general educational abilities,[18] (for example, reading, computation, change making, and the recognition and interpretation of street signs and traffic signals).

Work evaluation assesses specific work skills using a real or simulated work situation.[18] Work habits and attitudes are also observed and evaluated. Work evaluation may be carried out by the occupational therapist following the prevocational assessment. However, work evaluation may also be performed by a vocational evaluator.

The prevocational or work evaluations may reveal the need to develop the necessary physical, performance,

Table 2. Skills and abilities for prevocational evaluation in occupational therapy

Physical resources-capacities	General abilities	Work behavior and attitudes	Work skills
Strength	Computational skills	Interpersonal skills, relationships	Dexterity
ROM	Reading skills	Reaction to supervision	Work speed
Sensation-perception-cognition	Mechanical aptitude	Cooperation with co-workers	Quality of work
Speech-hearing	Self-care independence	Interest	Use of tools and machines
Vision	Hygiene, appearance	Motivation	Ability to follow instruc-
Ability and tolerance for	Transfer-transportation	Concentration/perseverance at task	tions
Sitting	abilities	Emotional reactions	Verbal
Standing		Family concerns	Written
Walking		Child care	Demonstrated
Running		Home management responsibili-	Designed
Lifting-carrying		ties affecting employment	Demonstrated aptitudes
Grasp-handling			
Pushing-pulling			
Climbing-crouching			
Presence of chronic pain			
Effect on performance			

or psychosocial skills required of a worker. The occupational therapist may then engage the client in a work adjustment program. This has as its goals the development of physical capacities, such as transfer skills or speed of motion; psychosocial skills, such as ability to be supervised or get along with co-workers; and work habits, such as punctuality and perseverance at a task.

The vocational counselor coordinates the vocational evaluation. The vocational counselor gathers data from pertinent medical, psychological, social, educational, and vocational histories; examines environmental and cultural aspects of the client's situation[18] as they relate to employment; receives reports of prevocational and work evaluation; may counsel the client and administer specific aptitude or interest tests; and sets appropriate vocational goals with the client. The vocational counselor may assist the client in securing sheltered or competitive employment as a final outcome of the vocational evaluation program.

Role of the occupational therapist

The occupational therapist can function at all levels of evaluation but her skills are most suitable for prevocational and work adjustment programs.

Before evaluation is started, the client should be at or near his maximum rehabilitation potential. The focus of the program will be different from that of the rehabilitation program because there is emphasis on work speed, quality of products, concentration on task with minimal socialization, promptness, and perseverance. The occupational therapist evaluates physical resources (capacities, deficits), ADL, social behavior for work, emotional maturity, vocational development, general intellectual abilities, and performance of real or simulated jobs. Table 2 is a list of the skills and abilities that may be evaluated by the occupational therapist. A wide variety of forms have been devised to record the results of evaluation (Fig. 2-56).

A report of the findings of the prevocational and work evaluations should be prepared for the vocational counselor, who will use it to help the client select appropriate goals and determine the next step in the vocationally oriented program.

Methods of evaluation

A variety of methods can be used to evaluate work potential. Occupational therapists may use crafts activities to assess such factors as use of tools, manual dexterity, work quality, computation, perceptual skills, and work speed. Work samples or simulated work stations may be used to evaluate specific work skills as well as work habits and attitudes. Commercial systems of evaluation are also available. Kester[18] lists and describes several such systems.

To develop work samples or work stations the vocational counselor or the occupational therapist may survey the community to determine the job market and types of industries and businesses that are supported there. Suitable jobs can be selected and analyzed for their performance requirements. Some employers may be willing to provide the necessary equipment and material for a work sample test or work station. Some possibilities are clerical jobs, assembly work, business machines operation, and garment construction. The *Dictionary of Occupational Titles* (DOT) is a helpful resource for job descriptions and requirements. It is published by the U.S. Department of Labor Employment and Training Administration and is available from the U.S. Government Printing Office.

More realistic work evaluation may be effected through assignment of the client to sheltered employment or a job within the health care facility or cooperating agency on a trial basis. Under these conditions the supervisor, who is someone other than the therapist or counselor, should be apprised of the client's skills and limitations, vocational goals, and specific aspects of performance that are to be observed and evaluated. The standards of evaluation should also be clear to the work supervisor, that is, is the client to perform at minimum standards required for the job or will lesser performance be acceptable at this stage in his rehabilitation?

Candidates for evaluation

Who is selected for prevocational evaluation? Generally employment should be a consideration for adolescents, young adults, and older adults who are involved in rehabilitation for physical dysfunction. This group will include those who have never worked, those who have worked and will be returning to the same or similar jobs, and those who have worked and must seek a change in occupation.

The candidate should have achieved or have the potential to achieve (1) adequate independence in self-care with or without attendant care, (2) adequate transportation to and from the work place with or without assistance, and (3) adequate physical performance, and psychosocial skills to perform in a work setting. Inadequate vocational development may be a problem for some clients, especially those in the adolescent and young adult groups. With these individuals the prevocational program may need to include development of work habits, identification as a worker, and vocational exploration and choice making.

Alternatives to work

The result of the prevocational evaluation may be that the client is not a candidate for employment. Age, severity of the dysfunction, or serious psychosocial limi-

PREVOCATIONAL EVALUATION

PATIENT PROGRESS REPORT*

Name_____ Address _____ Phone_____

Admission date_____ Schedule_____Days per week_____Hours per day_____

Type of transportation facility used_____ Driver's license_____

Diagnosis_____

Appliances used_____ Dominant hand_____

Period of evaluation: From_____ To_____

Jobs performed_____

OBSERVATIONS

	WORK TIME (%)	SUP.	AV.	LTD.	POOR
PHYSICAL ASPECTS					
Walking					
Standing					
Sitting					
Lifting (in lbs.)					
Carrying (in lbs.)					
Bending					
Climbing stairs					
Speech					
Hearing					
Vision					
Working speed					
Self-care					
Bimanual dexterity					
Finger dexterity					
Unaffected hand					
Affected hand					
INTELLECTUAL ASPECTS					
Learning speed					
Retention					
Reading ability					
Work accuracy					
Arithmetical ability					
Judgment					
Problem solving					
Writing ability					
PERSONALITY ASPECTS					
Neatness					
Adaptability					
Regularity					
Punctuality					
Reliability					
Interest					
Initiative					
Ability to work independently					
Personal habits					
Interpersonal relations					
Conformance to rules					
Cooperativeness					
Perseverance					
Desire for employment					

COMMENTS: Include <u>brief</u> explanation pointing up any of above ratings checked.
Include brief summary of machines operated and jobs done.
Include any precautions to be observed with patient.

*NOTE: Rating terms, as used, are to be interpreted as being applicable to
performance in regular, competitive employment. Sup. = Superior,
Av. = Average, and Ltd. = Limited.

Fig. 2-56. Prevocational evaluation patient progress report. (Adapted from The Hartford Easter Seal Rehabilitation Center, 1964, Hartford, Conn.)

tations can make the goal of employment unrealistic. What are the alternatives for such individuals?

Occupational therapists can play a primary role in helping to select alternatives and in actively developing or working in alternative programs. The occupational therapist should not overlook the client's leisure needs and should evaluate performance of potential avocational pursuits that can be done independently at home. This is an area that therapists have neglected and relegated to a lesser status in their professional work. Yet avocational pursuits are an integral part of each person's occupational performance and contribute to health and well-being.

The occupational therapist can facilitate support, maintenance, or activities groups or day-care programs within the health care facility, if funding allows, or seek alternative community programs for the disabled. Examples of these are arthritis or stroke clubs that have been organized in many communities. Some disabled individuals are able to take part in senior citizen and adult education programs that are offered to all residents of a community.

It is necessary for the occupational therapist to explore the alternatives and evaluate the client for his ability to participate. It is often necessary for the occupational therapist, or a friend or family member whose help has been enlisted, to accompany the client to community programs the first few times to facilitate the client's adjustment and solve any problems that prohibit full participation.

Summary

The occupational therapist has an important role to play in prevocational evaluation. Together with the vocational counselor, social worker, and other pertinent members of the health care team, occupational therapy can facilitate the client's progress toward self-sufficiency through employment.

If employment goals are not a feasible outcome of the prevocational evaluation, occupational therapy can offer alternatives that can give meaning and satisfaction to the client's life.

REVIEW QUESTIONS
Motor evaluation

1. Describe general rules for positioning the goniometer when measuring joint ROM.
2. With which diagnoses would joint measurement be a primary evaluation procedure?
3. List and discuss four purposes of joint measurement.
4. Is formal joint measurement necessary for every client? If not, how may ROM be evaluated quickly?
5. Describe the steps in the procedure for joint measurement.
6. How is joint ROM measurement recorded on the evaluation form?
7. List the average normal ROM for elbow flexion, shoulder flexion, finger MP flexion, hip flexion, knee flexion, and ankle dorsiflexion.

8. Define the muscle grades: normal (5), good (4), fair− (3−), fair (3), poor (2), poor− (2−), trace (1), and zero (0).
9. What are the criteria used to determine muscle grades?
10. In relation to the floor as a horizontal plane, describe what is meant by with gravity assisting, with gravity eliminated, against gravity, and against gravity and resistance.
11. What does the manual muscle test measure?
12. What does the manual muscle test not evaluate about motor function?
13. List the steps in the muscle testing procedure.
14. How can you differentiate between muscle weakness and joint limitation?
15. If there is joint limitation, can muscle strength be measured accurately? How?
16. For which types of physical dysfunctions is the manual muscle test most appropriate and useful?
17. Considering the criteria used to grade muscle function in the manual muscle test and the characteristic motor behavior of patients with hemiplegia, why are Brunnstrom's Hemiplegia Evaluation and the Functional Muscle Examination more appropriate for measuring their motor function?
18. Is it always necessary to perform the manual muscle test to determine level of strength? If not, what alternative may be used to make a general assessment of strength? Very generally, describe the procedure.
19. What is evaluated in Brunnstrom's Hemiplegia Evaluation?
20. Describe the procedure for evaluating for recovery stage 4.
21. What are the criteria for achievement of each recovery stage?
22. What is the purpose of the Functional Muscle Examination? Why was it designed?
23. Describe the components of a comprehensive hand evaluation.
24. Why should the physical evaluation precede the functional evaluation?
25. What should the therapist observe when evaluating hand function?
26. Name two standardized functional evaluations for the hand.
27. Describe the quick clinical tests for radial, median, and ulnar nerve dysfunction and give the rationale for each in terms of motor function.
28. Describe the test for the type I swan-neck deformity.
29. Describe the test for the type II boutonnière deformity.
30. List the reflexes that are integrated in each of the CNS levels described in the text.
31. Describe or demonstrate the procedures and give the norms for each of the following reflexes or reactions: extensor thrust, ATNR, TLR, neck righting, optical righting, and equilibrium reactions.
32. How is the sucking reflex different from the rooting reflex?
33. Describe Landau's reflex.

Sensory and perceptual evaluation

1. Why is sensory and perceptual evaluation necessary and important to occupational therapy?
2. What types of disabilities should be routinely given sensory evaluation?
3. How is light touch sensitivity evaluated? Describe.
4. If the patient recognizes that he was touched but cannot localize the stimulus, what grade would be given on the test for light touch?
5. What are the alternatives for responses in the position sense test?
6. Why is it important to grasp the fingers and wrist laterally during the test for position sense?
7. What are some methods for occluding the patient's vision? What are the alternatives to blindfolding or asking the patient to keep his eyes closed?

8. Define "stereognosis," and describe how it can be evaluated.
9. Define "body scheme," and describe three ways it can be evaluated.
10. Define "motor planning."
11. Describe the clinical test for form perception and spatial relationships.
12. How can you evaluate for presence of a visual field defect?

Performance evaluation

1. Describe the "daily schedule," and tell its purpose in the performance evaluation of the client.
2. List the steps in the activities of home management evaluation.
3. What is the purpose of the home evaluation?
4. List the steps in the home evaluation.
5. Who should be involved in a comprehensive home evaluation?
6. What kinds of things are assessed in a home evaluation?
7. How does the therapist record and report results of the home evaluation and make the necessary recommendations?
8. Describe the differences between prevocational evaluation, work adjustment, and vocational evaluation.
9. What is the role of the occupational therapist in vocationally oriented programs?
10. List three criteria the client should meet before embarking on a vocational evaluation.
11. What are three methods that may be used to assess vocational potential?
12. List the evaluation tools you would use to measure dysfunction in clients with joint limitation (for example, arthritis), LMN disability (for example, peripheral nerve injury), UMN disability (for example, hemiplegia), and amputation (for example, upper extremity).

REFERENCES

1. American Academy of Orthopedic Surgeons: Joint motion: method of measuring and recording, Chicago, 1965, American Academy of Orthopedic Surgeons.
2. Anonymous: How to measure range of motion of the upper extremities, Downey, Calif., Rancho Los Amigos Hospital. Mimeographed.
3. Anonymous: Procedures for gross sensory evaluation, Downey, Calif., Rancho Los Amigos Hospital. Mimeographed.
4. Anonymous: The technique of goniometry, Richmond, Va., Baruch Center of Physical Medicine, Medical College of Virginia. Mimeographed.
5. Banus, B.S., editor: The developmental therapist, Thorofare, N.J., 1971, Charles B. Slack, Inc.
6. Bobath, B.: Adult hemiplegia: evaluation and treatment, London, 1970, William Heinemann Medical Books Ltd.
7. Burton, R.I., et al.: The hand: examination and diagnosis, Aurora, Colo., 1978, The American Society for Surgery of the Hand.
8. Brand, P., and Wood, H.: Hand volumeter instruction sheet, United States Public Health Service Hospital, Carville, La.
9. Brunnstrom, S.: Movement therapy in hemiplegia, New York, 1970, Harper & Row, Publishers, Inc.
10. Carroll, D.: A quantitative test of upper extremity function, J. Chron. Dis. 18:479, 1965.
11. Chusid, J.G.: Correlative neuroanatomy and functional neurology, ed. 15, Los Altos, Calif., 1973, Lange Medical Publications.
12. Creelman, G.: Post Office Box 146, Idyllwild, Calif. 92349. Commercially available volumeter and pamphlet.
13. Dellon, A.L., Curtis, R.M., and Edgerton, M.T.: Reeducation of sensation in the hand after nerve injury and repair, Plast. Reconstr. Surg. 53:297, 1974.
14. Esch, D., and Lepley, M.: Evaluation of joint motion: methods of measurement and recording, Minneapolis, 1974, University of Minnesota Press.
15. Fiorentino, M.R.: Reflex testing methods for evaluating CNS development, Springfield, Ill., 1973, Charles C Thomas, Publisher.
16. Hunter, J.M., et al.: Rehabilitation of the hand, St. Louis, 1978, The C.V. Mosby Co.
17. Jebsen, R.H., et al.: An objective and standardized test of hand function, Arch. Phys. Med. Rehabil. 50:311, 1969.
18. Kester, D.L.: Prevocational and vocational assessment. In Hopkins, H.L., and Smith, H.D., editors: Willard and Spackman's occupational therapy, ed. 5, Philadelphia, 1978, J.B. Lippincott Co.
19. Landen, B.R., and Amizich, A.D.: Functional muscle examination and gait analysis, J. Amer. Phys. Ther. Assoc. 43:39, 1963.
20. Lages, W.: Rheumatic diseases, lectures, San Jose, Calif., 1974-1978, Department of Occupational Therapy, San Jose State University.
21. Lister, G.: The hand: diagnosis and indications, London, 1977, Churchill Livingstone.
22. Melvin, J.L.: Rheumatic disease: occupational therapy and rehabilitation, Philadelphia, 1977, F.A. Davis Co.
23. Moberg, E.: Objective methods for determining the functional value of sensibility of the hand, J. Bone Joint Surg. 40:454-476, 1958.
24. Moberg, E.: Aspects of sensation in reconstructive surgery of the upper extremity, J. Bone Joint Surg. 46:817-825, 1964.
25. Pardoe, R.: Burns and wound healing, lectures, San Jose, Calif., 1974-1978, Department of Occupational Therapy, San Jose State University.
26. Peiper, A.: Cerebral function in infancy and childhood, New York, 1963, Consultants Bureau Enterprises.
27. Semans, S.: Developmental reactions, Stanford, Calif., 1968, Division of Physical Therapy, Stanford University. Mimeographed.
28. Smith, H.D., and Tiffany, E.: Evaluation overview. In Hopkins, H.L., and Smith, H.D., editors: Willard and Spackman's occupational therapy, ed. 5, Philadelphia, 1978, J.B. Lippincott Co.
29. Trombly, C.A., and Scott, A.D.: Occupational therapy for physical dysfunction, Baltimore, 1977, The Williams & Wilkins Co.
30. Von Prince, K.: Hand rehabilitation after burn injury, lecture, San Jose, Calif., 1970, Department of Occupational Therapy, San Jose State College.
31. Watanabe, S.: Regional institute on the evaluation process, Final Rep. RSA-123-T-68, New York, 1968, American Occupational Therapy Association.
32. Williams, L.A.: A suggested method for evaluating proprioception, stereognosis, and body scheme in adult patients with cerebral vascular accident for occupational therapists, Master's project, San Jose, Calif., 1964, Department of Occupational Therapy, San Jose State College. Unpublished.
33. Yaekel, M.: Hand rehabilitation, lecture. San Jose, Calif., 1971, Department of Occupational Therapy, San Jose State College.

SUPPLEMENTARY READING

American Occupational Therapy Association Council on Practice: Evaluation procedures in occupational therapy, 1969, Illinois Occupational Therapy Association and American Occupational Therapy Association.
Bell, E., Jurek, K., and Wilson, T.: Hand skill measurement: a gauge for treatment, Am. J. Occup. Ther. 30:80, 1976.
Gurgold, G.D., and Harden, D.H.: Assessing the driving potential of the handicapped, Am. J. Occup. Ther. 32:41, 1978.
Hasselkus, B.R., and Safrit, M.J.: Measurement in occupational therapy, Am. J. Occup. Ther. 30:429, 1976.

Lewko, J.H.: Current practices in evaluating motor behavior of disabled children, Am. J. Occup. Ther. **30**:413, 1976.

MacBain, K.P., and Hill, R.H.: A functional assessment for juvenile rheumatoid arthritis, Am. J. Occup. Ther. **27**:326, 1973.

Maloney, F.P., et. al.: Use of the Goal Attainment Scale in the treatment and ongoing evaluation of neurologically handicapped children, Am. J. Occup. Ther. **32**:505, 1978.

Moore, J.W.: The initial interview and interaction analysis, Am. J. Occup. Ther. **31**:29, 1977.

Okoye, R.: Functional evaluation of the adult with CNS dysfunction, New York, 1976, New York State Occupational Therapy Association, Long Island District.

Phelps, P.E., and Walker, E.: Comparison of the finger wrinkling test results to established sensory tests in peripheral nerve injury, Am. J. Occup. Ther. **31**:565, 1977.

Silverman, E.H., and Elfant, I.L.: Dysphagia: an evaluation and treatment program for the adult, Am. J. Occup. Ther. **33**:382, 1979.

Smith, H.B.: Smith hand function evaluation, Am. J. Occup. Ther. **27**:244, 1973.

Werner, J.L., and Omer, G.E., Jr.: Evaluating cutaneous pressure sensation of the hand, Am. J. Occup. Ther. **24**:347, 1970.

Willard, H.S., and Spackman, C.S., editors: Occupational therapy, ed. 4, Philadelphia, 1971, J.B. Lippincott Co.

Zimmerman, M.E.: The functional motion test as an evaluation tool for patients with lower motor neuron disturbances, Am. J. Occup. Ther. **23**:49, 1969.

Chapter 3

Treatment planning

A treatment plan is the design or proposal for a therapeutic program. It includes specific treatment objectives and methods for reaching those objectives and indicates how the program should progress.

The importance of writing a treatment plan cannot be overstated. It is necessary to have specific objectives set down in an orderly and sequential manner. These, then, will be clear to the therapist, the client, and other concerned personnel. The treatment plan helps the therapist know how to proceed efficiently and provides a standard for measuring the progress of the client and thus the effectiveness of the plan of action.

Therapists who do not write treatment plans often work in a trial and error manner, wasting precious time and money. They may be poorly prepared to defend their course of action to themselves, the client, or the rehabilitation team. They may tend to lack confidence in reporting about the clients assigned to their care. The failure to have a well-written treatment plan available will also present many problems to other staff members who may have to apply treatment in the absence of the assigned therapist. Experienced therapists who think they no longer need to write treatment plans will find that their mental plans are not as clear or as comprehensive as they imagined when they attempt to set them on paper.

Perhaps one of the most important purposes for writing a treatment plan, then, is that it allows the therapist to plan and analyze the proposed course of action. In so doing the therapist should ask many questions. Some of these are (1) What are the client's capabilities and assets? (2) What are the client's limitations and deficits? (3) What does occupational therapy have to offer this client? (4) What are specific short-range objectives? (5) What are some long-range objectives? (6) Are the treatment objectives consistent with the client's needs and personal objectives? (7) If objectives are not compatible, how do they need to be modified? (8) What treatment methods are available to meet these objectives? (9) What is the best theoretical framework for treatment of this client? (10) When should the client have met the objectives? (11) What standards shall be used to determine when the client has reached an objective?

(12) How shall the effectiveness of the treatment plan be evaluated?

The treatment plan affirms therapist's competence and the professionalism of occupational therapy. It can provide a systematic method for gathering research data and documents the purposes and effectiveness of occupational therapy services. The treatment plan can enhance the quality of service and its effectiveness.

THE TREATMENT PLANNING PROCESS
Data gathering

After the client is referred for occupational therapy services, the therapist must gather data to develop an appropriate treatment plan. Sources for these data are the referral form; the medical record; social, educational, vocational, and play histories; interview of the client or family and friends; and the results of evaluation procedures completed by occupational therapy and other services.

Data analysis and problem identification

After data have been gathered, they are analyzed to identify functions and dysfunctions, and it is determined if occupational therapy can be employed to alleviate the problems. From a careful analysis of all of the data gathered,[6] a list of problems should be developed, which forms the basis of the treatment plan. Those physical, psychosocial, cognitive, and performance skills deficits that may be amenable to occupational therapy intervention should be noted. Limitations that require intervention by other professional services should be communicated through the appropriate referral process.

Selecting and writing treatment objectives

After the data have been gathered and analyzed, the next step in the treatment planning process is the setting down of objectives. These should reflect the client's needs and should be consistent with the more general objectives stated on the referral, although they need not be limited to these, if the referral agent approves. The occupational therapy objectives should complement objectives of ancillary services. Whenever possible the therapist should select objectives and plan the treatment program in conjunction with the client.

A treatment objective is a statement of intent describing a proposed change in a client. The statement conveys clearly the physical function, performance skill, or behavior pattern the client will demonstrate when the treatment procedure or program has been successfully completed.

The therapist must select objectives that the client is to reach by the end of a treatment program so that treatment procedures relevant to those objectives may also be selected. Progress and evaluation of the client's performance will be based on the objectives selected.

When no clearly defined objectives have been stated, there is no sound basis for selecting appropriate treatment methods, and it is impossible to evaluate the effectiveness of the treatment program. It is important to state objectives to be able to evaluate the degree to which the client is able to perform in the desired manner.

A meaningful objective conveys to others a picture of what the client will be like when the objective has been achieved. The picture conveyed is identical to the one the therapist has in mind. Thus it succeeds in communicating the therapist's intent and describes the terminal behavior of the client well enough to preclude misinterpretation. A comprehensive treatment objective has the following three qualities:

1. Conditions. The circumstances that will allow terminal behavior to take place, for example, environment, special devices, data, or degree of training and assistance required for the client to perform the desired terminal behavior.
2. Statement of terminal behavior. The physical changes, kind of behavior, or performance skill that the client is expected to display.
3. Criteria. The level of acceptable performance or degree of competence the client is expected to achieve to have successfully accomplished the terminal behavior.[8]

The following are examples of comprehensive treatment objectives and their analysis:

Given instruction, daily practice, and assistive devices the client's performance of dressing and feeding skills will be improved so that they are performed independently in no more than twice the time it takes nondisabled individuals to perform the same activities.

> CONDITIONS: Given instruction, daily practice, and assistive devices.
> TERMINAL BEHAVIOR: The client's performance of dressing and feeding skills will be improved.
> CRITERIA: Independently in no more than twice the time it takes nondisabled individuals.

Given demonstration, instruction, and practice in principles of joint protection and energy conservation the client will use these principles in self-care, school, and play activities so that deformity is prevented and activity tolerance is increased from 2 to 4 hours.

> CONDITIONS: Given demonstration, instruction, and practice in principles of joint protection and energy conservation.
> TERMINAL BEHAVIOR: The client will use these principles in self-care, school, and play activities.
> CRITERIA: So that deformity is prevented and activity tolerance is increased from 2 to 4 hours.

After guided participation in a structured activity group at the center the client will be able to initiate and sustain social interaction in a community activity program 50% of the time.

> CONDITION: After guided participation in a structured activity group at the center.
> TERMINAL BEHAVIOR: The client will be able to initiate and sustain social interaction in a community activity program.
> CRITERIA: 50% of the time.

Given a program of daily exercise and activity the ROM of right shoulder flexion will increase from 110° to 160° so that the client can resume bowling within 1 year.

> CONDITIONS: Given a program of daily exercise and activity.
> TERMINAL BEHAVIOR: The ROM of right shoulder flexion will increase.
> CRITERIA: From 110° to 160° so that the client can resume bowling within 1 year.

There are many variables and unknown factors in the growth and development or recovery of clients with physical dysfunction. Therefore the degree to which they can benefit from or participate in or succeed in habilitation and rehabilitation programs cannot be predicted with certainty. This often makes it difficult for therapists to write comprehensive treatment objectives. However, the therapist should attempt to write such objectives, using past experience with similar patients and knowledge gained from gathering pertinent data to describe desired terminal behavior, conditions, and criteria for each treatment objective. If this is not possible, it is recommended that a specific statement of terminal behavior should suffice until applicable conditions and criteria become apparent. The stated terminal behaviors can then be modified to become comprehensive objectives.

The following are examples of specific statements of terminal behavior:

1. The joint ROM of the left elbow will increase.
2. The client will become proficient in operating the control systems of the left above-elbow prosthesis.
3. The client will be able to dress independently.
4. The strength of the client's left deltoid and biceps muscles will increase.
5. The client will become proficient in the use of the mobile arm supports.
6. The client will develop feelings of self-worth and acceptance of disability.

Selecting treatment methods

When objectives have been selected, the treatment methods that will help the client achieve them are chosen. This is probably one of the most difficult steps in the treatment planning process. A treatment principle or assumption that is applied to the cause of an identified problem should underlie the selection of an appropriate treatment method.[3] For example, after peripheral nerve injury and repair, when nerve regeneration is progressing, a principle would be that use of reinnervated muscles will maintain or increase their tone and strength. Therefore graded therapeutic activity or exercise may be the method of choice to effect the desired goals. Many other factors will affect the selection of treatment methods. Some of the factors that should be considered in the selection of treatment methods are (1) What is the goal for the client? (2) What are the precautions or contraindications that affect the occupational therapy program? (3) What is the prognosis for recovery? (4) What were the results of evaluations in occupational therapy and other services? (5) What other treatment is the client receiving? (6) What are the goals of other treatment programs, and are the occupational therapy goals consonant with these? (7) How much energy does the client expend in other therapies? (8) What is the state of the client's general health? (9) What are the client's interests, vocational skills, and psychological needs? (10) What roles will the client assume in the community? (11) What kinds of activities or exercise will be most useful to the client?[11] (12) How can treatment be graded to meet the client's changing needs as progression or regression occurs? (13) What special equipment or adaptations of therapeutic equipment are needed for the client to perform maximally?

When treatment methods are selected, it should be clear to others reading the treatment plan exactly how the methods will be used to reach specific objectives. Sometimes several methods may be needed to achieve one objective, or it may happen that the same methods may be used to reach several objectives.

Implementing the treatment plan

When at least one objective and one or more treatment methods have been selected, the treatment plan is implemented. The client engages in the procedures that have been designed to ameliorate the problems and capitalize on strengths and capabilities. A comprehensive treatment plan may evolve over a period of time. While a lengthy evaluation is in progress, for example, Activities of Daily Living assessment, the client may have commenced a program of therapeutic activity to strengthen specific muscle groups. Thus as a comprehensive evaluation is being completed, an increasing number of problems may be identified and additional objectives and methods may be added to the treatment plan.

Reevaluating the client and the initial treatment plan

Once the treatment plan is implemented, its effectiveness is evaluated on an ongoing basis. The therapist must be an alert observer and ask (1) Are the objectives suitable to the client's needs and capabilities? (2) Are the methods the best ones for fulfilling the treatment objectives? (3) Does the client relate to the treatment methods and see them as worthwhile and meaningful? (4) Are the treatment objectives realistic, and are they consonant with the client's personal objectives?

Scrutinizing the treatment plan in this way will enable the therapist to modify the plan as the need arises. The criterion for determining the effectiveness of the plan is the progress of the client toward the stated objectives in the time set for reaching those objectives. Therefore periodic reevaluation of the client, using the same tests and observations that were used to determine baseline function, can provide objective evidence of maintenance or progress, which validates the treatment plan.

Revising the treatment plan

The information gained from observations and reevaluation of the client, as outlined earlier, may necessitate some revision or modification of the initial treatment plan. The client's progress may be significant enough to increase such factors as duration, complexity, or resistance of activity. In degenerative diseases where maintenance of optimum function is often a primary objective, resistance, duration, and complexity of activity may need to be decreased to accommodate the gradual inevitable decline of physical resources. The client's motivation or inability to see the therapeutic program as helpful or meaningful may necessitate change in treatment approaches and methods.

When the initial plan is revised according to the client's needs and progress, it is once again implemented. This process of reevaluation, revision, and reimplementation of the treatment plan is continuous throughout the course of the therapeutic program (Fig. 3-1).

A TREATMENT PLAN MODEL

The treatment plan model is an adaptation of one that was used at the Hartford Easter Seal Rehabilitation Center in Hartford, Connecticut.[4] It is useful for teaching treatment planning during academic preparation, and it may be modified for clinical use.

The student is presented with a hypothetical case study, or a real client if a practicum experience is available, and is directed to complete the treatment plan, using the Treatment Planning Guide. If given a hypothetical client the student is directed to complete the Results of Evaluation segment of the treatment plan according to his or her knowledge of the particular diagnosis and its resultant disability.

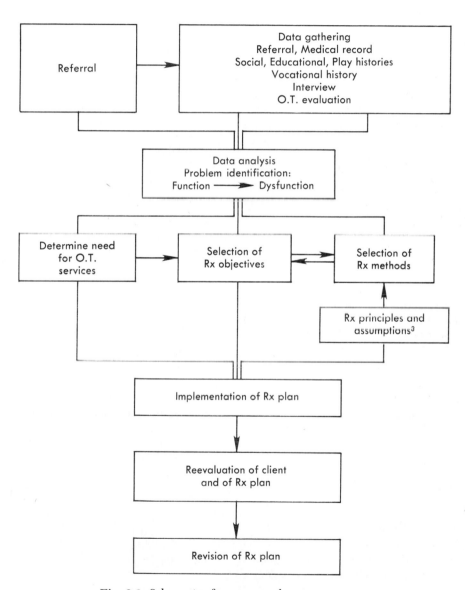

Fig. 3-1. Schematic of treatment planning process.

TREATMENT PLAN MODEL[4]

Case _____

Refer to questions and information on the treatment planning guide and fill out a treatment plan for the assigned case study. List information or use outline form only.

A. **Statistical data.**
   1. Name
      Age
      Diagnosis
      Disability
   2. Treatment aims as stated in referral.
B. **Other services.**
C. **OT evaluation.**
D. **Results of evaluation.** List function tested or observed in each category, and summarize the results of the OT evaluation.
   1. Evaluation data.
      a. Physical resources
      b. Sensory-perceptual functions
      c. Cognitive functions
      d. Psychosocial functions
      e. Prevocational potential
      f. Functional skills
   2. Problem identification. List the problems that have been identified that require occupational therapy intervention.

E Specific OT objectives	F Methods used to meet objectives	G Gradation of treatment

H. **Special equipment.**
   1. Ambulation aids. List ambulation aids required by the client, and give a short statement of justification for each choice.
   2. Splints. List splints required by client with a short statement of justification for each choice. Describe how and when client is to use splints.

3. Assistive devices. List devices needed for increased independence in self-care, home management, or travel, and give a short statement of justification for each choice.

Treatment plan guide

A. **Statistical data.** Fill in the requested information from the information given in the case study.
B. **Other services.** What other services would be active with this patient? List and give a brief statement of the role of the services listed.
   Medical service
   Nursing
   Social service
   Speech therapy
   Physical therapy
   Vocational counseling
   Sheltered employment
   Psychology-psychiatry
   Community social groups
   Educational services
   Spiritual counselor
C. **OT evaluation.** From the list below select the performance components and performance skills that should be evaluated. Indicate whether assessment would be by testing or by observation.
   1. Physical resources.
      Muscle strength
      ROM
      Physical endurance
      Standing tolerance
      Walking tolerance
      Sitting balance
      Involuntary movement
      Speed of movement
      Level of motor development
      Equilibrium and protective mechanisms
      Coordination—muscle control
      Stage of recovery, synergy patterns (stroke patients only)
      Available functional movements
      Hand function

TREATMENT PLAN MODEL—cont'd

C. OT evaluation—cont'd
2. Sensory-perceptual functions.
    Sensation—touch, pain, temperature, smell, taste
    Body scheme
    Stereognosis
    Proprioception
    Visual perception
      Visual fields
      Spatial relations
      Position in space
      Figure-ground
      Perceptual constancy
      Visual-motor coordination
      Depth perception
      Verticality
    Motor planning—gross and fine
3. Cognitive functions.
    Judgment
    Safety awareness
    Motivation
    Memory
    Sequencing
    Anticipation
    Problem solving
    Rigidity
    Basic language skills for function
      Comprehension
      Expression
      Reading
      Writing
4. Psychosocial functions.
    Maturity (development)
    Interpersonal skills
    Adjustment to disability
    Reality functioning

5. Prevocational potential.
    Work habits and attitudes
    Potential work skills
    Work tolerance
6. Functional skills.
    Self-care
    Homemaking
    Home evaluation
    Community travel
      Public transportation
      Private transportation
D. **Results of evaluation.** Summarize findings from tests and observations, and identify the problems that require occupational therapy intervention.
E. **Treatment objectives.** List specific objectives of treatment. Write them in comprehensive form as described on pp. 89 to 91.
F. **Treatment methods.** List the activities or exercises that might be appropriate for this client. Show how they will fulfill stated treatment objectives. Describe them specifically enough so another student or therapist could carry out the procedures easily.
G. **Grading.** Describe or list ways in which methods have to be graded for this client.
H. **Special equipment.**
    1. Ambulation aids. List ambulation aids required by the client, and give a short statement of justification for each choice.
    2. Splints. List splints required by client with a short statement of justification for each choice. Describe how and when the client is to use splints.
    3. Assistive devices. List devices needed for increased independence in self-care, home management, or travel, and give a short statement of justification for each choice.

SAMPLE TREATMENT PLAN

Case study

Mrs. R. is 49 years old. She has two sons. One is age 26 and married and the other is age 17. Mrs. R. is divorced. She and her younger son make their home with her married son, his wife, and 4-year-old son. Prior to the onset of her illness Mrs. R. lived in an apartment with her younger son.

Mrs. R. has had Guillain-Barré syndrome. She has been left with residual weakness of all four extremities. Leg strength is in the poor to fair plus range, and arm strength is fair to good. There may be some further recovery, but muscle strength is not expected to reach normal level. Mrs. R. can ambulate with the aid of a walker but often uses a standard wheelchair for safety and energy conservation.

Mrs. R. appears thin and frail. She speaks in a weak voice and appears to be passive and discouraged. She feels she cannot accomplish anything. The home situation is poor. Mrs. R. does not communicate with her daughter-in-law, and there are conflicts between the couple and Mrs. R. concerning the management of the teenaged son. Mrs. R. feels unable to assert her authority as his mother or to express her needs and feelings. The disability has brought about the loss of her independence and has changed her role in relation to her younger son.

Her daughter-in-law reported that Mrs. R. is dependent for self-care, never attempts to help with homemaking, and isolates herself in her room much of the time. She believes that her mother-in-law is capable of more activity "if only she would try." She says she is willing to allow Mrs. R. to do some of the household work.

Mrs. R. was referred for occupational therapy services as an outpatient for physical restoration (or maintenance) and training toward increased independence.

Treatment plan[2]

Refer to questions and information on the treatment planning guide, and fill out a treatment plan for the assigned case study. List information or use outline form only.

A. **Statistical data.**
1. Name: Mrs. R.
   Age: 49
   Diagnosis: Guillain-Barré syndrome
   Disability: Residual weakness, upper and lower extremities
2. Treatment aims as stated in referral:
   Physical restoration or maintenance
   Training toward increased independence

B. **Other services.**
Medical service: Medication prescription, supervision of rehabilitation program, general health maintenance
Physical therapy: Muscle restoration
Social service: Family counseling and group therapy for psychological support
Group therapy: Psychological support

C. **OT evaluation.**
Muscle strength: Manual muscle test
Passive ROM: Test
Physical endurance: Observe
Walking tolerance (with walker): Observe
Sitting balance: Observe
Speed of movement: Observe
Coordination: Test and observe
Available functional movements: Test and observe
Sensation: Test[1,5]
Motivation: Observe
Maturity, interpersonal skills, adjustment to disability: Observe
Self-care: Observe
Homemaking: Observe
Home evaluation: Observe[9]

D. **Results of evaluation.**
1. Evaluation data.
   a. Physical resources.
      (1) Strength: All muscles same grade bilaterally.
          Scapula: All muscles G
          Shoulder: All muscles G
          Elbow: Flexors F+, extensors F
          Forearm: Supinators F, pronators F+
          Wrist: Flexors F, extensors F
          Hand: All muscles F, except finger flexors F+
          Trunk: All muscles G
          Hip: All muscles F+, except adductors and external rotators F
          Knee: Extensors and flexors F
          Ankle: Dorsiflexors P+, plantar flexors F
          Foot: Invertors P, evertors F−
          Toes: Flexors F−, extensors P
      (2) ROM: All joints within functional to normal range.
      (3) Physical endurance, ambulation: Mrs. R.'s physical endurance is low. She can ambulate with a walker but fatigues quickly. For safety and energy conservation she often uses a wheelchair. She has slight incoordination of her legs and cannot perform fine movements using the hands because of muscle weakness.

SAMPLE TREATMENT PLAN—cont'd

D. Results of evaluation—cont'd
Evaluation data—cont'd
  b. Sensory-perceptual functions.
    (1) Primary sensation
      Touch: Intact
      Pain: Intact
      Temperature: Intact
    (2) Somesthetic perception
      Proprioception: Intact
      Stereognosis: Intact
  c. Cognitive functions. All within normal functional limits for a 49-year-old adult.
  d. Psychosocial functions. Mrs. R. has not adjusted well to her disability. She appears to be passive and discouraged and feels she cannot accomplish anything. Much of each day she isolates herself in her room.
  The home situation is poor. Prior to the onset of her illness Mrs. R. lived in an apartment with her younger son, who is age 17. They now make their home with the older son, age 26, his wife, and 4-year-old son. Mrs. R. does not communicate with her daughter-in-law, and there are conflicts between the couple and Mrs. R. concerning the management of the teenage son. The disability has brought about the loss of her independence and has changed her role in relation to her younger son. She feels unable to assert her authority as his mother or to express her needs and feelings.
  e. Prevocational potential. Not applicable because Mrs. R. is not a candidate for future employment.
  f. Functional skills. Mrs. R. is dependent in self-care activities. She manages some light personal care, such as washing her face, brushing her hair, and brushing her teeth with an adapted toothbrush, but needs assistance in getting on and off the toilet, to and from the shower, and drying herself.
  Mrs. R. can put on a blouse, cardigan, and loose dress but cannot fasten buttons or zippers. She does not dress any part of the lower extremities except for putting on loose socks.
  Mrs. R. does not do any of the house cleaning, kitchen work, laundry, or gardening, although she is capable of some light activities such as dusting and folding clothes.
2. Problem identification.
  a. Self-care dependence
  b. Muscle weakness
  c. Low physical endurance
  d. Incoordination due to muscle weakness
  e. Home management dependence
  f. Depression
  g. Self-isolation
  h. Lack of self-assertiveness
  i. Reduced social interaction
  j. Poor family communication
  k. Changed role as mother

E Specific OT objectives	F Methods used to meet objectives	G Gradation of treatment

Given 2 weeks of training Mrs. R. will be able to dress herself within a half hour in most types of clothing	Putting on slacks, panties, stockings, skirts, shifts, blouses, pullover shirts, brassiere, and shoes
	Fastening buttons
	Teaching energy-saving techniques:
	  Buttoning house dresses before slipping over head
	  Deciding which articles to put on before transferring to wheelchair, example, socks or slacks
	  Placing these articles within reach of bed before retiring each night
	Teaching methods of dressing:
	  Rolling hips to put on slacks
	  Stabilizing body while standing to let dress fall over hips
		Start with easier tasks—house dresses, large pullover shirts, and loafers
		Go to more difficult tasks as muscle strength increases and client becomes proficient in easier tasks—stockings, slacks, tie, and shoes

Continued.

SAMPLE TREATMENT PLAN—cont'd

E Specific OT objectives	F Methods used to meet objectives	G Gradation of treatment
After 1 week of training Mrs. R. will be able to perform light household activities so that she realizes she can accomplish things and will be more open to communication with her daughter-in-law	Dusting up to levels reachable from wheelchair Folding clothes and washing fine clothes in bathroom sink Washing dishes—sitting on high chair with legs under sink Setting napkins and silverware on table[1] Interacting more with daughter-in-law through planning together and dividing household tasks	
Through exercise and activity muscle strength will increase in both hands and wrists from F to G (finger flexors, F+ to G) and coordination of the hands will improve so that Mrs. R. can perform homemaking activities in less time and with less fatigue	Teaching active isotonic exercise for F muscles and progressive resistive exercise for finger flexors through the following activities: Breaking up lettuce Washing small clothes Beating eggs Painting	Add weights; advance to progressive resistive isotonic exercise when muscles reach F+ Increase complexity of exercise as coordination increases Use activities requiring more strength coordination: Cutting vegetables Wringing out clothes Sifting flour Watercolor with large brush; paint with acrylic paint using small brush
Through regular performance of daily activities muscle strength of shoulders, elbows, and forearms will increase so that activities can be performed more quickly and efficiently Shoulders: G to N Elbow extensors: F to G Flexors: F+ to G Supinators: F to G Pronators: F+ to G	Making orange juice (wheelchair side to side with waist-level table; use pronators and supinators; alternate sides) Washing glasses Rolling out pastry Wiping table and counter Setting plates and glasses on table Removing plates and glasses from cupboard where they are slightly above waist level Braid-weaving project	Client must remove more and more meat of oranges Use a heavier pin and heavier, more elastic dough Change to tasks requiring more strength—scrubbing wall Remove more plates at one time; placement of plates at higher level; add weight to upper arm
Given 3 week of training and practice Mrs. R. will be independent in using the toilet and will not take more than 10 minutes to transfer on and off toilet.	Teaching nonweight-bearing front transfer, not only using arms but also scooting hips and turning trunk[7]	Assistance in bringing body forward until elbow extensors F+; assistance in bringing body backwards until knee muscles F+ and elbow extensors F+; supervision until patient performs task in safest and easiest manner
With adequate endurance Mrs. R. will use the strength she regains in her lower extremities around the home so that she reaches her maximum level of functioning	Dressing—standing to pull slacks over hips and zipper up slacks instead of using bed Transferring Using walker instead of wheelchair	Balance of activities—watch for fatigue At start use returning lower extremity strength only for dressing and transferring Increase use of walker commensurately with returning strength

SAMPLE TREATMENT PLAN—cont'd

E Specific OT objectives	F Methods used to meet objectives	G Gradation of treatment
By end of treatment Mrs. R. will be a more active, participating member of the family, communicating freely with all members of the family so that she no longer isolates herself in her room and asserts herself without hesitation	Increasing confidence by becoming more independent Forming closer relationship with daughter-in-law resulting from change in attitude as client gains confidence and realizes potential Aiding family in understanding psychological aspects of client's disability and rehabilitation Family providing encouragement and praising client's accomplishments and attempts Encouraging client to express her feelings and needs Not letting client get away with statements such as "Yes, I'm doing fine," when she does not look it[10]	Less and less encouragement from therapist and family
By end of treatment Mrs. R. will no longer depend on her family and therapies for her interests, social interaction, and psychological support. She will show interest in and attend neighborhood church meetings, interact with neighbors, and go out with friends	Evening strolls and interacting with neighbors Attending nearby church Visiting friends in former neighborhood Taking up old and new hobbies Watching grandson at park	Start with less demanding activities, such as evening strolls. Build up to more demanding ones Initially therapist will accompany Mrs. R. to a meeting or on a community outing; later recruit friend to accompany her until she is able to travel independently and is motivated to do so

II. **Special equipment**
1. Ambulation aids.
   Walker for support during ambulation
   Electric wheelchair or regular wheelchair accompanied by assistant for outings into community to conserve time and energy
2. Splints.
   None required
3. Assistive devices.
   a. Button fastener and loops of ribbon on ends of zippers: To facilitate self-care activities
   b. Installation of a low dowel in closet that is reachable from wheelchair to hang blouses: To make it possible for Mrs. R. to reach clothing from sitting position
   c. Flannel mitt: To facilitate dusting by eliminating static grasp of dust cloth
   d. Terry cloth mitt: For dish washing to eliminate static grasp of dishcloth
   e. Large sponge: For gross grasp and ease of handling
   f. Built-up handles on eggbeater and brush: For gross grasp and ease of handling
   g. 2½-inch rounded guardrail at each side of toilet (on side of shower, on wall)[7]: For safety in transfers
   h. Swinging, detachable footrests on wheelchair: To get as close as possible to toilet

REVIEW QUESTIONS

1. Define "treatment plan."
2. Why is it important to write a treatment plan?
3. List the steps in developing a treatment plan.
4. List and define the three qualities of a comprehensive treatment objective. Give an example of each.
5. If it is not possible to write a comprehensive objective, which one quality would be *most* important to set down first?
6. List at least six factors to consider when selecting treatment methods.
7. Is it necessary to develop a complete comprehensive treatment plan before treatment can commence? How is the plan developed?
8. Is it ever necessary to change the initial treatment plan?
9. How is a treatment plan evaluated for its effectiveness?
10. How does the therapist know when to modify or change the treatment plan?

EXERCISES

1. Analyze the following objectives by asking which characteristics of a comprehensive objective each contains and which ones each lacks. Then rewrite and state each one more comprehensively.
   a. Joint ROM at the left elbow will be improved from 40° to 135° to 15° to 135°.
   b. The client will become more self-assertive among her peers.
   c. The client will become proficient in control and use of the left below-elbow prosthesis.
2. Read the following case study and write three treatment objectives, relative to improving strength, for this patient. Incorporate all of the qualities of a comprehensive treatment objective for each.

Case study

Mr. P. is a 35-year-old electronics assembler. He completed the tenth grade in school. He is right-handed, married, and the father of two children under 8 years old. He suffered an injury of the right radial nerve at midforearm level with minor involvement of the median nerve. The injury occurred 2 months ago and partial to full recovery is expected to occur within 10 months.

Mr. P. is now supporting his family with insurance compensation payments but fears these will terminate before recovery has occurred, and he is back on the job. He is worried and depressed about this.

The client is an outpatient and has been referred to occupational therapy for physical and functional restoration.

Muscle grades (consider all those not listed as normal)
Extensor carpi radialis longus and brevis: P
Extensor carpi ulnaris: P+
Extensor digitorum communis: F
Supinator: P+
Extensor pollicis longus and brevis: F+
Opponens pollicis: G
Flexor policis: F+
Pronator: G

3. Using the directions for writing a treatment plan and the Treatment Planning Guide, write a brief treatment plan for the client described in the case study with emphasis on improvement of muscle function.

REFERENCES

1. American Occupational Therapy Association: The objectives and functions of occupational therapy, New York, 1958, American Occupational Therapy Association.
2. Balwinski, C.M.: Treatment plan for lower motor neuron dysfunction. Unpublished paper presented in partial fulfillment of the requirements for OT 167, San Jose, Calif., Spring 1977, San Jose State University.
3. Day, D.: A systems diagram for teaching treatment planning, Am. J. Occup. Ther. **27**:239-243, 1973.
4. Hartford Easter Seal Rehabilitation Center: Adaptation from Treatment plan model, 1968, Hartford, Conn. Unpublished.
5. Holvey, D.N., and Talbott, J.H.: The Merck manual of diagnosis and therapy, ed. 12, Rahway, N.J., 1972, Merck & Co., Inc.
6. Illinois Occupational Therapy Association Committee on Practice: Evaluation procedures in occupational therapy, New York, 1969, American Occupational Therapy Association.
7. Ince, L.: The rehabilitation medicine services, Springfield, Ill., 1974, Charles C Thomas, Publisher.
8. Mager, R.F.: Preparing objectives for programmed instruction, San Francisco, 1962, Fearon · Pittman Publishers, Inc.
9. Nichols, P.J.R.: Rehabilitation of the severely disabled, Borough Green, Sevenoaks, Kent, England, 1971, Butterworth & Co. Ltd.
10. Pedretti, L.W.: Manual for advanced physical disability procedures, San Jose, Calif., 1973, San Jose State University.
11. Willard, H.S., and Spackman, C.S., editors: Occupational therapy, ed. 4, Philadelphia, 1971, J.B. Lippincott Co.

Chapter 4

Treatment methods for physical dysfunction

Early in the history of occupational therapy the psychological effects of the performance of purposeful activity were considered primary in the treatment of persons with physical dysfunction. It was later recognized that physical benefits accrued from the performance of activity, and kinesiological considerations were also applied in the selection of appropriate therapeutic activities.

Occupational therapy was founded on the concept that it is natural for humans to be engaged in activity, and the process of being occupied contributes to the health and well-being of the organism.[3] Activity is valuable for the maintenance of health in the healthy individual and for the restoration of health after illness and disability. By engaging in relevant, meaningful, and purposeful activity an individual is able to effect changes in behavior and performance from dysfunctional toward more functional patterns. The occupational therapist acts as facilitator of the change process.[4] Therefore physical dysfunction can be ameliorated when the client participates in goal-directed activity.[3] The value of therapeutic activity lies in the client's mental and physical involvement in an activity that provides the exercise needed to help develop purposeful use of the affected parts[9] and an opportunity to meet emotional, social, and personal gratification needs.[3]

The uniqueness of occupational therapy lies in its emphasis on the extensive use of purposeful activity. This emphasis gives occupational therapy the theoretical foundation for its broad application to both psychosocial and physical dysfunction, as well as to health maintenance. In the context of occupational therapy purposeful activity is defined as activity that has an autonomous goal beyond the motor function required to perform the task. For example, sawing wood may have the autonomous objective of securing parts for construction of a bookshelf, while the therapeutic objectives may be to strengthen shoulder and elbow musculature or to provide for release of aggression. Therefore purposeful motor function is the use of the neuromuscular system to accomplish the inherent or autonomous goal of the activity being performed. By this definition the conscious effort of the client performing the activity is focused on the ultimate objective of the movement and not on the movement itself.[3] The client directs and is in control of his movement. As he becomes absorbed in the performance of the activity, he uses the affected parts more naturally and with less fatigue.[9] This notion is supported by neurophysiological experiments that have shown that concentration on motion has a detrimental effect on that motion and that muscles controlled by conscious attention and focused effort fatigue rapidly. Therefore it is neurologically more sound to focus attention on the activity and its autonomous goal than on the muscles or motions being used to accomplish the activity. The inherent goal of the activity may be so obvious that the unsophisticated observer may fail to see the more subtle therapeutic objectives. Likewise the client engaged in the activity may have difficulty comprehending its importance to his ultimate well-being.[3]

Traditionally occupational therapy has been associated with the use of arts and crafts as therapeutic modalities. Arts and crafts are still in use as treatment methods and constitute an effective and substantial portion of many occupational therapy programs. But occupational therapy is not restricted to the use of arts and crafts, and the scope of its treatment methods has changed and broadened considerably over the years. Other purposeful activities used in treatment programs include ADL (for example, self-care, travel, communications, and home management activities). In prevocational programs simulated work activities or actual job samples are used to evaluate potential work skills of clients. Leisure or avocational activities may be used for exercising, physical conditioning, and establishing or maintaining the physical and psychosocial functions of the individual.

In addition to these purposeful, goal-oriented activities therapists have become increasingly skillful in the use of therapeutic exercise and in sensorimotor approaches to treatment, both traditionally belonging to the field of physical therapy. These methods are justified for use by some occupational therapists because they are necessary for the development of the individual's ability to perform activities that will increase the level of independent functioning, a primary aim of occupational therapy. For occupational therapists to apply and practice sensorimotor approaches to treatment effectively, specialized training and a sound understanding of the underlying neurophysiological principles are essential.

Information on therapeutic exercise, therapeutic activities, ADL, and an orientation to three sensorimotor approaches to treatment have been included in this chapter.

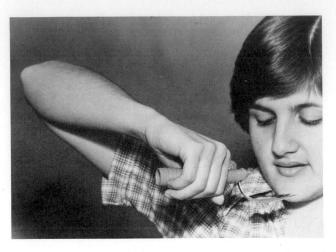

Fig. 4-1. Shoulder abduction is used to compensate for weak elbow flexion.

SECTION ONE
Therapeutic exercise

Therapeutic exercise is the specialized application of passive and active body movements or muscle contractions to maintain or restore maximum musculoskeletal function.[6] Many of its principles are applicable to therapeutic activity, and many occupational therapists use it in treatment programs. If used by occupational therapists its purposes should be to prepare the client for performance of functional activities and to augment therapeutic activity and performance skills phases of the occupational therapy program. When used as a treatment procedure, it is the most efficient means available for improving the strength of specific muscles or muscle groups. Therapeutic activities provide more general than specific exercise and accomplish strengthening objectives less rapidly than therapeutic exercise.[8]

GENERAL PRINCIPLES OF THERAPEUTIC EXERCISE

After partial or complete denervation of muscle and during inactivity or disuse, muscle strength decreases. When strength is inadequate, substitution patterns are likely to develop. A substitution is the attempt to achieve a functional goal by using muscle groups and patterns of motion not ordinarily used because of loss or weakness of the muscles normally used to perform the movements.[1] An example is using shoulder abduction to achieve a hand-to-mouth movement if elbow flexors cannot perform against gravity (Fig. 4-1). When muscle loss is permanent, some substitution patterns may be desirable as a compensatory measure to improve performance of functional activities. However, many are not desirable, and it is often the aim of therapeutic exercise to prevent or correct substitution patterns.

A muscle must contract to its maximum capacity to effect an increase in strength. Therefore strengthening exercises are not effective if the contraction is insufficient. Excess strengthening, on the other hand, may result in muscle fatigue, pain, and temporary reduction of strength.[7] If a muscle is overworked, it will fatigue and will not be able to contract. Selection of the type of exercise must suit the muscle grade and the client's fatigue tolerance level. Fatigue level varies from individual to individual, and threshold for muscle fatigue decreases in pathological states. Many clients may not be sensitive to fatigue or may push themselves beyond tolerance in the belief that this will hasten recovery. This means that the therapist must make a careful assessment of the client's muscle power and capacity for exercise. The therapist must also supervise the client closely and observe for signs of fatigue.[8] These signs may be slowed performance, distractibility, perspiration, increase in rate of respiration, performance of exercise pattern through a decreased ROM and inability to complete the prescribed number of repetitions.

PURPOSES OF THERAPEUTIC EXERCISE

The general purposes of exercise are (1) to develop awareness of normal movement patterns and improve voluntary, automatic movement responses; (2) to develop strength and endurance in patterns of movement that are acceptable and necessary and will not produce deformity; (3) to improve coordination, regardless of strength; (4) to increase specific power of desired isolated muscles or muscle groups; (5) to aid in overcoming ROM deficits; (6) to increase strength of muscles that will power hand splints, mobile arm supports, and other devices; (7) to increase work tolerance and physical endurance through increased strength; and (8) to prevent or eliminate contractures developing due to imbalanced muscle power by strengthening the antagonistic muscles.[2]

PREREQUISITES FOR THE USE OF THERAPEUTIC EXERCISE

For therapeutic exercise to be effective the client must meet certain criteria. It is most effective in the treatment of orthopedic disorders such as fractures and arthritis and lower motor neuron disorders that produce weakness and flaccidity. Examples of these are peripheral nerve injuries and diseases, poliomyelitis, Guillain-Barré syndrome, infectious neuronitis, and spinal cord injuries and diseases.

Therapeutic exercise is contraindicated for clients who have poor general health or inflamed joints or who have had recent surgery.[1] As defined and described here, it cannot be used effectively with those who have spasticity and lack voluntary control of isolated motion or those who cannot control dyskinetic movement. These latter conditions are likely to occur in upper motor neuron disorders. It may not be useful where there is severely limited joint ROM due to well-established, permanent contractures.[8]

The candidate for therapeutic exercise must be medically able to participate in the exercise regime, able to understand the directions for the exercise and its purposes, and interested and motivated to perform the exercise. The client must have available motor pathways, as demonstrated by muscle power on demonstrated muscle testing, and the potential for recovery or improvement of strength, ROM, coordination, or movement patterns, as the goal may be. It is important that some sensory feedback is available to the client. This means that sensation must be at least partially intact so that the client can perceive motion and position of the exercised part and have some sense of superficial and deep pain. Muscles and tendons must be intact, stable, and free to move. Joints must be able to move through an effective ROM for those types of exercise that use joint motion as part of the procedure. The client should be relatively free of pain during motion and should be able to perform isolated, coordinated movement. If there is any dyskinetic movement, the client should be able to control it so that the exercise procedure can be performed as prescribed.[1]

PRECAUTIONS FOR THERAPEUTIC EXERCISE

Generally joints should be worked through pain-free ROM only. Weak muscles should not be overstretched in the exercise procedure. Weak muscles that are overstretched will function less efficiently even if full rein-

nervation occurs. Excess fatigue of muscles should be avoided. Muscles around sites of recent surgery, such as tendon transplants, tendon grafts, skin grafts, and joint and bone reconstruction, should not be exercised until medical clearance has been obtained.[8] Unless directed by the physician the therapist should not exercise inflamed joints with active or resistive techniques. Sometimes isometric contractions are advised to maintain muscle strength while not moving the inflamed joint.

TYPES OF MUSCLE CONTRACTION USED IN THERAPEUTIC EXERCISE[5,7]
Isometric contraction

During an isometric contraction there is no joint motion, and the muscle length remains the same. A muscle and its antagonist may be contracted at any point in the ROM to stabilize a joint. This may be without resistance or against some outside resistance such as the therapist's hand or a tabletop. An example of isometric exercise of triceps against resistance is pressing against the tabletop with the ulnar border of the forearm while the elbow remains at 90°.

Isotonic or concentric contraction

During an isotonic contraction there is joint motion and the muscle shortens. This may be done with or without resistance. Isotonic contractions may be performed in positions with gravity assisting or gravity eliminated or against gravity, according to the client's muscle grade and the goal of the exercise. An example of isotonic contraction of the biceps is lifting a fork to the mouth during eating. If a filled cup is lifted to the mouth, the biceps contracts against resistance.

Eccentric contraction

When muscles contract eccentrically, the tension in the muscle increases or remains constant while the muscle lengthens. This may be done with or without resistance. An example of an eccentric contraction performed against no resistance is the slow lowering of the arm to the table. The biceps is contracted eccentrically in this instance. An example of eccentric contraction against resistance is the controlled return of a pail of sand lifted from the ground. Here, the biceps is contracting eccentrically to control the rate and coordination of the elbow extension in setting the pail on the ground.

EXERCISE CLASSIFICATION

The type of exercise selected will depend on muscle grade, muscle endurance, joint mobility, diagnosis and physical condition, treatment goals, position of the patient, and desirable plane of movement.

Passive exercise

The purpose of passive exercise is to maintain ROM, thereby preventing contractures and adhesions. It is used when absent or minimal muscle strength (grades O-T) precludes active motion or when active exercise is contraindicated because of the client's physical condition. During the exercise procedure the joint or joints to be exercised are moved through their normal ranges manually by the therapist or client or mechanically by an external device such as a pulley or counterbalance sling. The joint proximal to the joint being exercised should be stabilized during the exercise procedure[5] (Fig. 4-2).

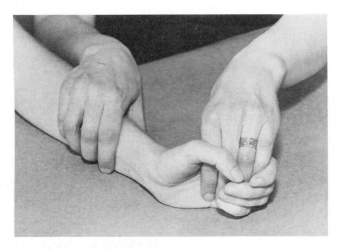

Fig. 4-2. Therapist is performing passive exercise of wrist.

Passive stretch

The purpose of passive stretch or forced exercise is to increase ROM. Essentially this is passive exercise, as just described, with a gentle, firm push or pull at the end of the joint motion. If the client's muscle grades are adequate, he can move the part actively through the available ROM, and the therapist can take it a little further thus forcing or stretching the soft structures around the joint.

The procedure requires a good understanding of joint anatomy and muscle function. It should be carried out cautiously under good medical supervision. Muscles to be stretched should be in a relaxed state.[7] The therapist should never force muscles when pain is present unless she has been ordered by the physician to work through pain. Gentle, firm stretching held for a few seconds is more effective and less hazardous than quick, short stretching. The parts around the area being stretched should be stabilized and compensatory movements should be prevented. Incorrect stretching procedures can produce muscle tearing, joint fracture, and inflammatory edema.[6]

Active-assisted exercise

The goal of active-assisted exercise is to increase strength of trace to poor muscles while maintaining ROM as well. In active-assisted exercise the client moves the part actively through the range possible, and the remainder of the range is completed by manual or mechanical assistance (Fig. 4-3). Mechanical assistance may be supplied by slings, pulleys, weights, springs, or elastic bands (Fig. 4-4). In the case of trace muscles the client merely contracts the muscle, and the thera-

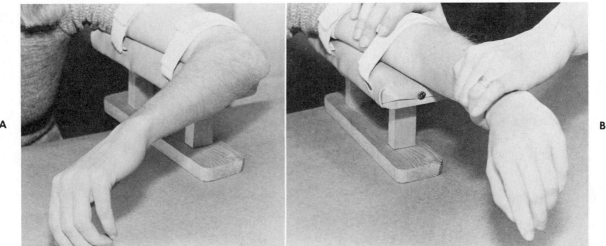

Fig. 4-3. **A,** Client extends elbow from full flexion toward extension in gravity-eliminated plane to degree possible actively. **B,** Therapist assists client to complete ROM.

pist completes the entire ROM. This exercise is graded by decreasing the amount of assistance until the client can perform active exercise.[5,7]

Active exercise

Active motion through the complete ROM with gravity eliminated or against gravity may be used for poor to fair muscles for the purpose of improving strength, with the added benefit of maintaining ROM as well. It may be used with higher muscle grades for the maintenance of strength and ROM when resistance is contraindicated. In this type of exercise the client moves the part through the complete ROM independently. If the exercise is performed in a gravity-eliminated plane, a powdered surface, skateboard, deltoid aid, or free-moving suspension sling may be used to reduce the resistance offered by friction. It is graded by adding resistance as strength improves.[5,7]

Resistive exercise

Resistive exercise is primarily for increasing strength of fair plus to normal muscles but may also be helpful for producing relaxation of the antagonistic muscles of the contracting muscles. This latter purpose can be useful if increased range is desired for stretching or relaxing spastic muscles.

The client performs muscle contraction against resistance and moves the part through the full ROM. The resistance applied should be the maximum that the muscle is capable of contracting against. Resistance may be applied manually or be weights, springs, elastic bands, sandbags, or special exercise devices. It is graded by progressively increasing the amount of resistance[5,7] (Fig. 4-5).

One specialized type of resistive exercise is the De-Lorme method of progressive resistive exercise (PRE). PRE is based on the fact that "strength can be increased significantly only by contracting against a degree of resistance that calls forth maximal effort,"[2] and muscles perform more efficiently if given a "warm-up" period. During the exercise procedure small loads are used initially. These are increased gradually after each set of 10 repetitions of the desired movement. The muscle is thus warmed up to prepare to exert its maximum power for the final 10 repetitions. The exercise procedure consists of three sets of 10 repetitions each, with resistance applied as follows: (1) First set, 10 repetitions at 50% of maximum resistance; (2) second set, 10 repetitions at 75% of maximum resistance; and (3) third set, 10 repetitions at maximum resistance. The client is instructed to inhale during the shortening contraction and exhale during the relaxation or eccentric contraction.

An example of a PRE is a triceps extending the cl-

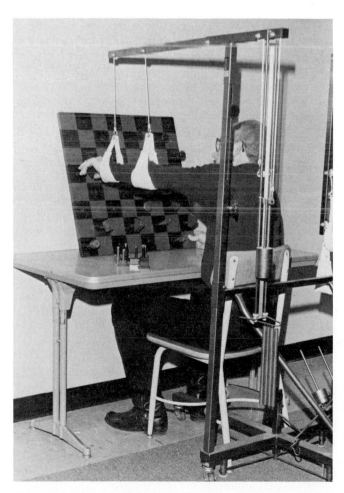

Fig. 4-4. Active-assisted exercise with deltoid aid assisting shoulder flexion in reaching activity.

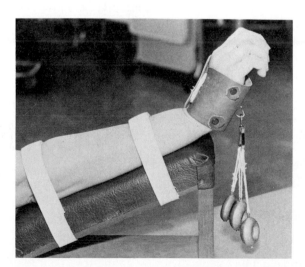

Fig. 4-5. Resistive exercise to wrist extensors, using forearm stabilizer and handcuff to compensate for inadequate grasp.

bow against a 12-pound maximum, performing 10 repetitions against 6 pounds of resistance, 10 repetitions against 9 pounds, and the final 10 repetitions against 12 pounds.

Maximal resistance, the amount of resistance the muscle can lift through the ROM 10 times, is determined by contracting the muscle and moving the part through the full ROM against progressively increasing loads for sets of 10 repetitions until the maximal load that can be lifted 10 times is reached.

At the beginning of the treatment program it is often difficult for the therapist to determine the maximum resistance that the client is capable of taking. This may be because (1) the client may not know how to exert his maximum effort, (2) the client may be reluctant to exercise strenuously for fear of pain or reinjury, (3) the client may be unwilling or unable to endure discomfort, and (4) the client may have difficulty with timing of exercises.

Experience of the therapist and trial and error will aid in determining maximum resistance when this is difficult. The therapist should estimate the amount of resistance the client can take and then add or subtract resistance (for example, weight or tension) until the client can perform the sets of repetitions adequately.

The exercises should be performed once daily four or five times weekly and rest periods of 2 to 4 minutes should be allowed between each set of 10 repetitions. Modifications of the exercise procedure may be made to suit individual needs. Some possibilities are 10 repetitions at 25% of maximum resistance, 10 repetitions at 50%, 10 repetitions at 75%, and 10 repetitions at maximum. Another possibility is 5 repetitions at 50% and 10 repetitions at maximum. Still another possibility is to omit the second set of exercises. Adjustments in the first two sets of exercises may be made to suit the capacity of the individual. The greatest gains may be made in the early weeks of the treatment program with smaller increases occurring at a slower pace in the subsequent weeks or months. During performance of the exercise the therapist should be aware of joint alignment of exercise device; proper fit and adjustment of device; ruling out substitute movements; and clear instructions of speed, ROM, and proper breathing.[2,6]

Isometric exercise

In isometric exercises a muscle or group of muscles is actively contracted and relaxed without producing motion of the joint that it ordinarily mobilizes. The contractions may be performed against no outside resistance by asking the client to "set" the muscle or resistance may be applied manually or by asking the client to hold against a wall, the edge of a table, or his own hand.

The purpose of isometric exercise with no resistance is to maintain muscle strength when active motion is not possible. It may be used with any muscle grade above trace but is especially useful for patients in casts or with arthritis or burns when joint motion is not possible or is contraindicated.

The purpose of resistive isometric exercise is to increase muscle strength of fair plus to normal muscles when joint motion is not possible or not desirable. It is graded by increasing the amount of outside resistance or the degree of force the client holds against.

Isometric exercises should be performed for one exercise session per day 5 days a week. Maximum resistance should be applied for 5 to 6 seconds per contraction. A tension gauge should be used to accurately monitor the amount of resistance applied. It has been shown that daily single, brief isometric exercises are at least as effective and sometimes more effective than isotonic exercises for increasing strength. Isometric exercises also increase the endurance to a higher level than isotonic resistive exercises. However, brief isometric exercises performed at resting length are not always superior to isotonic exercises. There are many situations in which movement through complete ROM is a desirable aspect of the exercise program, for example, for increasing joint ROM, preventing contracture, and preparing for use of prosthetic devices. Isometric exercise has several specific applications, as in arthritis, when joint motion may be contraindicated, but muscle strength must be increased or maintained.[2,5,6]

Coordination exercises[6]

It may be desirable to teach control of individual prime movers when they are so weak that they cannot be used normally. The purpose of the exercise is to improve muscle strength and muscle coordination into normal motor patterns. To achieve these ends the individual must learn precise control of the muscle. This is an essential step in the development of optimum coordination for persons with neuromuscular disease. To achieve these goals Kottke[6] described a procedure that he called *neuromuscular reeducation*. To participate successfully in this type of exercise the client must be rational and be able to learn and follow instructions, cooperate, and concentrate on the muscular retraining. Before beginning the client should be comfortable and securely supported. The exercises should be carried out in a nondistracting environment. It is important that the client be alert, calm, and not tired. He should have good proprioception and an adequate pain-free arc of motion of the joint on which the muscle acts. Neuromuscular reeducation can begin when there is at least 30° of pain-free motion.

The client's awareness of the desired motion and muscles that effect it are first increased by passive lengthening and relaxing of the muscle to stimulate the proprioceptive stretch reflex. This passive movement may be repeated several times. The client's awareness may be enhanced if the therapist also demonstrates the desired movement and if the movement is performed by the analogous unaffected part. The skin over the muscle belly may be stimulated to enhance the effect of the stretch reflex.

The therapist should explain the location and function of the muscle, its origin and insertion, line of pull, and action on the joint. The therapist should then demonstrate the motion, and instruct the client to think of the pull of the muscle from insertion to origin. The skin over the muscle insertion can be stroked in the direction of the pull while the client concentrates on the sensation of the motion during the passive movement performed by the therapist.

The exercise sequence then begins with instructing the client to think about the motion while the therapist carries it out passively and strokes the skin over the insertion in the direction of the motion. The client then is instructed to assist by contracting the muscle while the therapist performs passive motion and stimulates the skin as before. Next the client moves the part through the ROM with assistance and cutaneous stimulation while the therapist emphasizes contraction of the prime mover only. Finally the client carries out the movement independently, using the prime mover.

Coordination exercises must be initiated against minimal resistance if activity is to be isolated to prime movers. If the muscle is very weak (trace to poor), the procedure may be carried out entirely in an active-assisted manner, so that the muscle contracts against no resistance and can function without activating synergists.

Progression from one step to the next depends on successful performance of the step without substitutions. Each step is carried out three to five times per training session for each muscle to be exercised, depending on the client's exercise tolerance.

Coordination is the combined activity of many muscles into smooth patterns and sequences of motion. Coordination is an automatic response monitored primarily through proprioceptive sensory feedback. To achieve a high degree of coordination proprioceptive mechanisms must be intact. Visual and tactile sensory feedback may be used to compensate or substitute for limited proprioception, but the coordination achieved will never be as great as when proprioception is intact.

The development of coordination depends on the repetitious performance of the desired precise patterns of motion to effect integration of the sensory stimuli and motor response. Initially the rate of performance may be slow. As a habit pathway is established, the activity can be performed with less effort and concentration and

with increasing speed. A high degree of coordination and speed does not develop until the pattern of motion becomes automatic and does not require the constant awareness of the performer. Coordination training should begin with simple movement patterns and progress to more complex patterns. Resistance should be minimal.[6]

Occupational therapists, often in conjunction with physical therapists, may initiate coordination training with neuromuscular reeducation and progress to repetitious activities requiring desired coordinated movement patterns. Examples of exercise-like activities that demand repetitious patterns of nonresistive movement are placing small blocks, marbles, cones, paper cups, or pegs. These can later be translated to more purposeful activities, such as leather lacing, mosaic tile work, needlecrafts, or weaving.

If CNS impulses irradiate to muscles not involved in the movement pattern, incoordinated motion will result. Constant repetition of an incoordinated movement pattern will reinforce it, resulting in a persistent incoordination. Factors that increase incoordination are fear, poor balance, too much resistance, pain, fatigue, strong emotions, and prolonged inactivity.[6]

CONCLUSION

Several types of exercise have been described. These may be applied by the occupational therapist and may be used in conjunction with purposeful activity. They are more expertly applied by the physical therapist, who is extensively trained in their use. In many treatment facilities the physical therapist is responsible for the formal exercise program, and the occupational therapist helps the client to apply newly gained strength, range, and coordination in therapeutic activities and daily living skills. The respective therapists' roles may not be that sharply defined, with each sharing in exercise and activity aspects of the treatment program according to their skills, interests, and agreed-on division of labor.

REVIEW QUESTIONS
Treatment methods: therapeutic exercise

1. Define "therapeutic exercise."
2. What is meant by "substitution patterns"? Why do they occur?
3. What demand must be made on a muscle for its strength to increase?
4. What happens to a muscle that is fatigued?
5. List four signs of fatigue from excess exercise.
6. List at least four purposes of therapeutic exercise.
7. With which types of disabilities would you use therapeutic exercise? Which disabilities is it less useful for? Why?
8. To participate in a therapeutic exercise program the client must possess certain characteristics. List and discuss at least four of these requirements.
9. List four precautions or contraindications to therapeutic exercise, and explain why each can preclude the use of therapeutic exercise.

10. Define three types of muscle contraction, and give an example of how each occurs in daily activity.
11. What type of exercise should be used if muscle grades are fair plus to good? Why?
12. What type of exercise should be used if muscle grades are zero and trace? Why?
13. If a patient has joint pain and inflammation with good muscle strength, what type of exercise should be used? Why?
14. How is passive stretching different from passive exercise?
15. Describe the procedure and precautions for passive stretching.
16. When beginning PRE, how is the client's maximum resistance determined?
17. Describe the procedure for PRE to strengthen fair plus wrist extensors.
18. Describe the steps in coordination exercises.
19. Describe how the client would be instructed in coordination exercises for palmar prehension.
20. What is the name that Kottke used for coordination exercises?

SECTION TWO
Therapeutic activities

Therapeutic activities here are defined as arts, crafts, recreational, sports, leisure, and work activities that may be used or adapted for use to meet one or more of the following therapeutic objectives: (1) to develop or maintain strength, endurance, work tolerance, ROM, and coordination; (2) to use newly mastered voluntary, automatic movement in goal-directed tasks; (3) to provide for purposeful use of and general exercise to affected parts; (4) to explore vocational potential or train in work adjustment skills; (5) to improve sensation, perception, and cognition; and (6) to improve socialization skills and enhance emotional growth and development.

Cynkin[1] in *Occupational Therapy: Toward Health Through Activities* maintains that occupational therapy deals with the activities of everyday life. The activities that form the pattern to one's life are taken for granted until some dysfunction occurs to disrupt the activities pattern. Occupational therapy was founded on the premise that performance of activities promotes physical and mental well-being. From this idea came the use of activities as therapeutic media for persons with mental or physical dysfunction. This implies that dysfunction can be modified, altered, or reversed toward function through engagement in activities.

When occupational therapists began to look to medicine, biological sciences, and psychiatry for theoretical bases, their study of therapeutic activities fell behind. It was difficult to define the very nature of activities and to classify and categorize them into "standard procedures" expected of a profession in an age devoted to science and technology. Activity analyses that were attempted tended to be mechanical and difficult to apply, and many omitted the analysis of important elements in the client-activity interaction.

Occupational therapists have continued to look to the sciences for theoretical foundations and rationale for being in an effort to gain credibility and respectability in the medical community. In recent years occupational therapists have adopted several of the newer sensorimotor or neurophysiological approaches to treatment (for example, neurodevelopmental, sensory integration, and movement therapy) and therapeutic exercise that were introduced and are practiced or shared in practice by other disciplines. There has been emphasis on specialized techniques, resulting in proliferation of academic knowledge to keep pace with bases for rationalizing those techniques. At the same time stress on activities in academic programs has diminished. Activities have been modified and their purposes distorted to fit in with the current trend toward more technological practice. The outcome is a trend toward the disavowal of activities as the core of occupational therapy, now evident in many occupational therapy intervention programs.[1]

The uniqueness of occupational therapy rests with activities, in the belief (1) that activities are characteristic of and essential to human existence; (2) that culturally specific activities patterns can be detected and described by studying the manifest activities, values, and norms of different sociocultural groups; (3) that acceptable or unacceptable idiosyncratic variations can be found by studying the individual activities patterns of those groups; (4) that the individual leads a most satisfying way of life if able to carry out a set of activities approved by the group but also fulfilling personal needs and wants; (5) that such activity patterns can be equated with function; and (6) that activities themselves, systematically selected and combined in patterns tailored to each individual, are means for the development or restoration of function.*

Despite the efforts of several outstanding professionals in occupational therapy who advocate activities as the prime focus of occupational therapy and have sought integrative theories for activities or conceptual schemes for activity analysis, a pervasive "activities" frame of reference is not yet apparent in educational institutions, clinical practice, and the general attitudes of practicing professionals.[1] Actions taken by the Representative Assembly of the American Occupational Therapy Association, in its meeting in April 1979, may serve to reverse these trends and to reestablish activities as the common core of occupational therapy. The Representative Assembly adopted the following philosophical base of occupational therapy:

Man is an active being whose development is influenced by the use of purposeful activity. Using their capacity for

---

*From Cynkin, S.: Occupational therapy: toward health through activities, Boston, 1979, Little, Brown & Co.

intrinsic motivation, human beings are able to influence their physical and mental health and their social and physical environment through purposeful activity. Human life includes a process of continuous adaptation. Adaptation is a change in function that promotes survival and self-actualization. Biological, psychological, and environmental factors may interrupt the adaptation process at any time throughout the life cycle. Dysfunction may occur when adaptation is impaired. Purposeful activity facilitates the adaptive process.

Occupational therapy is based on the belief that purposeful activity (occupation) including its interpersonal and environmental components, may be used to prevent and mediate dysfunction, and to elicit maximum adaptation. Activity as used by the occupational therapist includes both intrinsic and therapeutic purpose.*

Besides the adoption of this philosophical base the Representative Assembly affirmed that there should be universal acceptance and implementation of the active participation of the patient-client in occupation for the purpose of improving performance as the common core of occupational therapy. It further specified that "facilitation procedures" are acceptable as occupational therapy only when used to prepare the client or patient for better performance and prevention of disability through self-participation in occupation.[4]

Cynkin makes several assumptions about activities that relate to their nature, human nature, and change; these are summarized here. Activities fulfill many of an individual's needs and wants, and they are essential to physical and psychosocial growth and development and the achievement of mastery and competence. Activities are socioculturally regulated by the values and beliefs of the culture that defines acceptable behavior for groups of individuals in the culture. A society may be rigid or flexible in its interpretation of acceptable behaviors for various groups. In either case there is a point where deviations in behavior or activities patterns are deemed unacceptable. Changes in activities patterns can move or change from dysfunctional toward more functional. Individuals can change and desire change. Change takes place through motor, cognitive, and social learning.

Cynkin concludes from these assumptions that activities must be analyzed for "their inherent properties, socioculturally acquired characteristics, their meaning to individuals, and their potential as instruments of change."[1] A careful analysis by the occupational therapist is essential to use activities for therapeutic purposes. An analysis should yield information about the usefulness and application of therapeutic activities as intervention strategies for physical dysfunction and health maintenance.

---

*From Occupational therapy newspaper, Rockville, Md., June 1979, American Occupational Therapy Association.

PRINCIPLES OF ACTIVITY ANALYSIS

If activities are to be used as the core of occupational therapy, their usefulness as therapeutic modalities must be defined, analyzed, and classified.[1] Activities selected for therapeutic purposes should (1) be goal-directed, (2) have some significance and meaning to the client to meet his individual needs in relation to his social roles, (3) require the mental or physical participation of the client, (4) be designed to prevent or reverse dysfunction, (5) develop skills to enhance performance in life roles, (6) relate to the client's interests, (7) be adaptable, gradable, and age appropriate, and (8) be selected through knowledge and professional judgment of the occupational therapist in concert with the client.[2]

In the treatment of physical dysfunction if improvement of motor performance is the goal of the therapeutic activity, then an important aspect of the activity analysis is on muscles, joints, and motor patterns required to perform the activity. This is usually done by observation, palpation, joint measurement, and knowledge of kinesiology. Trombly and Scott[5] maintain that electromyographical studies and use of biofeedback apparatus can yield more accurate analysis of muscle function during performance of therapeutic activities. These modalities are rarely used in occupational therapy practice today. They would be excellent means to document the effect of activities on motor function and thus establish a stronger theoretical base for the use of activities in the treatment of physical dysfunction.[5]

An activity should be analyzed under the specific circumstances that it is to be performed. Steps of the activity must be identified and broken down into the motions required to perform each step. ROM, degree of muscle strength, and type of muscle contraction to perform each step should be identified.

In developmental and upper motor neuron disorders activities also should be analyzed for their effect on the reinforcement, inhibition, or elicitation of primitive reflexes, equilibrium reactions, and normal and abnormal movement patterns. Stability or mobility requirements of the trunk, neck, and extremities should be analyzed. Required concentration and attention are also noted. Whether cortical or subcortical (automatic) control of movement is necessary should be determined. The sensory input and feedback provided by the activity should be observed for its potential effect on facilitation or inhibition of movement and performance. The client's cognitive functions, such as memory and ability to learn the activity process, and the value and meaning of the activity to him must also be considered before selection of activity.[5]

Selecting appropriate and meaningful activities for the client should begin with obtaining and analyzing the individual's Activities Configuration Protocol. This model by Cynkin includes information about the client's values, educational history, work history, and vocational interests and plans. Additional information on social, community, and family roles would be helpful. This information may be obtained from interviews with the client and significant friends and family members. The reader is referred to the original source for the complete Activities Configuration Protocol.[1]

A carefully detailed account of the client's daily schedule can be very helpful in analyzing the client's activities pattern. The procedure for obtaining the daily schedule is described in Chapter 2.

ADAPTATION OF ACTIVITY

Activities may be adapted to suit the particular needs of the individual. If the required movement patterns or degree of resistance, for example, cannot be obtained when the activity is performed in the usual manner, simple adaptations or modifications may be made. These are usually accepted by the client if they are not complex and do not require motions that are strained and unnatural to the performance of the activity. The novice is cautioned that the value of the activity to the client may be diminished if it is designed to be performed in some contrived manner to achieve the desired movement patterns. Such methods require that the client focus on movements rather than on the process or end product.[5] This reduces satisfaction and defeats one of the primary purposes and benefits of purposeful activity described at the beginning of this chapter.

An example of a simple adaptation is positioning a large checkerboard in a vertical position to achieve the desired range of shoulder flexion while playing the game (Fig. 4-6). Positioning an object such as a mosaic tile project at increasing or decreasing distances from the client on the tabletop can affect the range needed to reach the materials. Handles may be extended to effect increased range such as on a loom (Fig. 4-7).

Weights may be added to the client or to the equipment to increase the resistance required to perform the activity. A wrap sandbag with a Velcro fastener attached to the wrist could be used to increase resistance to arm movements during macrame or weaving. A pulley and weight system can be attached to the beater of the floor loom to increase resistance to the biceps or triceps, depending on whether the weight is attached to the back or the front of the loom (Fig. 4-8). Springs or elastic devices may be used to increase resistance on smaller pieces of equipment.[5]

Tool handles may be increased in size by using a larger dowel or padding the handle with foam rubber to accommodate limited ROM or facilitate grasp. Grasp mitts

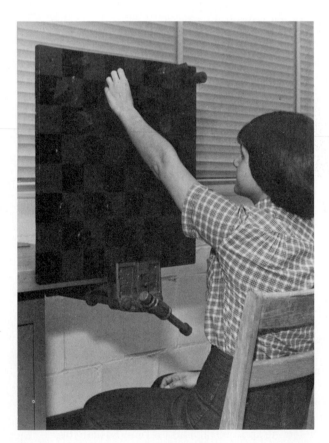

Fig. 4-6. Checkerboard is positioned vertically to increase ROM of shoulder flexion while playing game.

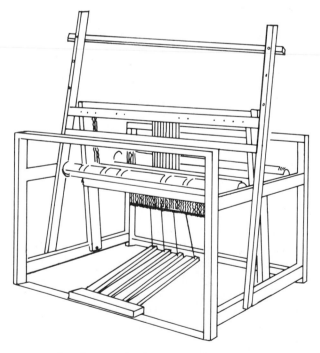

Fig. 4-7. Floor loom with adjustable vertically extended beater bar to require increasing ranges of shoulder flexion.

may be used when arm motion is desirable but grasp strength is inadequate to hold onto a tool or equipment handle. Adaptation of activity can be a challenge to the creativity and ingenuity of the occupational therapist. She should remember that for the adaptations to be used effectively, the client must be able to use them in a good, comfortable position. The client must understand the need and purpose of the activity and the adaptations and be willing to perform the activity with the simple modifications. Peculiar and complicated adaptations that require frequent adjustment and modification should be avoided.[6]

GRADATION OF ACTIVITY

Gradation of activity means that the activity should be appropriately paced and modified to demand the client's maximum capacities at any point in his progress or regress. There are many ways in which activities may be graded to suit the client's individual needs and the treatment objectives. Resistance may be increased by adding

weights to the equipment or to the client, changing the texture of the materials, or changing to another more or less resistive activity. Endurance may be graded by moving from light to heavy work and increasing the length of the work period. Joint ROM may be graded by positioning materials to demand greater reach or excursion of joints or adapting equipment with lengthened handles. Standing and walking tolerance may be graded by increasing the length of time spent standing to work, perhaps at first in a stand-up table (Fig. 4-9), and increasing the time and distance spent in activities requiring walking. These may include home management and workshop activities. Coordination and muscle control may be graded by decreasing amount of gross resistive movements and increasing fine controlled movements required in the therapeutic activities. An example is progressing from sawing wood with a crosscut saw to using a coping saw to using a jewelers' saw to using chip-carving tools. Dexterity and speed of movement may be graded by practice, at increasing speeds, once

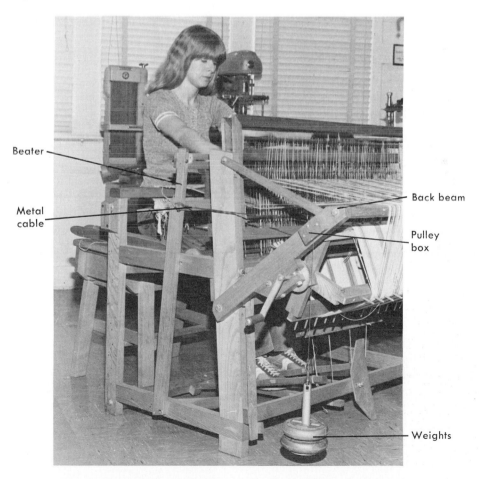

Fig. 4-8. Floor loom adapted with metal cable attached from beater through pulley on back beam from which weights are hung. Weights provide resistance to elbow flexors and shoulder extensors, as arranged.

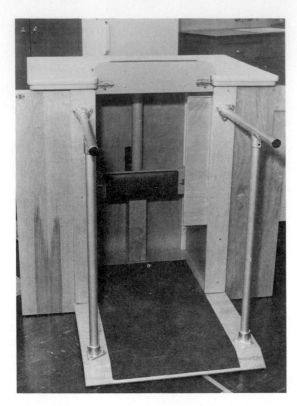

Fig. 4-9. Stand-up table with sliding door, padded knee support, and backrest.

movement patterns have been mastered through coordination training and neuromuscular reeducation. Activities may also be graded for number of steps, complexity, problem solving, independent decision making, and social interaction requirements.

SELECTION OF ACTIVITY

In the treatment of physical dysfunction, activities are usually selected for their potential to improve physical performance skills, as well as their potential psychosocial benefits. Activities selected for improvement of physical performance should provide desired exercise or purposeful use of affected parts. They should enable the client to transfer the motion, strength, and coordination gained to useful, normal daily activities.

If activities are to meet requirements for physical restoration, they must meet three basic criteria: (1) Activities should provide action rather than position of in-volved joints and muscles, that is, they should allow alternate contraction and relaxation of the muscles being exercised and allow the joints to course through their available ROM. (2) Activities should provide repetition of motion. This means that activities should allow for an indefinite but controllable number of repetitions of the desired movement patterns sufficient to be of benefit to the client. (3) Activities should allow for one or more kinds of gradation, such as for resistance, range, coordination, endurance, or complexity.[2,6]

The type of exercise that is needed must be considered. Active and resistive exercise are most often used in the performance of therapeutic activity.[6] Requirements for passive and assistive exercise are less easily applied to therapeutic activities, although not impossible.

Other important considerations in the selection of activity are (1) properties of the materials and equipment; (2) preparation and completion time; (3) complexity; (4) type of instruction and supervision required; (5) structure and controls in the activity; (6) learning requirements; (7) independence, decision making, and problem solving required; (8) social interaction potential; (9) communication skills required, and (10) potential gratification to the individual.

Prevocational activities must be selected for their ability to evaluate or develop work-related skills. Crafts, job samples, or work simulations may be selected for their similarities to skills required in the actual job. Physical skills required, work speed, concentration, ability to follow instructions and accept supervision, and work habits and attitudes may be assessed or developed through the use of such activities.[2]

The activity selected should have a reasonable goal or end product. Sanding wood or hammering numerous nails for no purpose other than to perform the associated movement patterns are poor activities[5] and might be replaced better by therapeutic exercise. These are examples of a tendency on the part of some occupational therapists to convert activities to exercise, an interesting phenomenon in light of the practice trends cited earlier.

An activity analysis model and a completed sample activity analysis follow, which offer the student or therapist a systematic approach to looking at activities for their therapeutic potential. This model includes the important factors that must be considered in the selection of activity that have been outlined.

Text continued on p. 109.

ACTIVITY ANALYSIS MODEL

A. **Activity or process under analysis:** _____
   1. Describe the activity and its component steps.
   2. Describe the necessary equipment and materials and positioning of the worker in relation to the equipment and materials.
B. **Criteria for use of the activity as an exercise.**
   1. Action rather than position of muscles and joints.
      a. To which joints is movement localized?
      b. Which joints are in static or holding positions?
      c. Which muscle groups are used to perform the movements of the joints in motion? What types of muscle contraction are used?
      d. How much muscle strength is required to perform the activity/parts of activity (indicate muscle groups and estimated muscle grade needed for each)?
      e. Estimate amount of normal ROM that moving joints are coursing through. List and indicate minimal, moderate, and full.
   2. Repetition of motion.
      a. Is the same movement/movement pattern performed repeatedly? Describe patterns.
      b. Is the number of repetitions controllable, that is, can the activity be stopped at any time without negating the goal of the activity or ruining the end product?
      c. Is the number of repetitions sufficient to effect the desired treatment goals?
   3. Gradation.
      a. Is the activity gradable? How?
      b. How can the activity be graded if increased/decreased ROM is desired?
      c. How can the activity be graded if increased/decreased strength (resistance) is desired?
      d. How can the activity be graded if increased coordination (gross to fine movement patterns) is desired?
      e. What other types of gradation are possible?
C. **Sensory-perceptual-cognitive demands of the activity.**
   1. Sensory input from materials and performance.[3]
      a. Tactile
      b. Proprioceptive
      c. Vestibular
      d. Visual
      e. Olfactory
      f. Gustatory
      g. Pain
      h. Thermal
      i. Pressure
      j. Visceral

   2. Sensory integration processes.[3]
      a. Tactile-proprioceptive-vestibular functions.
         (1) Equilibrium and protective reactions: What are the sitting and standing balances required?
         (2) Postural and bilateral integration: Are postural adjustments and coordinated use of both body sides required?
         (3) Does the activity require tactile discrimination? Describe.
         (4) How essential is proprioceptive feedback to adequate performance?
         (5) Are the required motor planning skills simple or complex?
      b. Visual functions.
         (1) Does the activity require visual scanning? How much? Describe.
         (2) What types of differentiation and recognition are required?
            (a) Color
            (b) Size
            (c) Shape and form
         (3) Does the activity require simple or complex perception of position in space and spatial relationships? Describe.
            (a) Fitting parts
            (b) Matching, fitting shapes or forms
            (c) Differentiating patterns
            (d) Observing, changing positions of parts
         (4) Is the figure-background perception required simple or complex? Describe.
         (5) Does the activity require gross or fine visual-motor coordination? Describe.
         (6) Does the activity require simple or complex sequencing or ordering of visual patterns (for example, arranging from top to bottom, left to right, or first to last)? Describe.
      c. Auditory functions.
         (1) Is hearing essential to the performance of the activity, that is, could activity be performed if one could not hear?
         (2) Is sound discrimination essential to adequately perform the activity? Why? Describe.
      d. Cognitive demands of the activity.
         (1) How critical is long-term memory (more than 2 days) to the performance of the activity?

Continued.

ACTIVITY ANALYSIS MODEL—cont'd

C. **Sensory-perceptual-cognitive demands of the activity—cont'd**
  2. Sensory integration processes—cont'd
    (2) How critical is short-term memory (1 hour to 2 days) to the performance of the activity?
    (3) Does the activity require the logical sequencing or ordering of steps or stages? Does the completion of one step depend on the anticipation of the next step and readiness for it?
    (4) Does the activity require analysis of problems and problem-solving skills (for example, recognizing errors, analyzing problems, determining solutions, and using the correct procedures to effect the solutions)?
    (5) Does the activity require the ability to do any of the following?
      (a) Read
      (b) Write
      (c) Speak
      (d) Comprehend oral instructions
      (e) Comprehend written instructions
      (f) Comprehend demonstrated instructions
      (g) Comprehend diagrams
      (h) Learn another system of symbols
    (6) What level of concentration does the activity require?
    (7) Does the activity require generalization of learning from past experience or for future use?
D. **Safety factors.**
  1. Is there danger of cutting, piercing, or burning the skin?
  2. Is there danger of losing control of tools or machinery?
E. **Interpersonal aspects of the activity.**[1]
  1. What is the number of people required or possible for participation?
  2. What is the nature of interpersonal transactions?
    a. Dependent
    b. Independent
    c. Cooperative
    d. Collaborative
    e. Competitive
F. **Sociocultural symbolism of the activity.**
  1. What does the activity symbolize in the culture?
  2. What does the activity symbolize in any specific subgroup within the culture?
  3. Does the activity connote sex role identification in the culture or to most individuals?

G. **Psychological-emotional responses to the activity.**
  1. What feelings does the activity evoke in the worker (for example, aggression, peace, or boredom)?
  2. Does the worker derive personal gratification from the performance of the activity?
H. **Therapeutic use of the activity.**
  1. List the autonomous or inherent objectives of the activity.
  2. List the possible therapeutic objectives.
    a. Physical
    b. Sensory integrative
    c. Psychosocial
    d. Vocational

Sample activity analysis

A. **Activity or process under analysis:** Pinch process in pinch pottery.
  1. A hole is made with the thumb in a ball of clay 3 to 4 inches in diameter (Fig. 4-10, *A*). The thumb and first two fingers then pinch around and around the hole from base to top of the ball of clay to gradually thin and spread the walls of the clay to produce a small, round clay pot (Fig. 4-10, *B* and *C*).
  2. The activity requires a ball of soft ceramic clay and a wooden table surface or a wooden work board on a metal or formica table. The table should be 30 to 32 inches high or a comfortable height for the worker when he is in an erect, sitting position at the table.
B. **Criteria for use of the activity as an exercise.**
  1. Action rather than position of muscles and joints.
    a. Movement is localized to flexion and extension of the MP and IP joints of digits one and two, opposition and abduction of the CMC joint of the thumb, and flexion and extension of the MP and IP joints of the thumb.
    b. Static or holding positions are maintained at the wrist during the pinch process. However, the wrist makes many minor adjustments into radial and ulnar deviation and flexion and extension as the hand moves around and up and down the pot. The back and neck are stabilized. There is only slight movement at the shoulder and elbow to make adjustments in the position of the hand as it moves around the pot.
    c. The opponens pollicis, flexors pollicis longus and brevis, and flexors digitorum profundis and superficialis are acting in concentric contraction. Palmar interossei are in isometric contraction to maintain adduction of the fin-

ACTIVITY ANALYSIS MODEL—cont'd

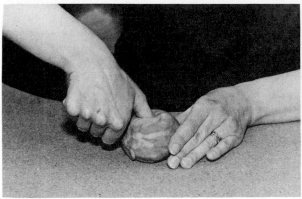

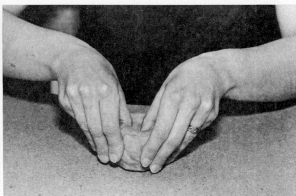

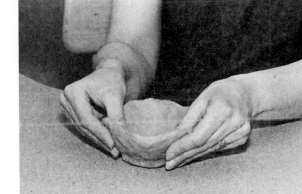

Fig. 4-10. A, Opening pinch pot with thumb. **B,** Walls of pot are gradually spread with pinching motion of fingers. **C,** Pinching continues in circular direction until desired size of pot is reached.

gers. Lumbricales are acting concentrically to flex the MP joints and maintain extension of the IP joints of the fingers during the pinch process. The extensor digitorum communis, extensor indicis proprius, extensors pollicis longus and brevis, and abductor pollicis are in eccentric contraction, which accounts for their controlled lengthening during the pinch process and concentric contraction during the release from pinch.

d. The muscle strength required in the flexor groups and the opponens pollicis is at least fair plus, because the muscles must overcome the slight resistance of the clay. Poor strength is adequate for the extensors and thumb abductors, since they act to release the pinch, and there is no resistance to these motions. Muscle endurance must be adequate to repeat the movement pattern around the pot at least once before a rest is required.

e. Joints course through a minimal ROM. MP joints are in 60° to 90° of flexion, and IP joints are in nearly full extension during the pinch process.

2. Repetition of motion.
   a. The pinching motion with the thumb in opposition to the first two digits is repeated until the pot has reached the desired height and thickness.
   b. The number of repetitions is controllable, since the process may be stopped and the project damp-stored for future use at any time.
   c. The number of repetitions is adequate for one or two treatment sessions. If more pinching activity is desirable, similar projects may be used.

3. Gradation. The activity cannot be graded for increasing ROM. It can be graded slightly for increasing strength by increasing the stiffness of the clay. It may also be graded for sitting tolerance by increasing the length of the work periods and for sitting balance by decreasing the amount of support for sitting.

Continued.

ACTIVITY ANALYSIS MODEL—cont'd

Sample activity analysis—cont'd

C. **Sensory-perceptual-cognitive demands of the activity.**

  1. Sensory input from materials and performance. There are tactile, proprioceptive, visual, slight olfactory, thermal, and pressure stimuli received from working with clay.

  2. Sensory integration processes.[3]

    a. Tactile-proprioceptive-vestibular functions.

      (1) The activity requires good sitting balance or trunk stabilization if balance is not adequate. Good head and neck control are required.

      (2) The activity requires the ability to make slight postural adjustments of trunk and proximal upper extremity joints and the use of both hands, one for supporting and moving the pot and the other for the pinching process.

      (3) Fine tactile discrimination is required to feel the texture, moisture content, and thickness of the clay. Visual functions may substitute to some extent.

      (4) Proprioceptive feedback is necessary for adequate performance to determine position of hand and fingers and degree of strength of pinch, so as not to progress too rapidly or break the clay by squeezing too hard.

      (5) The motor planning skills required are relatively simple, since the same motor pattern and a familiar one already learned are repeated over and over. The motor pattern can be easily learned from visual or proprioceptive learning techniques.

    b. Visual functions.

      (1) The activity requires minimal visual scanning. Gaze is fixed on the object at the center of the work area.

      (2) Differentiation and recognition.

        (a) The activity does not require color differentiation.

        (b) Size discrimination of the height and thickness of the walls is required. It can be obtained partially through tactile and proprioceptive feedback.

        (c) Shape and form perception through visual and tactile feedback is required to maintain the round shape of the pot.

      (3) Requirements for position in space and spatial relationships are simple, since there is only one object and no fitting, matching of parts or shapes, or differentiating patterns.

      (4) Figure-background perception required is simple, since there is only one object on a significantly contrasting background.

      (5) The activity requires moderate to fine visual-motor coordination, since fine muscles are acting in a controlled manner in response to visual, tactile, and proprioceptive information.

      (6) Some simple visual sequencing is required to progress with the pinching in a circular manner and from bottom to top.

    c. Auditory functions.

      (1) Hearing is not essential to the performance of pinch pottery except to receive instructions. Demonstrated and written/illustrated instructions may be substituted.

      (2) Sound discrimination is not required.

    d. Cognitive demands of the activity.

      (1) Long-term memory is not required.

      (2) Short-term memory is essential if the project is to be completed in 2 to 3 days without reinstruction and continuous supervision.

      (3) The activity requires sequencing of steps, and the completion of one step is necessary before the next can be started.

      (4) The activity requires simple problem-solving skills for recognition of changes in shape and thickness of walls. Knowledge of the behavior of clay and its properties for analysis or of when to seek assistance to correct these problems is essential to the successful outcome of the end product.

      (5) The activity requires the ability to comprehend oral or demonstrated instructions.

      (6) The activity requires the ability to generalize from previous experience with pinch movements, soft materials, and round objects.

D. **Safety factors.**

  1. There is no danger of cutting, piercing, or burning the skin.

  2. There is no danger of losing control of tools or machinery, since none are used.

E. **Interpersonal aspects of the activity.**

  1. The activity may be done alone or in a group of people performing the same or similar activities.

  2. Interpersonal transactions may be independent if the worker is working alone or with others and needs little supervision and assistance; dependent if more assistance, supervision, prodding, or reassurance is required; and competitive

---

ACTIVITY ANALYSIS MODEL—cont'd

if all group members are making the same or similar objects, and there is a sense of competition, for example, for degree of attractiveness, use of the end product, speed of work, or admiration of supervisors.

F. **Sociocultural symbolism of the activity.**
   1. The activity in American culture symbolizes the artistic, "hippie," or perhaps liberal or naturalistic groups of individuals in the society.
   2. The activity is seen as a leisure rather than a work skill and may be associated with child's play by some individuals.
   3. The activity may have a more feminine than a masculine identification to the older or more conservative segments of the society.

G. **Psychological-emotional responses to the activity.**
   1. The soft, moist, pliable, and plastic properties of the clay may evoke peace and pleasure in many persons. Others may regard it as "messy" and dirty.
   2. The potential for gratification is good, since the end product is easy to achieve, is creative, is as personal as the worker's own fingerprints, and is useful.

H. **Therapeutic use of the activity.**
   1. The autonomous objectives of the activity are to derive pleasure and sense of worth from producing a creative object, produce a useful product, and interact with others with similar interests.
   2. Therapeutic objectives.
      a. The physical objectives of the activity are to increase strength of opponens pollicis and flexor muscles of the fingers and thumb and improve coordination.
      b. The sensory integrative objectives are to increase tactile, proprioceptive, and thermal sensory input to the hands and improve concentration and sequencing skills and form perception.
      c. The psychosocial objectives are to improve self-esteem and interaction skills, reduce anxiety, and provide an outlet for self-expression.
      d. There is little potential for vocationally related objectives in this activity.

REVIEW QUESTIONS
Treatment methods: therapeutic activities

1. List four objectives of therapeutic activities.
2. Name four classifications of activities that could be used for therapeutic objectives.
3. Discuss Cynkin's premises about activities in occupational therapy.
4. List at least five requirements that activities need to meet if they are to be used for therapeutic purposes.
5. How can activities be adapted to meet specific therapeutic objectives and allow for gradation of the therapeutic program?
6. List four ways in which activities may be graded.
7. What are the three criteria an activity must meet to be useful for exercise purposes?
8. Name and discuss at least five factors that should be considered in the selection of activities.
9. Can therapeutic activity and therapeutic exercise be used simultaneously in a treatment program? How and why?
10. Select one of the following activities, and complete an activity analysis according to the model provided.
    a. Sawing wood
    b. Pulling the beater on the floor loom
    c. Knitting
    d. Pulling leather lacing
    e. Rolling out dough
    f. Using a push broom

SECTION THREE
Activities of daily living

Activities of daily living (ADL) are tasks of self-maintenance, mobility, communication, and home management that enable an individual to achieve personal independence in his environment. Evaluation of and training in the performance of these important life tasks have long been important aspects of occupational therapy programs in virtually every type of health facility. Loss of ability to care for one's personal needs and manage the environment can result in loss of self-esteem, a deep sense of dependency, or even feelings of infantilism and can profoundly affect the role and function of the caretakers of the individual who has lost these performance skills.[7]

The role of occupational therapy in ADL, then, is to assess ADL performance skills, determine problems that interfere with independence, determine treatment objectives, and provide training or equipment to enhance the achievement of a higher level of independence. The occupational therapist may also be involved in ameliorating physical, cognitive, social, and emotional functions that are interfering with ADL performance. The need to learn new methods or use assistive devices to perform ADL may be temporary or permanent, depending on the particular dysfunction and the prognosis for recovery.

Definition of ADL

ADL include mobility, self-care, management of environmental hardware and devices, communication, and home management activities. These major classifications are further defined as follows: (1) mobility includes movement in bed, wheelchair mobility and transfers, indoor ambulation with special equipment, outdoor ambulation with special equipment, and management of public or private transportation; (2) self-care includes dressing, feeding, toileting, bathing, and grooming activities; (3) management of environmental hardware and devices includes the ability to use telephones, keys, faucets, light switches, windows, doors, scissors, and street control signals; (4) communication skills include the ability to write, read, type, or use the telephone, a tape recorder, or a special communications device; (5) home management activities include marketing, meal planning and preparation, cleaning, laundry, child care, and the ability to manage household appliances, such as vacuum cleaners, can openers, ranges, refrigerators, electric mixers, and hand-operated utensils.

Factors to consider in ADL evaluation and training

Before commencing ADL performance evaluation and training the occupational therapist must assess performance components and consider several factors about the client and his environment. Physical resources, such as strength, ROM, coordination, sensation, and balance, should be evaluated to determine potential skills and deficits in ADL performance and possible need for special equipment. Perceptual and cognitive functions should be evaluated to determine potential for learning ADL skills. General mobility in bed or wheelchair or ambulation should be assessed.

In addition to these relatively concrete and objective evaluations the occupational therapist should be familiar with the client's culture and its values and mores in relation to self-care, the sick role, family assistance, and independence. The values of the client, his peer group, and his culture should be important considerations in selecting objectives and initial activities in the ADL program. The balance of activities in the client's day, which demand his time and energy, may influence how many ADL may be performed independently. The environment to which the client will return is an important consideration. Will he return to live alone or with his family or a roommate? Will he be going to a skilled nursing facility or to a board and care home permanently or temporarily? Will he be returning to work and community activities? The type and amount of assistance available in the home environment must be considered if the appropriate caretaker is to receive orientation and training in the appropriate supervision and assistance required. The finances available for assistant care, special equipment, and home modifications are important considerations. For example, a wheelchair-bound client who is wealthy may be willing and able to make major modifications in the home, such as installing an elevator, lowering kitchen counters, widening doorways, and replacing deep pile carpeting to accommodate a wheelchair life-style. His less well-off counterpart may need the assistance of the occupational therapist in making less costly modifications, such as removing scatter rugs and door sills, installing a plywood ramp at the entrance, replacing the bathroom door with a curtain, and attaching a hand-held shower head to the bathtub faucet.

The ultimate goal of any ADL training program is for the client to achieve *his* maximum level of independence. It is important to note that the "maximum level of independence" is defined differently for each client. For the client with mild muscle weakness in one arm due to a peripheral neuropathy, complete independence in ADL may be his "maximum," while for the high-level quadriplegic feeding and oral hygiene activities with devices and assistance may be the maximum level of independence that can be expected. Therefore the potential for independence should be based on each client's unique personal needs, values, capabilities, limitations, and environmental resources.

Independence is a strong value in the American culture. It should not be pursued for its own sake on that basis or because it is a value of the rehabilitation personnel or family or friends of the client.

ADL EVALUATION
General procedure

When some data have been gathered about the client's physical, psychosocial, and environmental resources, the feasibility of ADL evaluation or training should be determined by the occupational therapist in concert with the client, supervising physician, and other members of the rehabilitation team. In some instances ADL should be delayed because of limitations of the client or in favor of more immediate treatment objectives that require the client's energy and participation.

Evaluation of ADL performance is often initiated with an interview, using an ADL checklist as a guide for questioning the client about his capabilities and limitations. Several types of ADL checklists are available, but they cover similar categories and performance tasks. The ADL interview may serve as a screening device to determine need for further assessment by observation of performance. This is determined by the therapist's professional judgment based on knowledge of the client, the dysfunction and results of previous evaluations. A partial or complete performance evaluation is invaluable in assessing ADL performance. The phrase "one look is worth a thousand words" applies well here. The ADL interview alone, as a measure of performance, can be inaccurate, because the client may recall his performance prior to the onset of the dysfunction, may have some confusion or memory loss, and may overestimate or underestimate his abilities, because he has had little opportunity to perform routine ADL since the onset of the physical dysfunction.

Ideally the occupational therapist should conduct the performance evaluation at the time and in the environment in which the activities to be evaluated usually take place. For example, a dressing evaluation could be arranged for early in the morning when the client usually is dressed by nursing personnel. Feeding evaluation should occur at regular meal hours. If this is not possible because of schedules, personnel, or environmental constraints in the treatment facility or client's home, the evaluation may be conducted during regular treatment sessions in the occupational therapy clinic under simulated conditions. This is not as good, since it requires that the client perform or reperform routine self-maintenance tasks at irregular times in an artificial environment and can contribute to a lack of carry-over for those clients who have difficulty generalizing learning.

The therapist should begin by selecting relatively simple and safe items from the ADL checklist for the client to perform and should progress to more difficult and complex items. The evaluation should not be completed all at once, since this would be fatiguing and somewhat artificial. Those items that would be unsafe or that very obviously cannot be performed should be omitted and the appropriate notation made on the evaluation form.

During the performance evaluation the therapist should observe the methods that the client is using or attempting to use to accomplish the task and try to determine causes of performance problems. Some of these might be weakness, spasticity, involuntary motion, perceptual deficits, or low endurance. If problems and their causes can be identified, the therapist has a good foundation for establishing training objectives, priorities, and methods and need for assistive devices. Other very important aspects of this evaluation that should not be overlooked are the client's need for respect and privacy and the ongoing interaction between the client and therapist. The client's feelings about having his body viewed and touched should be respected. Privacy should be maintained for toileting, grooming, and dressing tasks. The therapist with whom the client is most familiar and comfortable may be the most appropriate person to conduct the ADL evaluation and training. As the therapist interacts with the client during the performance of ADL, it may be possible to elicit the client's attitudes and feelings about the particular tasks, his priorities in training, dependence and independence, and cultural, family, and personal values and customs about performance of daily living activities.

Recording results of the ADL evaluation. During the interview and performance evaluation the therapist makes the appropriate notations on the ADL checklists. These may include separate checklists for self-care, home management, mobility, and home environment evaluations. The information is then summarized succinctly for inclusion in the client's permanent records where interested professional co-workers can refer to it.

ADL TRAINING

If, after evaluation, it is determined that ADL training is to be initiated, it is important to establish appropriate short- and long-term objectives, based on the evaluation and on the client's priorities for independence. Trombly and Scott[11] suggest the following sequence of training for self-care activities: feeding, grooming, continence, transfer skills, toileting, undressing, dressing, and bathing. This sequence is based on the normal development of self-care independence in children.

This sequence provides a good guide but may need to be modified to accommodate the specific dysfunction and the capabilities, limitations, and personal priorities of the client. One client was known to deem smoking a more important skill than feeding. Although the hand-to-mouth movement pattern in both activities is similar, and feeding was objectively estimated as a priority over smoking, the client was content to be fed by an assistant but became very involved in achieving smoking independence using mobile arm supports and assistive devices. Only after some independence was achieved here was feeding an acceptable activity.

The occupational therapist should estimate which ADL are possible and which are impossible for the client to achieve. She should explore with the client the use of alternate methods of performing the activities and the use of any assistive devices that may be helpful. She should determine for which tasks the client will require assistance and how much should be given. It may not be possible to estimate these factors until the training program is underway.

The ADL training program may be graded by beginning with a few simple tasks and gradually increasing the number and complexity of tasks to be performed. Training should progress from dependent to assisted to supervised to independent, with or without assistive devices.[11] The rate at which grading can occur will depend on the client's recovery, endurance, skills, and motivation.

Methods of teaching ADL

The methods of teaching the client to perform daily living tasks must be tailored to suit each client's learning style and ability. The client who is alert and grasps instructions quickly may be able to perform an entire process after a brief demonstration and verbal instruction. Clients who may have perceptual problems, poor memory, and difficulty following instructions of any kind will require a more concrete, step-by-step approach, reducing the amount of assistance gradually as success is achieved. For such persons it is important to break the activity down into small steps and progress through them slowly, one at a time. Slow demonstration of the task or step in the same plane and in the same manner in which the client is expected to perform is very helpful. Verbal instructions to accompany the demonstration may or may not be helpful, depending on the client's receptive language skills and ability to process and integrate two modes of sensory information simultaneously.

Touching body parts to be moved, dressed, bathed, or positioned or passive movement of the part through the desired pattern to achieve a step or a task are helpful tactile and kinesthetic modes of instruction. These can be used to augment or substitute for demonstration and verbal instruction, again depending on the client's best avenues of learning. It is necessary to perform a step or complete task repetitiously to achieve skill, speed, or retention of learning. Tasks may be repeated several times during the same training session, if time and the client's physical and emotional tolerance allow, or they may be repeated on a daily basis until desired retention or level of skill is achieved. Trombly and Scott describe the process of "backward chaining" in teaching ADL skills. In this method the therapist assists the client until the last step of the process is reached. The client then performs this step independently, which affords a sense of success and completion. When the last step is mastered, the therapist assists until the last two steps are reached and the client then completes these two steps. The process continues with the therapist offering less and less assistance and the client performing successive steps of the task, from last to first, independently. This method is particularly useful in training patients with brain damage.[11]

Before beginning training in any ADL the therapist must make some preparations. The therapist should provide adequate space and arrange equipment, materials, or furniture for maximum convenience and safety. The therapist should be thoroughly familiar with the task to be performed and any special methods or assistive devices that will be used in its performance. She should be able to perform the task, as she expects the client to perform it, skillfully. After the preparation the activity is presented to the client, usually in one or more modes of demonstration and verbal instruction described earlier. The client then performs the activity either along with the therapist or immediately after being shown, with the amount of supervision and assistance required. Performance is modified and corrected as needed and the process is repeated to ensure learning. In the final phase of instruction when the client has mastered the task or several tasks, he is placed on his own to perform them independently. The therapist should follow up by checking on performance in progress and later arrange to check on adequacy of performance and carry-over of learning with nursing personnel, caretaker, or the supervising family members.[4]

Recording progress in ADL performance

The ADL checklists used to record performance on the initial evaluation usually have one or more spaces for recording changes in abilities and results of reevaluation during the training process. The sample checklist given later in this chapter is so designed and filled out. Progress is usually summarized for inclusion in the medical record. The progress report should summarize changes in the client's abilities and current level of independence and estimate the client's potential for further independence, his attitude and motivation for ADL training, and future goals for the ADL program.

When describing levels of independence occupational therapists often use terms like *moderate independence*, *maximal assistance*, and *minimal skill*. These quantitative terms have little meaning to the reader unless they are defined or supporting statements are used in progress summaries to give specific meaning for each. It also needs to be specified whether the level of independence refers to a single activity, a category of activities such as dressing, or all ADL. In designating levels of independence an agreed-on performance scale should be used to mark the ADL checklist. General categories and their definitions might be the following:

1. Independent. Can perform the activity or activities without cueing, supervision, or assistance, with or without assistive devices, at normal or near normal speeds
2. Partially dependent. Can perform at least 50% of the activity or activities independently; may

be considerably slower than normal performance, use assistive devices, and require some level of assistance
  a. Minimal assistance: Supervision, cueing, or less than 20% physical assistance
  b. Moderate assistance: Supervision, cueing, and 20% to 50% physical assistance
  c. Maximal assistance: Supervision, cueing, and 50% to 80% physical assistance
3. Dependent. Can perform only one or two steps of the activity or very few activities independently; may fatigue easily and perform very slowly; may require elaborate equipment and devices to perform basic skills such as feeding; needs more than 80% physical assistance

These definitions are broad and general. They can be modified to suit the program plan and approach of the particular treatment facility.

A sample case study, ADL and home management checklists, and summaries of an initial evaluation and progress report are included on pp. 114-121 (Figs. 4-11 and 4-12). The reader should keep in mind that the evaluation and progress summaries relate to the ADL portion of the treatment program only.

SAMPLE CASE STUDY

J.V. is a 48-year-old married woman who suffered a cerebral thrombosis resulting in a CVA 6 months ago. She lives in a modest home with her husband and teenage daughter and was a full-time homemaker before the onset of her stroke. She was a cheerful and active woman who enjoyed cooking, baking, gardening, and visiting her neighbors and friends. The stroke resulted in the disturbance of cerebellar and brain stem functions. J.V. has a severe motor apraxia for speech, cannot close her mouth, drools, and walks with a broad-based ataxic gait. Since the onset of her disability J.V. has been very depressed, weeps frequently, is dependent for much of her self-care, and sits idly for long periods of time. She was referred to occupational therapy for evaluation and training in ADL, adjustment to disability, and development of drooling and swallowing control to facilitate feeding.

SAMPLE ADL PROGRESS REPORT

J.V. has attended occupational therapy three times weekly for 3 weeks since the initial evaluation. Further evaluation of self-care skills revealed that J.V. is capable of some hygiene skills, except a tub bath, nail care, hair care, and makeup application. However, at home she remains almost entirely dependent on Mr. V. for self-care, whining, crying, and complaining of feeling weak.

Home management evaluation revealed considerable difficulty with most tasks except table setting, dusting, dish washing, and sweeping, which she can perform if given cues and supervision. Performance of more complex tasks is limited by psychomotor retardation, incoordination, distractibility, inability to sequence a process, and apraxia for fine hand activities. It was necessary to supervise J.V. closely and give step-by-step instructions while she performed household tasks. A few simple homemaking tasks were performed for several training sessions, but performance did not improve.

J.V. appears to be very depressed and lacks intrinsic motivation. It was suggested to her family that they offer less assistance for self-care, and involve her with them in household tasks that she can perform, under their supervision, if possible.

The occupational therapy program will continue with greater emphasis on achieving control of mouth musculature, a primary goal of J.V. ADL training will be delayed until J.V. is moving toward the achievement of this primary goal.

SPECIFIC ADL TECHNIQUES

In many instances specific techniques to solve specific ADL problems are not possible. Rather the occupational therapist may have to explore a variety of methods or assistive devices to reach a solution. It is sometimes necessary for the therapist to design a special device, method, splint, jig, or piece of equipment to make a particular activity possible for the client to perform. Many of the assistive devices available today through rehabilitation equipment companies were first conceived of and made by occupational therapists and clients. Many of the special methods used to perform specific activities also evolved through trial and error approaches of the therapists and their clients. Clients often have good suggestions for therapists, since they live with the limitation and are confronted regularly with the need to adapt the performance of daily tasks. The purpose of the following summary of techniques is to give the reader some general ideas about how to solve ADL problems for specific classifications of dysfunctions. The reader is referred to the references and supplementary reading list at the end of this section for more specific instruction in ADL methods.

Limited ROM[1,4,8,9,11]

The major problem for persons with limited joint ROM is to compensate for the lack of reach and joint excursion through such means as environmental adaptation and assistive devices. Some adaptations and devices are outlined here.

Dressing activities. The following are general suggestions for facilitating dressing:
1. Use front-opening garments, one size larger than needed and made of fabrics that have some stretch.
2. Use dressing sticks (Fig. 4-13 on p. 122) with a garter on one end and neoprene-covered coat hook on the other for pushing and pulling garments off and on feet and legs. A pair of dowels with a cup hook on end of each can be used to pull socks on if a loop tape is sewn to the tops of the socks.
3. Use larger buttons or zippers with a loop on the pull tab.
4. Replace buttons, snaps, hooks, and eyes with Velcro (for those clients who cannot manage traditional fastenings).
5. Eliminate the need to bend to tie shoelaces or use

Text continued on p. 122.

OCCUPATIONAL THERAPY DEPARTMENT

ACTIVITIES OF DAILY LIVING EVALUATION

Name __J. V._____ Age __48__ Diagnosis __CVA_____ Dom. __Right_____

Mode of ambulation __Independent_____ Disability __Bilateral incoordination, ataxia, apraxia of mouth musculature__

Grading key: I = Independent D = Dependent
MiA = Minimal assistance NA = Not applicable
MoA = Moderate assistance 0 = Not evaluated
MaA = Maximal assistance

TRANSFERS AND AMBULATION

	Date	Independent	Assisted	Dependent
Tub or shower	8/1			D
Toilet	8/1		MiA	
Wheelchair	NA			
Bed and chair		I		
Ambulation			MiA	
Wheelchair management	NA			
Car			MiA	

BALANCE FOR FUNCTION

	Adequate	Inadequate
Sitting	I	
Standing	I	
Walking		MiA

SUMMARY OF EVALUATION RESULTS

Date __8/1_____

Intact	Impaired		REMARKS
		SENSORY STATUS	
X		Touch	
X		Pain	
X		Temperature	
	X	Position sense	More marked on left
	X	Olfaction	
	X	Stereognosis	More marked on left
	X	Visual fields (hemianopsia)	
		PERCEPTUAL/CONCEPTUAL TESTS	
X		Follow directions	Verbal
X		Visual spatial (form)	
	X	Visual spatial (block design)	Minimal impairment
X		Make change	
	X	Geometric figures (copy)	Some difficulty with the triangle and diamond
		Square, circle, triangle, diamond	
	X	Praxis	Mild apraxia evident on fine hand activities
		FUNCTIONAL RANGE OF MOTION	
X		Comb hair—two hands	
X		Feed self	
X		Button collar button	
X		Tie apron behind back	
X		Button back buttons	
X		Button cuffs	
X		Zip side zipper	
	X	Tie shoes	Poor balance limits
	X	Stoop	reach and bending for these
	X	Reach shelf	activities

Fig. 4-11. ADL evaluation. (Adapted from Activities of daily living evaluation form OT 461-1, Hartford, Conn., 1963, The Hartford Rehabilitation Center.)

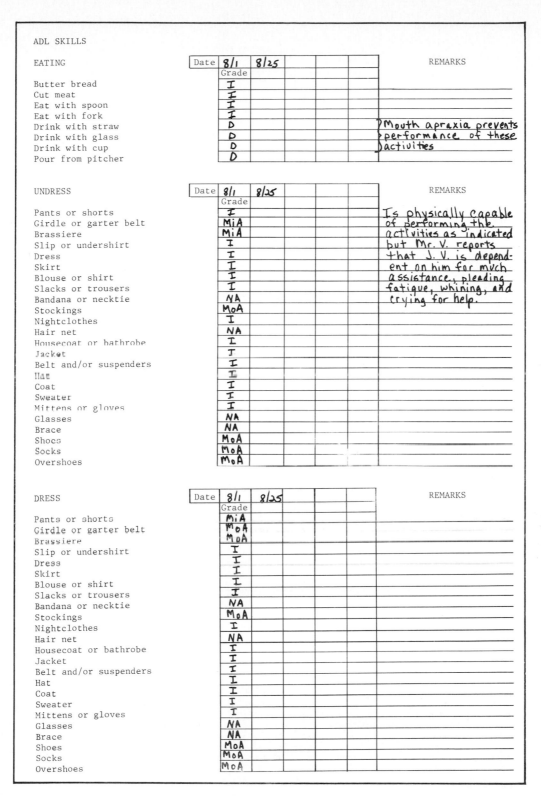

ADL SKILLS

EATING	Date	8/1	8/25				REMARKS
	Grade						
Butter bread		I					
Cut meat		I					
Eat with spoon		I					
Eat with fork		I					
Drink with straw		D					?Mouth apraxia prevents
Drink with glass		D					performance of these
Drink with cup		D					activities
Pour from pitcher		D					

UNDRESS	Date	8/1	8/25				REMARKS
	Grade						
Pants or shorts		I					Is physically capable
Girdle or garter belt		MiA					of performing the
Brassiere		MiA					activities as indicated
Slip or undershirt		I					but Mr. V. reports
Dress		I					that J. V. is depend-
Skirt		I					ent on him for much
Blouse or shirt		I					assistance, pleading
Slacks or trousers		I					fatigue, whining, and
Bandana or necktie		NA					crying for help.
Stockings		MoA					
Nightclothes		I					
Hair net		NA					
Housecoat or bathrobe		I					
Jacket		I					
Belt and/or suspenders		I					
Hat		I					
Coat		I					
Sweater		I					
Mittens or gloves		I					
Glasses		NA					
Brace		NA					
Shoes		MoA					
Socks		MoA					
Overshoes		MoA					

DRESS	Date	8/1	8/25				REMARKS
	Grade						
Pants or shorts		MiA					
Girdle or garter belt		MoA					
Brassiere		MoA					
Slip or undershirt		I					
Dress		I					
Skirt		I					
Blouse or shirt		I					
Slacks or trousers		I					
Bandana or necktie		NA					
Stockings		MoA					
Nightclothes		I					
Hair net		NA					
Housecoat or bathrobe		I					
Jacket		I					
Belt and/or suspenders		I					
Hat		I					
Coat		I					
Sweater		I					
Mittens or gloves		I					
Glasses		NA					
Brace		NA					
Shoes		MoA					
Socks		MoA					
Overshoes		MoA					

Fig. 4-11, cont'd. ADL evaluation.   *Continued.*

FASTENINGS	Date	8/1	8/25				REMARKS
	Grade						
Button		I					
Snap		MoA					
Zipper		MiA					
Hook and eye		MoA					
Garters		D					
Lace		D					
Untie shoes		D					
Velcro		MiA					

HYGIENE	Date	8/1	8/25				REMARKS
	Grade						
Blow nose		O	I				
Wash face, hands		O	I				
Wash extremities, back		O	MoA				
Brush teeth or dentures		O	I				
Brush or comb hair		O	I				
Set hair		O	D				
Shave or put on makeup		O	MiA				
Clean fingernails		O	ID				
Trim fingernails, toenails		O	D				
Apply deodorant		O	I				
Shampoo hair		O	D				
Use toilet paper		O	I				
Use tampon or sanitary napkin		O	NA				

COMMUNICATION	Date	8/1	8/25				REMARKS
	Grade						
Verbal		D					
Read		I					
Hold book		I					
Turn page		I					
Write		I					Writes name and few words
Use telephone		D					
Type		D					

HAND ACTIVITIES	Date	8/1	8/25				REMARKS
	Grade						
Handle money		O					
Handle mail		O					
Use of scissors		O					
Open cans, bottles, jars		O					
Tie package		O					
Sew (baste)		O					
Sew button, hook and eye		O					
Polish shoes		O					
Sharpen pencil		O					
Seal and open letter		O					
Open box		O					

Fig. 4-11, cont'd. ADL evaluation.

COMBINED PERFORMANCE
    ACTIVITIES

Date	8/1	8/25				REMARKS
	Grade					

Open-close refrigerator — 0 / I
Open-close door — 0 / I
Remove and replace object — 0 / I
Carry objects during locomotion — D / D
Pick up object from floor — 0 / D
Remove, replace light bulb — 0 / D
Plug in cord — 0 / D

Date						REMARKS
	Grade					

OPERATE

Light switches — 0 / I
Doorbell — 0 / I
Door locks and handles — 0 / D
Faucets — 0 / I
Raise-lower window shades — D / D
Raise-lower venetian blinds — 0 / D
Raise-lower window — 0 / D
Open and close drawer — 0 / I
Hang up garment — 0 / I

Fig. 4-11, cont'd. ADL evaluation.

OCCUPATIONAL THERAPY DEPARTMENT

ACTIVITIES OF HOME MANAGEMENT

Name _J. V._____ Date _8/25_____

Address _Anytown, USA_____

Age _48_____ Weight _135 lb___ Height _5'5"_____ Role in family _Wife, Mother_

Diagnosis _CVA_____ Disability _Bilateral ataxia, apraxia of mouth musculature_

Mode of ambulation _Independent, no aides, mild ataxic gait_____

Limitations or contraindications for activity_____

DESCRIPTION OF HOME

1. Private house _____✓_____
    No. of rooms _6 — Kitchen, dining room, living room 3 bedrooms_
    No. of floors _2_
    Stairs _14 — Bedrooms on second floor_
    Elevators _0_

2. Apartment house _____
    No. of rooms _____
    No. of floors _____
    Stairs _____
    Elevators _____

3. Diagram of home layout (attach to completed form)

Will patient be required to perform the following activities? If not, who will perform?

Meal preparation	No	Daughter
Baking	No	Daughter (J.V. used to bake a lot.)
Serving	Yes	
Wash dishes	Yes	
Marketing	No	Husband
Child care (under 4 years)	No	
Washing	Yes	
Hanging clothes	NA	Has dryer
Ironing	No	Daughter
Cleaning	Yes	Light cleaning
Sewing	No	Does not sew
Hobbies or special interest	Yes	Baking and gardening would be desirable activities

Does patient really like housework?   Yes_____ No_ X _

Fig. 4-12. Activities of home management. (Adapted from Occupational Therapy Department, University Hospital, Ohio State University, Columbus, Ohio.)

ACTIVITIES OF HOME MANAGEMENT

Sitting position: Chair___X___ Stool___X___ Wheelchair___NA___
Standing position: Braces___NA___ Crutches___NA___ Canes___NA___
Handedness: Dominant hand__Right__ Two hands__X__ One hand only_____ Assistive_____

Grading key: I = Independent   MaA = Maximal assistance
             MiA = Minimal assistance   D = Dependent
             MoA = Moderate assistance   O = Not evaluated

CLEANING ACTIVITIES	Date	8/25					REMARKS
		Grade					
Pick up object from floor		D					
Wipe up spills		D					
Make bed (daily)		D					
Use dust mop		I					
Shake dust mop		D					
Dust low surfaces		I					
Dust high surfaces		D					
Mop kitchen floor		D					
Sweep with broom		I					
Use dust pan and broom		MiA					
Use vacuum cleaner		D					
Use vacuum cleaner attachments		D					
Carry light cleaner tools		I					
Use carpet sweeper		I					
Clean bathtub		D					
Change sheets on bed		D					
Carry pail of water		D					

MEAL PREPARATION	Date	8/25					REMARKS
		Grade					
Turn off water		I					
Turn off gas or electric range		I					
Light gas with match		D					
Pour hot water from pan to cup		D					
Open packaged goods		I					
Carry pan from sink to range		D					
Use can opener		D					
Handle milk bottle		I					
Dispose of garbage		D					
Remove things from refrigerator		D					
Bend to low cupboards		D					
Reach to high cupboards		D					
Peel vegetables		D					
Cut up vegetables		D					
Handle sharp tools safely		D					
Break eggs		D					
Stir against resistance		D					
Measure flour		D					
Use eggbeater		D					
Use electric mixer		D					
Remove batter to pan		D					
Open oven door		I					
Carry pan to oven and put in		D					
Remove hot pan from oven to table		D					
Roll cookie dough or piecrust		D					

Fig. 4-12, cont'd. Activities of home management. *Continued.*

ACTIVITIES OF HOME MANAGEMENT—cont'd

MEAL SERVICE

	Date	8/25				REMARKS
		Grade				
Set table for four		I				
Carry four glasses of water to table		D				
		D				
Carry hot casserole to table		I				
Clear table		I				
Scrape and stack dishes		I				
Wash dishes (light soil)		I				
Wipe silver		I				
Wash pots and pans		MiA				
Wipe up range and work areas		MoA				
Wring out dishcloth		I				

LAUNDRY

	Date	8/25				REMARKS
		Grade				
Wash lingerie (by hand)		D				
Wring out, squeeze dry		D				
Hang on rack to dry		I				
Sprinkle clothes		I				
Iron blouse or slip		D				
Fold blouse or slip		D				
Use washing machine		D				

SEWING

	Date	8/25				REMARKS
		Grade				
Thread needle and make knot		D				
Sew on buttons		D				
Mend rips		D				
Darn socks		D				
Use sewing machine		NA				
Crochet		NA				
Knit		NA				
Embroider		NA				
Cut with shears		D				

HEAVY HOUSEHOLD ACTIVITIES WHO WILL DO THESE?

	Date	8/25				REMARKS
		Grade				
Wash household laundry		D				Daughter
Hang clothes		D				Has dryer
Clean range		D				Husband
Clean refrigerator		D				Daughter
Wax floors		D				Husband
Marketing		D				Husband
Turn mattresses		D				Husband
Wash windows		D				Husband
Put up curtains		D				Daughter

Fig. 4-12, cont'd. Activities of home management.

WORK HEIGHTS

SITTING/STANDING

Best height for   Wheelchair_____ Chair _X_ Stool _X_

Ironing   17½" seated

Mixing   26" on high stool at counter

Dish washing   26" on high stool at counter

General work   _____

Maximum depth of counter area (normal reach) 25"

Maximum useful height above work surface 33" if standing

Maximum useful height without counter surface 68" if standing

Maximum reach below counter area 20" if standing

Best height for chair 17½" — Can be used at adjustable ironing board

Best height for stool with back support 24" — Can be used at sink or food preparation counter

SUGGESTIONS FOR HOME MODIFICATION

Remove scatter rugs in bedroom.

Install guard rail on both sides of toilet.

Install grab bars on wall next to bath tub.

Place nonskid strips on bottom of bath tub.

Fig. 4-12, cont'd. Activities of home management.

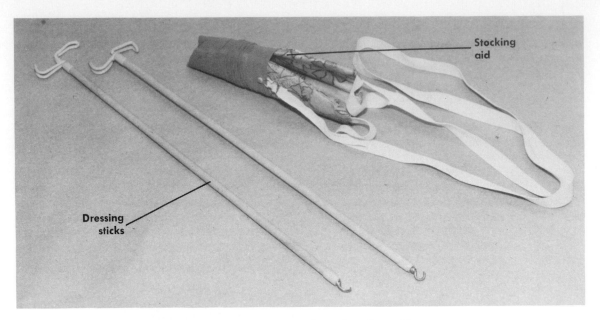

Fig. 4-13. Dressing sticks and stocking aid.

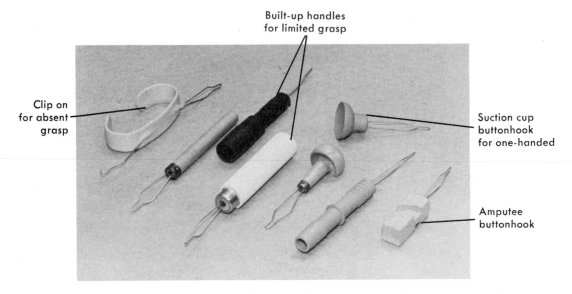

Fig. 4-14. Buttonhooks to accommodate limited or special types of grasp or amputation.

the finger joints in this fine activity by using elastic shoelaces or other adapted shoe fasteners.

6. Facilitate donning stockings without bending to the feet by using stocking aids made of garters attached to long webbing straps or buying those that are commercially available (Fig. 4-13).

7. Use one of several types of commercially available buttonhooks if finger ROM is very limited (Fig. 4-14).

8. Use scissor reachers for picking up socks and shoes,

arranging clothes, removing clothes from hangers, and picking up objects on the floor (Fig. 4-15).

Feeding activities. The following are assistive devices that can facilitate feeding:

1. Built-up handles on eating utensils can accommodate limited grasp or prehension (Fig. 4-16).

2. Elongated or specially curved handles on spoons and forks may be needed to reach the mouth. A swivel spoon or spoon-fork combination can compensate for limited supination (Fig. 4-17).

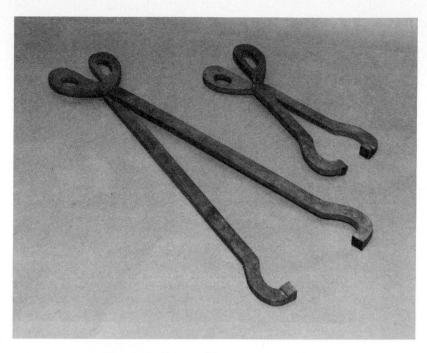

Fig. 4-15. Short and long scissor reachers.

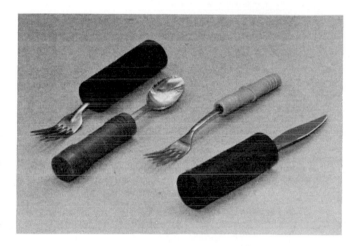

Fig. 4-16. Eating utensils with built-up handles.

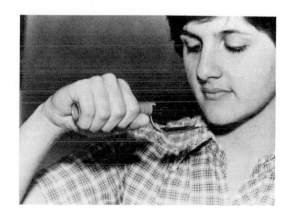

Fig. 4-17. Swivel spoon is used to compensate for limited supination.

3. Long plastic straws and straw clips on glasses or cups can be used if neck, elbow, or shoulder ROM limits hand-to-mouth motion or if grasp is inadequate to hold the cup or glass.
4. Universal cuffs or utensil holders can be used if grasp is very limited and even built-up handles do not work.
5. Plate guards or scoop dishes may be useful to prevent food from slipping off the plate.

Hygiene and grooming. Environmental adaptations that can facilitate bathing and grooming are as follows:

1. A hand-held shower head on flexible hose for bathing and shampooing hair can eliminate the need to stand in the shower and offers the user control of the direction of the spray. The handle can be built up or adapted for limited grasp.
2. A long-handled bath brush and sponge with a soap holder or long cloth scrubber can allow the user to reach legs, feet, and back. A wash mitt and soap on a rope can aid limited grasp (Fig. 4-18).
3. Long handles on comb, brush, toothbrush, lipstick, mascara brush, and safety or electric razor

may be useful for limited hand-to-head or hand-to-face movements.

4. Spray deodorant, hair spray, and spray powder or perfume can "extend" the reach by the distance the material sprays. Special adaptations may be required by some individuals to operate the spray mechanism.

5. Electric toothbrushes and Water Piks may be easier to manage for oral hygiene than a standard toothbrush.

6. A short reacher can extend reach for using toilet paper.

7. Dressing sticks can be used to pull garments up after using the toilet. An alternative is the use of

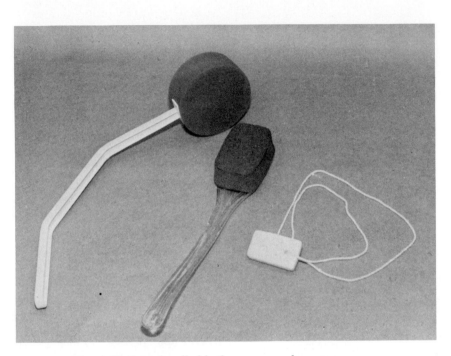

Fig. 4-18. Long-handled bath sponges and soap on a rope.

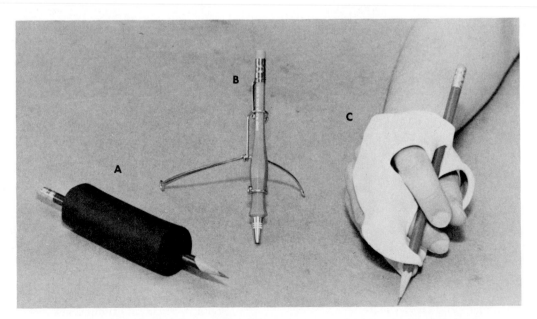

Fig. 4-19. Writing aids. **A,** Built-up pencil. **B,** Wire stand pencil holder. **C,** Thermoplastic custom-made writing device.

a long piece of elastic or webbing with garters on each end that can be hung around the neck and fastened to pants or panties, not allowing them to slip all the way to the floor during use of the toilet.

8. Safety rails can be used for bathtub transfers and safety mats or strips can be placed in the bathtub bottom to prevent slipping.

9. A bathtub seat, shower stool, or regular chair set in the bathtub or shower stall can eliminate the need to sit in the bathtub bottom or stand to shower and increases safety.

Communication and environmental hardware. The following are examples of environmental adaptations that can facilitate communication:

1. Extended or built-up handles on faucets can accommodate limited grasp.
2. Telephones should be placed within easy reach. A clip-type receiver holder, extended receiver holder, or speakerphone may be necessary. A dialing stick or push-button phone are still other adaptations.
3. Built-up pens and pencils to accommodate limited grasp and prehension can be used. A wire stand pencil holder and several other commercially available or custom fabricated writing aids are possible (Fig. 4-19).
4. Electric typewriters and book holders are aids that can facilitate communication for those with limited or painful joints.
5. Lever-type door knob extensions, car door openers, and adapted key holders can compensate for hand limitations.

Mobility and transfer skills. The individual who has limited ROM without significant muscle weakness may benefit from the following assistive devices:

1. A glider chair that is operated by the feet can facilitate transportation if there is limited hand and arm motion.
2. Platform crutches can prevent stress on hand or finger joints and accommodate limited grasp.
3. Enlarged grips on crutches or canes can accommodate limited grasp.
4. A raised toilet seat can be used if hip and knee motion is limited.
5. A walker with padded grips and forearm troughs can be used if there are marked hand, forearm, or elbow joint limitations.
6. A walker or crutch bags can facilitate the carrying of objects.

Home management activities.[5,9] Home management activities can be facilitated by a wide variety of environmental adaptations, assistive devices, energy conservation methods, and work simplification techniques. The principles of joint protection are essential

for those with rheumatoid arthritis. These are discussed in Chapter 9. The following are suggestions to facilitate home management for individuals with limited ROM:

1. Store frequently used items on the first shelves of cabinets just above and below counters or on counters where possible.
2. Use a high stool to work comfortably at counter height or attach a drop leaf table to the wall for planning and meal preparation area if a wheelchair is used.
3. Use a utility cart of comfortable height to transport several items at once.
4. Use reachers to get lightweight items (for example, cereal box) from high shelves.
5. Stabilize mixing bowls and dishes with nonslip mats.
6. Use lightweight utensils, such as plastic or aluminum bowls and aluminum pots.
7. Use electric can openers and electric mixers.
8. Use electric scissors.
9. Eliminate bending by using extended and flexible plastic handles on dust mops and brooms.
10. Facilitate sweeping by using dustpans and brushes with extended handles.
11. Eliminate bending by using wall ovens and counter top broilers.
12. Eliminate leaning and bending for ambulatory persons by using a top-loading automatic washer and elevated dryer. Wheelchair users can benefit from front-loading appliances.
13. Allow for sitting while ironing by using an adjustable ironing board.
14. Elevate the playpen and diaper table and use a Bathinette or plastic tub on the kitchen counter for bathing to reduce the amount of bending and reaching for the ambulatory mother during child care. The crib mattress can be raised, but this presents a safety factor when the child is more than a few months old.
15. Use larger and looser fitting garments with Velcro fastenings on children.

Problems of incoordination[1,6,11]

Incoordination in the form of tremors or ataxia or athetoid or choreiform movements can result from a variety of CNS disorders, such as Parkinson's disease, multiple sclerosis, cerebral palsy, and head injuries. The major problems encountered in ADL performance are safety and adequate stability of gait, body parts, and objects to complete the tasks.

The degree of incoordinated movement may be influenced by fatigue, emotional factors, and fears. The client must be taught appropriate energy conservation and work simplification techniques along with appropriate work pacing and safety methods to avoid the fatigue and apprehension that could increase incoordination and affect performance.

Dressing activities. Potential dressing difficulties can be reduced by using the following adaptations:

1. Front-opening garments that fit loosely can facilitate donning and removing garments.
2. Large buttons, Velcro, or zippers with loops on the tab can facilitate opening and closing fasteners. A buttonhook with a large, weighted handle may be helpful.
3. Elastic shoelaces, other adapted shoe closures, or slip-on shoes eliminate the need for bow tying.
4. Trousers with elastic tops for women or Velcro closures for men are easier to manage than those with hooks, buttons, and zippers.

5. Brassieres with front openings or Velcro replacements for the usual hook and eye may facilitate donning and removing this garment. A slipover elastic-type brassiere or bra-slip may also eliminate the need to manage the brassiere fastenings. Regular brassieres may be fastened in front at waist level, then slipped around to the back and the arms put into the straps, which are then worked up over the shoulders.
6. Clip-on ties can be used by men who use a tie.
7. Dressing should be performed while sitting on or in bed or in a wheelchair or chair with arms to avoid balance problems.

Feeding activities. Eating for clients with problems of incoordination can be quite a challenge. Lack of control during eating is not only frustrating to the individual

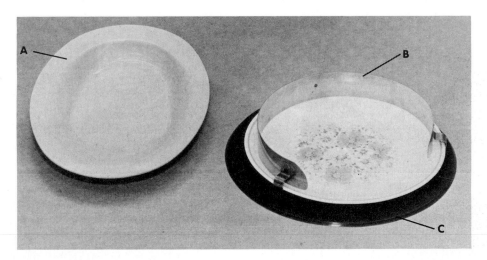

Fig. 4-20. *A*, Scoop dish. *B*, Plate with plate guard. *C*, Nonskid mat.

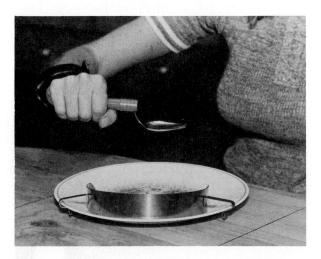

Fig. 4-21. Weighted wrist cuff and swivel utensil can sometimes compensate for incoordination or involuntary motion.

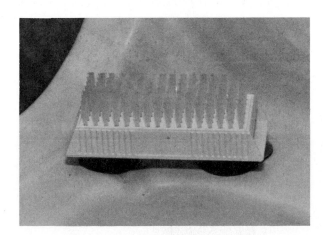

Fig. 4-22. Suction brush attached to bathroom sink.

but can produce embarrassment and social rejection. Therefore it is important to make eating safe, pleasurable, and as neat as possible. The following are some suggestions for achieving this goal:

1. Use plate stabilizers, such as nonskid mats, suction bases, or even wet dish towels.
2. Use a plate guard or scoop dish to prevent pushing food off the plate. The plate guard can be carried away from home and clipped to any ordinary dinner plate (Fig. 4-20).
3. Prevent spills during the plate-to-mouth excursion by using weighted or swivel utensils to offer some stability. Weighted cuffs may be placed on the forearm to decrease involuntary movement (Fig. 4-21).
4. Use long plastic straws with a straw clip on a glass or cup with a weighted bottom to eliminate the need to carry the glass or cup to the mouth thus avoiding spills. Plastic cups with covers and spouts may be used for the same purpose.
5. Use a resistance or friction-type arm brace similar to a mobile arm support, which was shown to help control patterns of involuntary movement during feeding activities of adults with cerebral palsy and athetosis by Holser et al.[3] Such a brace may help many clients with severe incoordination achieve some degree of independence in feeding.

Hygiene and grooming. Stabilization and handling of toilet articles may be achieved by the following suggestions:

1. Articles such as shaver, lipstick, and toothbrush can be attached to a cord if frequent dropping is a problem. An electric toothbrush may be more easily managed than a regular one.
2. Weighted wrist cuffs may be helpful during the finer hygiene activities, such as applying makeup, shaving, or hair care.
3. An electric razor rather than a blade razor offers stability and safety.
4. A suction brush attached to the sink or counter can be used for nail or denture care (Fig. 4-22).
5. Soap should be on a rope and can be worn around the neck or hung over a bathtub or shower fixture during bath or shower to keep it in easy reach.
6. An emery board or small piece of wood with fine sandpaper glued to it can be fastened to the tabletop for filing nails.
7. Large size roll-on deodorants are preferable to sprays or creams.
8. Sanitary napkins that stick to undergarments may be easier to manage than those that require clipping to a sanitary belt or tampons.
9. A bath mitt with a pocket to hold the soap can

be used for washing and eliminates the need for frequent soaping and rinsing and wringing a washcloth.

10. Nonskid mats should be used inside and outside the bathtub during bathing. Their suction bases should be securely fastened to the floor and bathtub before they are used. Safety grab bars should be installed on the wall next to the bathtub or fastened to the bathtub edge. A bathtub seat or shower chair provides more safety than standing while showering or transferring to bathtub bottom. Many incoordinated clients will require supervisory assistance during this hazardous activity. Sponge bathing while seated at a bathroom sink may substitute for bathing or showering several times a week.

Communication and environmental hardware. The following adaptations can facilitate communication for clients who have incoordination:

1. Doorknobs may be more easily managed if adapted with lever-type handles or covered with rubber or friction tape.
2. Managing dials or push buttons may be facilitated by using weighted cuffs or by stabilizing arms against body or on tabletop to control involuntary movement. A telephone receiver holder may be helpful.
3. Writing may be managed by using a weighted, enlarged pencil or pen. An electric typewriter with a keyboard guard is a very helpful aid to communication.
4. Keys may be managed by placing them on an adapted key holder that is rigid and offers more leverage for turning the key. However, inserting the key in the keyhole may be very difficult unless the incoordination is relatively mild (Fig. 4-23).
5. Extended lever-type faucets are easier to manage than turn knobs or push-pull spigots. To prevent burns during bathing and kitchen activities cold water should be turned on first and hot water added gradually.

Mobility and transfers. Clients with problems of in-

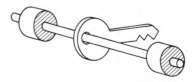

Fig. 4-23. Adapted key holder. Keys are slipped on small metal bar and rubber grommets or washers are slipped over ends to hold keys on. Similar adaptations are commercially available.

coordination may use a variety of ambulation aids, depending on the type and severity of incoordination. In degenerative diseases it is sometimes necessary to help the client recognize the need for and accept ambulation aids. This may mean graduation from a cane to crutches to a walker and finally to a wheelchair for some persons. Clients with incoordination can improve stability and mobility by the following suggestions:

1. Instead of lifting objects slide them on floors or counters.
2. Use suitable ambulation aids.
3. Use a utility cart, preferably a custom-made cart that is heavy and has some friction in the wheels.
4. Remove door sills, throw rugs, and shag carpeting.
5. Install banisters on indoor and outdoor staircases.
6. Substitute ramps for stairs wherever possible.

Home management activities.[5,6,11] It is important for the occupational therapist to make a careful assessment of homemaking activities performance to determine (1) which activities can be done safely, (2) which activities can be done safely if modified or adapted, and (3) which activities cannot be done adequately or safely and should be assigned to someone else. The major problems are stabilization of foods and equipment to prevent spilling and accidents and the safe handling of appliances, pots, pans, and household tools to prevent cuts, burns, bruises, electric shock, and falls. The following are suggestions for the facilitation of home management tasks:

1. Use a wheelchair and wheelchair lap board, even if ambulation is possible with devices. This will save energy and increase stability if balance and gait are unsteady.
2. If possible, use convenience and prepared foods to eliminate as many processes as possible, for example: peeling, chopping, slicing, and mixing.
3. Use easy-open containers or store foods in plastic containers once opened. A jar opener is also useful.
4. Use heavy utensils, mixing bowls, and pots and pans to increase stability.
5. Use nonskid mats on work surfaces.
6. Use electrical appliances such as crock pots, electric fry pans, and toaster-ovens, which are safer than using the range.
7. Use a blender and counter top mixer, which are safer than hand-held mixers and easier than mixing with a spoon or whisk.
8. If possible adjust work heights of counters, sink, and range to minimize leaning, bending, reaching, and lifting, whether the client is standing or using a wheelchair.
9. Use long oven mitts, which are safer than potholders.
10. Use pots, pans, casserole dishes, and appliances with bilateral handles, which may be easier to manage than those with one handle.
11. Use a cutting board with stainless steel nails to stabilize meats and vegetables while cutting. When not in use the nails should be covered with a large cork. The bottom of the board should have

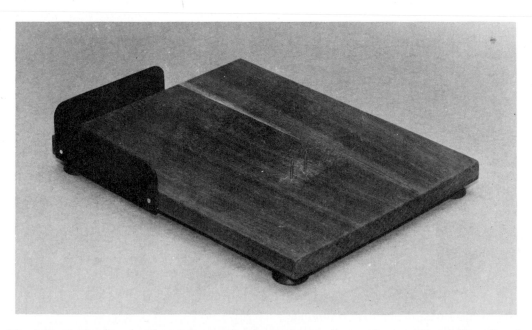

Fig. 4-24. Cutting board with stainless steel nails, suction cup feet, and corner for stabilizing bread is useful for clients with incoordination or who have one hand.

suction cups or be covered with stair tread, or the board should be placed on a nonskid mat to prevent slippage when in use (Fig. 4-24).

12. Use heavy dinnerware, which may be easier to handle, since it offers stability and control to the distal part of the upper extremity. On the other hand unbreakable dinnerware may be more practical if dropping and breakage are a problem.

13. Cover the sink, utility cart, and counter tops with protective rubber mats or mesh matting.

14. Use a serrated knife, which is easier to control, for cutting and chopping.

15. Use a steamer basket or deep fry basket for preparing boiled foods to eliminate the need to carry and drain pots with hot liquids in them.

16. Turn foods during cooking and when serving foods with tongs, which may offer more control and stability than a fork, spatula, or serving spoon.[5]

17. Vacuum with a heavy upright cleaner, which may be easier for the ambulatory client. The wheelchair user may be able to manage a lightweight tank-type vacuum cleaner or electric broom.

18. Use dust mitts when dusting.

19. Eliminate fragile knickknacks, unstable lamps, and dainty doilies.

20. Eliminate ironing by using no-iron fabrics or a timed dryer or by assigning this task to other members of the household.

21. Use front-loading washers, a laundry cart on wheels, and premeasured detergents, bleaches, and fabric softeners.

22. Sit while working and use foam rubber bath aids, an infant bath seat, and a wide, padded dressing table with safety straps with Velcro fastening to offer enough stability for bathing, dressing, and diapering an infant. Child care may not be possible unless the incoordination is mild.

23. Use disposable diapers with tape fasteners, which are easier to manage than cloth diapers and pins.

24. Do not feed the infant with a spoon or fork unless the incoordination is very mild or does not affect the upper extremities. This task may need to be performed by another household member.

25. Provide clothing for the child that is large, loose, with Velcro fastenings, and made of nonslippery stretch fabrics.

Hemiplegia or use of only one upper extremity[1,5,6,11]

The suggestions for performing daily living skills apply to persons with hemiplegia, unilateral upper extremity amputations, and temporary disorders, such as frac-

tures, burns, or peripheral neuropathy, which can result in the dysfunction of one upper extremity.

The hemiplegic individual will require specialized methods of teaching, and many will have greater difficulty in learning and performing one-handed skills than persons with orthopedic or lower motor neuron dysfunction. This is due to involvement of the trunk and leg, as well as the arm, and therefore possible ambulation and balance difficulties. Also, sensory, perceptual, cognitive, and speech disorders may be present from a mild to severe degree. These affect the ability to learn and retain learning and performance. Finally, the presence of motor and ideational apraxia sometimes seen in this group of clients can have a profound effect on the client's potential for learning new motor skills or remembering old ones.

Therefore the client with normal perception and cognition and the use of one upper extremity may learn the techniques quickly and easily. The hemiplegic client needs to be evaluated for sensory, perceptual, and cognitive deficits to determine potential for ADL performance and to establish appropriate teaching methods, already described, to facilitate learning.

The major problems for the one-handed worker are reduction of work speed and dexterity, stabilization to substitute for the role normally assumed by the nondominant arm, and, for the hemiplegic, balance and precautions relative to sensory loss.

Dressing activities. If balance is a problem, dressing should be done while seated in a locked wheelchair or sturdy armchair. Clothing should be within easy reach. Reaching tongs may be helpful for securing articles and assisting in some dressing activities. Assistive devices should be kept to a minimum for dressing and other ADL.

One-handed dressing techniques[*]

The following one-handed dressing techniques can facilitate dressing for persons with use of one upper extremity.

Front-opening shirts may be managed by any one of three methods. The first method can be used for jackets, robes, and front-opening dresses.

METHOD I
Donning shirt (Fig. 4-25)
1. Grasp shirt collar with normal hand and shake out twists (a).
2. Position shirt on lap with inside up and collar toward chest (b).

---

*Summarized from Activities of daily living for patients with incoordination, limited range of motion, paraplegia, quadriplegia, and hemiplegia, Cleveland, 1968, Highland View Hospital, Cuyahoga County Hospitals, Division of Occupational Therapy. Mimeographed, unpublished.

3. Position sleeve opening on affected side so it is as large as possible and close to affected hand, which is resting on lap (c).
4. Using normal hand place affected hand in sleeve opening and work sleeve over elbow by pulling on garment (d_1 – d_2).
5. Put normal arm into its sleeve and raise up to slide or shake sleeve into position past elbow (e).
6. With normal hand gather shirt up middle of back from hem to collar and raise shirt over head (f).
7. Lean forward, duck head, and pass shirt over it (g).
8. With normal hand adjust shirt by leaning forward and working it down past both shoulders. Reach in back and pull shirttail down (h).

9. Line shirt fronts up for buttoning and begin with bottom button (i). Button sleeve cuff of affected arm. Sleeve cuff of unaffected arm may be prebuttoned if cuff opening is large or button may be sewn on with elastic thread or sewn on a small tab of elastic and fastened inside shirt cuff.

Removing shirt
1. Unbutton shirt.
2. Lean forward.
3. With normal hand grasp collar or gather material up in back from collar to hem.
4. Lean forward, duck head, and pull shirt over head.
5. Remove sleeve from normal arm and then from affected arm.

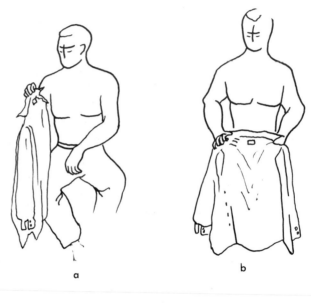

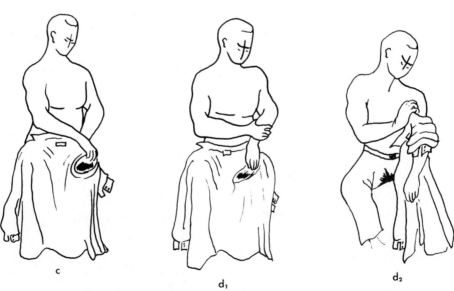

Fig. 4-25. Steps in donning shirt: method I. (Reproduced with permission of Mary S. Miller, Asst. Director of Occupational Therapy, Cuyahoga County Hospital, Cleveland, Ohio.)

METHOD II
Donning shirt

Method II may be used by clients who get shirt twisted or who have trouble sliding the sleeve down onto normal arm.

1. Position shirt as described in method I, steps 1 to 3.
2. With normal hand place involved hand into shirt sleeve opening and work sleeve onto hand, but do *not* pull up over elbow.
3. Put normal arm into sleeve and bring arm out to 180° of abduction. Tension of fabric from normal arm to wrist of affected arm will bring sleeve into position.
4. Lower arm and work sleeve on affected arm up over elbow.
5. Continue as in Steps 6 through 9 of method I.

Removing shirt

1. Unbutton shirt.
2. With normal hand push shirt off shoulders, first on affected side, then on normal side.
3. Pull on cuff of normal side with normal hand.
4. Work sleeve off by alternately shrugging shoulder and pulling down on cuff.
5. Lean forward, bring shirt around back, and pull sleeve off affected arm.

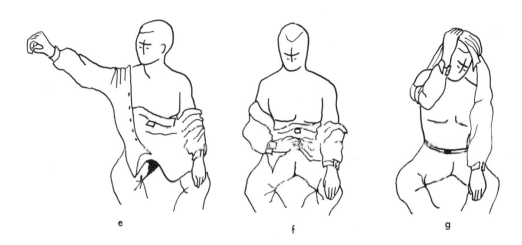

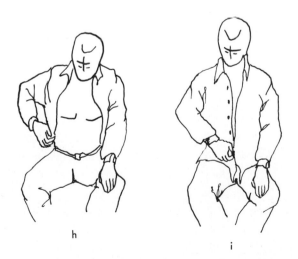

Fig. 4-25, cont'd. Steps in donning shirt: method I.

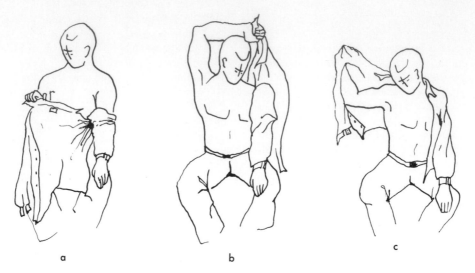

Fig. 4-26. Steps in donning shirt: method III. (Reproduced with permission of Mary S. Miller, Asst. Director of Occupational Therapy, Cuyahoga County Hospital, Cleveland, Ohio.)

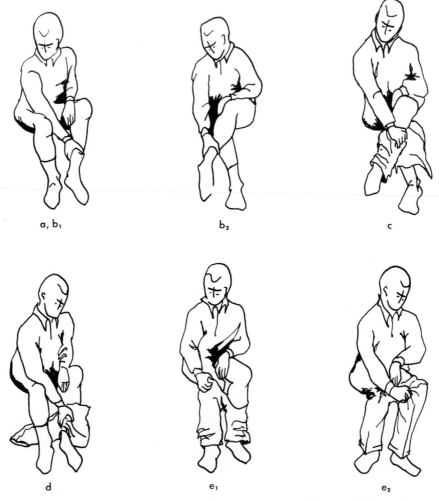

Fig. 4-27. Steps in donning trousers: method I. (Reproduced with permission of Mary S. Miller, Asst. Director of Occupational Therapy, Cuyahoga County Hospital, Cleveland, Ohio.)

METHOD III

Donning shirt (Fig. 4-26)

1. Position shirt and work on to arm as described in method I, steps 1 to 4.
2. Pull sleeve on affected arm up to shoulder (a).
3. With normal hand grasp tip of collar that is on normal side, lean forward, and bring arm over and behind head to carry shirt around to normal side (b).
4. Put normal arm into sleeve opening, directing it up and out (c).
5. Adjust and button as described in method I, steps 8 and 9.

Variation —donning pullover shirt

Pullover shirts can be managed by the following procedure:
1. Position shirt on lap, bottom toward chest and label facing down.
2. With normal hand roll up bottom edge of shirt back up to sleeve on affected side.
3. Position sleeve opening so it is as large as possible and use normal hand to place affected one into sleeve opening. Pull shirt up on to arm past elbow.
4. Insert normal arm into sleeve.
5. Adjust shirt on affected side up and on to shoulder.
6. Gather shirt back with normal hand, lean forward, duck head, and pass shirt over head.
7. Adjust shirt.

Variation —removing pullover shirt

Pullover shirts are removed by the following procedure:
1. Gather shirt up with the normal hand, starting at top back.
2. Lean forward, duck head, and pull gathered back fabric over head.
3. Remove from normal arm and then affected arm.

Trousers may be managed by one of the following methods. These may be adapted for shorts and women's panties as well. It is recommended that trousers have a well-constructed button fly front opening. This may be easier to manage than a zipper. Velcro may be used to replace buttons or zippers. Trousers should be worn in a size slightly larger than worn previously and should have a wide opening at the ankles. They should be donned after the socks have been put on but before the shoes are put on.

METHOD I

Donning trousers (Fig. 4-27)

1. Sit in sturdy armchair or in locked wheelchair (a).
2. Position normal leg in front of midline of body with knee flexed to 90°. Using normal hand reach forward and grasp ankle of affected leg or sock around ankle (b_1). Lift affected leg over normal leg to crossed position (b_2).
3. Slip trousers onto affected leg up to position where foot is completely inside of trouser leg (c). Do *not* pull up above knee or difficulty will be encountered in inserting normal leg.
4. Uncross affected leg by grasping ankle or portion of sock around ankle (d).
5. Insert normal leg and work trousers up onto hips as far as possible ($e_1 - e_2$). If wheelchair is used, place footrests in an up position.
6. If able to do so safely stand and pull trousers over hips. To prevent trousers from dropping place affected hand in pocket or place one finger of affected hand into belt loop $g_1 - g_3$).
7. Sit down to button front (h). If standing balance is good, remain standing to pull up zipper or button (g_3).

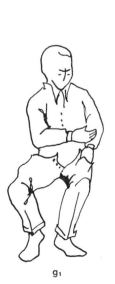 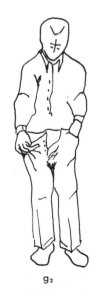 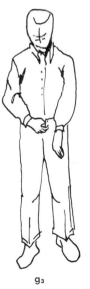 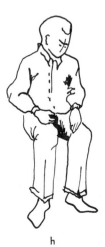

g₁   g₂   g₃   h

Fig. 4-27, cont'd. Steps in donning trousers: method I.

Removing trousers

1. Unfasten trousers and work down on hips as far as possible while seated.
2. Stand, letting trousers drop past hips or work them down past hips.
3. Sit and cross affected leg over normal leg, remove trousers, and uncross leg.
4. Remove trousers from normal leg.

METHOD II
Donning trousers

Method II is used for clients who are in wheelchairs with brakes locked or are in sturdy straight armchairs that are positioned with back against wall and for clients who cannot stand independently.

1. Position trousers on legs as in method I, steps 1 through 5.
2. Footrests remain in down position. Elevate hips by leaning back against chair and pushing down with normal leg. As hips are raised, work trousers over hips with normal hand.
3. Lower hips back into chair and fasten trousers.

Removing trousers

1. Unfasten trousers and work down on hips as far as possible while sitting.
2. With footrests in *down* position lean back against chair, push down with normal leg to elevate hips, and with normal arm work trousers down past hips.
3. Proceed as in method I, steps 3 and 4.

METHOD III
Donning trousers

Method III is for clients who are in a recumbent position. It is more difficult to perform than those method done sitting. If possible, bed should be raised to semireclining position for partial sitting.

1. Using normal hand place affected leg in bent position and cross over normal leg, which may be partially bent to prevent affected leg from slipping.
2. Position trousers and work onto affected leg, first, up to knee. Then uncross leg.
3. Insert normal leg and work trousers up onto hips as far as possible.
4. With normal leg bent press down with foot and shoulder to elevate hips from bed and with normal arm pull trousers over hips or work trousers up over hips by rolling from side to side.
5. Fasten trousers.

Removing trousers

1. Hike hips as in putting trousers on in method III, step 4.
2. Work trousers down past hips, remove unaffected leg, and then remove affected leg.

Clothing items, such as brassieres, neckties, socks, stockings, and braces, may be difficult to manage with one hand. The following methods are recommended.

BRASSIERE
Donning

1. Tuck one end of brassiere into pants, girdle, or skirt waistband, and wrap other end around waist. Hook brassiere in front at waist level and slip fastener around to back (at waistline level).
2. Place affected arm through shoulder strap, and then place normal arm through other strap.
3. Work straps up over shoulders. Pull strap on affected side up over shoulder with normal arm. Put normal arm through its strap and work up over shoulder by directing arm up and out and pulling with hand.
4. Use normal hand to adjust breasts in brassiere cups.

NOTE: It is helpful if brassiere has elastic straps and is one size larger than usually worn. If there is some function in affected hand, a fabric loop may be sewn to back of brassiere near fastener. Affected thumb may be slipped through this to stabilize brassiere while normal hand fastens it. All elastic brassieres, prefastened or without fasteners, may be donned by adapting method I for shirts described previously.

Removing

1. Slip straps down off shoulders, normal side first.
2. Work straps down over arms and off hands.
3. Slip brassiere around to front with normal arm.
4. Unfasten and remove.

NECKTIE
Donning

Clip-on neckties are attractive and convenient. If conventional tie is used, following method is recommended:

1. Place collar of shirt in up position and bring necktie around neck and adjust so that smaller end is at desired length when tie is completed.
2. Fasten small end to shirt front with tie clasp or spring clip clothespin.
3. Loop long end around short end (one complete loop) and bring up between V at neck. Then bring tip down through loop at front and adjust tie, using ring and little fingers to hold tie end and thumb and forefingers to slide knot up tightly.

Removing

Pull knot at front of neck until small end slips up enough for tie to be slipped over head. Tie may be hung up in this state and replaced by slipping it over head, around upturned collar, and knot tightened, as described in step 3 of donning necktie.

SOCKS OR STOCKINGS
Donning

1. Sit in straight armchair or in wheelchair with brakes locked.
2. With normal leg directly in front of midline of body cross affected leg over it.
3. Open top of stocking by inserting thumb and first two fingers near cuff and spreading fingers apart.
4. Work stocking onto foot before pulling over heel. Care should be taken to eliminate wrinkles.

5. Work stocking up over leg. Shift weight from side to side to adjust stocking around thigh.
6. Fasten stocking to garter. Velcro tabs may be substituted for garters.

NOTE: Stockings should be seamless and of soft, stretch-type fabric.

Removing

1. While sitting, unfasten garters.
2. Work socks or stockings down as far as possible with normal arm.
3. Cross affected leg over normal one as described in step 2 of donning socks or stockings.
4. Remove sock or stocking from affected leg. Dressing stick may be required by some clients to push sock or stocking off heel and off foot.
5. Lift normal leg to comfortable height or to seat level and remove sock or stocking from foot.

SHORT LEG BRACE
Donning (Fig. 4-28)

1. Sit in straight armchair or in wheelchair with brakes locked (a).
2. Bring normal leg to body midline. Cross hemiplegic leg over normal leg (b).
3. Pull tongue of shoe through laces and tuck under bottom part of lace, so that it does not push down into shoe as brace is donned (c).
4. Fold Velcro mesh flap back and hold back with calf band. With normal hand swing brace back and then forward so heel is between uprights. Swing shoe far enough forward so that toes can be inserted into shoe (d_1). Still holding onto upright bar of brace, turn shoe inward so that toes will go in at a slight angle, preventing catching toes at sides of shoe (d_2).
5. Pull brace up onto leg as far as possible (e_1). If difficulty is encountered in getting brace up far enough on leg, raise

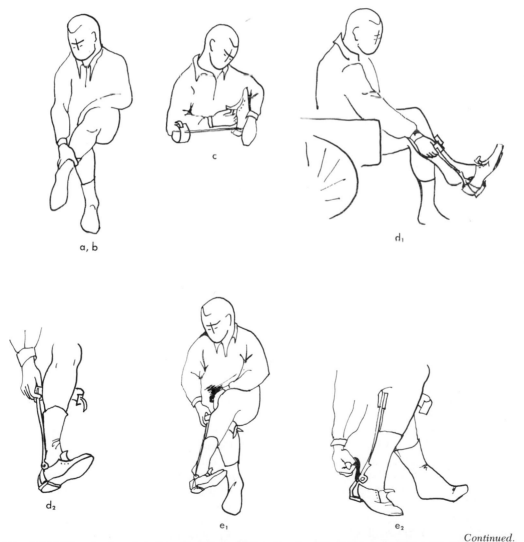

Continued.

Fig. 4-28. Steps in donning short leg brace. (Reproduced with permission of Mary S. Miller, Asst. Director of Occupational Therapy, Cuyahoga County Hospital, Cleveland, Ohio.)

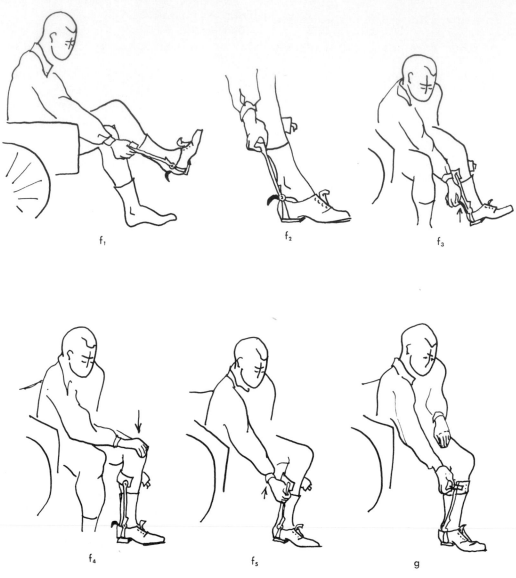

Fig. 4-28, cont'd. Steps in donning short leg brace.

affected leg by pulling up on crossbar, making foot easier to slip into shoe. Brace can now be held in position by pressure against crossbar between affected leg and normal leg, while shoehorn is inserted under heel in back (e₂). If there is difficulty is keeping brace on while inserting shoehorn, raise affected leg by pulling up on crossbar to position where ankle of affected leg is resting against knee of normal leg, with uprights on each side (e₂).

6. By holding uprights, uncross affected leg and position at 90° angle to floor (f₁ − f₂). Shoehorn is now in position where heel is pressing on it. Alternately, direct pressure downward on the knee and move shoehorn back and forth, using normal hand, until foot slips into shoe (f₃ − f₅).

7. Fasten laces and straps. One of many methods of one-handed bow tying may be used. Elastic shoelaces or other commercially available shoe fasteners may be required if unable to tie shoes (g).

Removing

Variation I

1. While seated as for donning, cross affected leg over normal leg.
2. Unfasten straps and laces with normal hand.
3. Push down on brace upright until shoe is off foot.

Variation II

1. Unfasten straps and laces.
2. Straighten affected leg by putting normal foot behind heel of shoe and pushing affected leg forward.
3. Push down on brace upright with hand and at same time push forward on heel of brace shoe with normal foot.

NOTE: Shoes may be donned by crossing legs, as described for stockings. Long-handled shoehorn may be helpful. Shoe tongue can have holes punched at top and shoelaces threaded through it to prevent tongue from being pushed into shoe

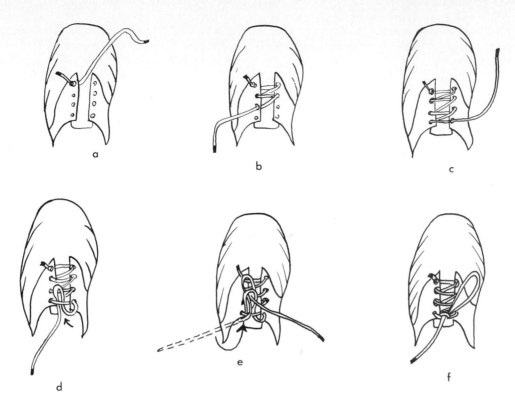

a b c

d e f

Fig. 4-29. One-hand shoe tying method. (Reproduced with permission of Mary S. Miller, Asst. Director of Occupational Therapy, Cuyahoga County Hospital, Cleveland, Ohio.)

when foot is forced in. Elastic shoelaces, buckles, or other adapted shoe closures are recommended for hemiplegic clients. Method for one-handed shoe tying is illustrated in Fig. 4-29 for those clients who prefer standard tie oxford.

Feeding activities. The only real problem encountered by the one-handed individual is managing a knife and fork simultaneously for meat cutting. This problem can be solved by the use of a rocker knife (Fig. 4-30) for cutting meat and other foods. It cuts with a rocking motion rather than a slicing back and forth action. The use of a rocking motion with a standard table knife or a sharp paring knife may be adequate to accomplish cutting tender meats and foods. If such a knife is used, the client is taught to hold the knife handle between the thumb and the third, fourth, and fifth fingers, and the index finger is extended along the top of the knife blade. The knife point is placed in the food in a vertical position, and then the blade is brought down to cut the food. The rocking motion, using wrist flexion and extension, is continued until the food is cut.

The occupational therapist should keep in mind that one-handed meat cutting involves learning a new motor pattern and may be difficult for clients with hemiplegia and apraxia.

Hygiene and grooming activities. With some assistive devices and the use of alternate methods hygiene and grooming activities can be accomplished by those with use of one hand or use of one side of the body. The following are suggestions for achieving hygiene and grooming with one hand.

1. Use an electric razor rather than a safety razor.
2. Use a bathtub seat or chair in the shower stall, wash mitt, long-handled bath sponge, safety rails on the bathtub or wall, soap on a rope or suction soap holder (Little Octopus), and suction brush for fingernail care.
3. Sponge bathe while sitting at the lavatory, using the wash mitt, suction brush, and suction soap holder. The uninvolved forearm and hand may be washed by placing a soaped washcloth on the thigh and rubbing the hand and forearm on the cloth.
4. Care for fingernails as described previously for clients with incoordination.
5. Use spray deodorants rather than creams or roll-ons, since they can be more easily applied to the uninvolved underarm.
6. Use a suction denture brush for care of dentures. The suction fingernail brush may also serve this purpose.

Communication and environmental hardware. The following are suggestions to facilitate writing, reading, and using the telephone:

1. The primary problem in writing is stabilization of the paper or tablet. This can be overcome by using a clip board or paper weight or by taping the paper to the writing surface. In some instances the affected arm may be positioned on the tabletop to stabilize the paper passively.
2. If dominance must be shifted to the nondominant extremity, writing practice may be necessary to improve speed and coordination. One-handed writing and typing instruction manuals are available.
3. Book holders may be used to stabilize a book while reading or holding copy for typing and writing practice.
4. The telephone is managed by lifting the receiver to listen for the dial tone, setting it down, dialing or pressing the buttons, then lifting the receiver to the ear. To write while using the telephone a telephone receiver holder that is on a stand or that rests on the shoulder must be used.

Mobility and transfers. Specific transfer techniques for clients with hemiplegia are described in Chapter 5.

Home management activities.[5] A wide variety of assistive devices is available to facilitate home management activities. Whether the client is disabled by the loss of function of one arm and hand, as in amputation or peripheral neuropathy, or whether both arm and leg are affected along with possible visual, perceptual, and cognitive dysfunctions, as in hemiplegia, will determine how many home management activities can realistically be performed, which methods can be used, and how many assistive devices can be managed. The reader is referred to the references and supplementary readings listed at the end of this chapter for details of home management with one hand. The following are some suggestions for one-handed homemakers:

1. Stabilization of items is a major problem for the one-handed homemaker. Stabilize foods for cutting and peeling by using a board with two stainless steel or aluminum nails in it. A raised corner on the board stabilizes bread while making sandwiches or spreading butter. Suction cups or a rubber mat under the board will keep it from slipping. Rubber stair tread may be glued to the bottom of the board.
2. Use sponge cloths, Dycem pads, wet dishcloths, or suction devices to keep pots, bowls, and dishes from turning or sliding during food preparation.
3. To open a jar, stabilize it between the knees or in a partially opened drawer while leaning against it or use a Zim jar opener (Fig. 4-31).
4. Open boxes, sealed paper, and plastic bags by stabilizing between the knees or in a drawer, as just described, and cutting open with a household shears.
5. Open an egg by holding it firmly in the palm of the hand, hitting it in the center against the edge of the bowl, and then using the thumb and index finger to push the top half of the shell up and the ring and little finger to push the lower half down. Separate whites from yolks by using an egg separator or a funnel.
6. Eliminate the need to stabilize the standard grater by using a grater with suction feet.
7. Stabilize pots on counter or range for mixing or stirring by using a pan holder with suction feet (Fig. 4-32).

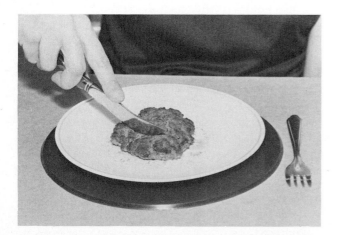

Fig. 4-30. Rocker knife for clients with one hand.

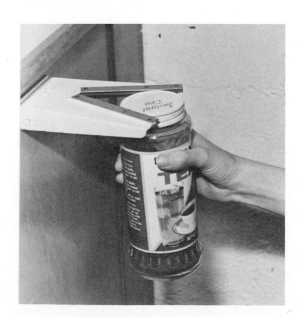

Fig. 4-31. Zim jar opener.

8. Eliminate the need to use hand-cranked or electric can openers requiring two hands by using a one-handed electric can opener.
9. Use a utility cart to carry items from one place to another. One that is weighted or constructed of wood may be used as a minimal support during ambulation for some clients.
10. Transfer clothes to and from the washer or dryer by using a clothes carrier on wheels.
11. Use electrical appliances, such as a lightweight electrical hand mixer, blender, and food processor, which can be managed with one hand and save time and energy. Safety factors and judgment need to be evaluated carefully when electrical appliances are considered.
12. Floor care becomes a greater problem if ambulation and balance, as well as one arm, are affected. For those clients with involvement of one arm only, a standard dust mop, carpet sweeper, or upright vacuum cleaner should present no problem. A self-wringing mop may be used if the mop handle is stabilized under the arm and the wringing lever operated with the normal arm. Clients with balance and ambulation problems may manage some floor care from a sitting position. Dust mopping or using a carpet sweeper may be possible if gait and balance are fairly good without the aid of a cane.

These are just a few of the possibilities to solve home management problems for one-handed individuals. The occupational therapist must evaluate each client to determine how the dysfunction affects performance of homemaking activities. One-handed techniques take more time and may be difficult for some clients to master. Activities should be paced to accommodate the client's physical endurance and tolerance for one-handed

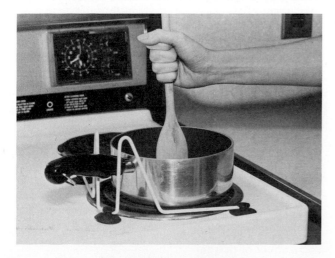

Fig. 4-32. Pan stabilizer.

performance and use of special devices. Work simplification and energy conservation techniques should be employed.

New techniques and devices should be introduced on a graded basis as the client masters one technique and device and then another. Family members need to be oriented to the client's skills, special methods used, and work schedule. The therapist with the family and client may facilitate the planning of homemaking responsibilities to be shared by other family members and the supervision of the client, if that is needed.

If special equipment and assistive devices are needed for ADL, it is advisable to acquire these through the health agency, if possible. The therapist can then train the client in their use and demonstrate to a family member before sending these items home.

ADL for wheelchair-bound individuals with good to normal arm function (paraplegia)

Clients who are confined to a wheelchair need to find ways to perform ADL from a seated position, transport objects, and adapt in an environment designed for standing and walking. Given normal upper extremity function, the wheelchair ambulator can probably perform independently.

Dressing activities.* It is recommended that wheelchair-bound clients put on clothing in this order: stockings, undergarments, braces (if worn), trousers or slacks, shoes, shirt, or dress.

TROUSERS
Donning

Trousers and slacks are easier to fasten if they button or zip in front. If braces are worn, zippers in side seams may be helpful. Wide bottom slacks of stretch fabric are recommended. Procedure for putting on trousers, shorts, slacks, and underwear is as follows:

1. Use side rails or trapeze to help pull self up to sitting position.
2. Sit on bed and reach forward to feet or sit on bed and pull knees into flexed position.
3. Holding top of trousers flip pants down to feet.
4. Work pant legs over feet and pull up to hips. Crossing ankles may help get pants on over heels.
5. In semireclining position roll from hip to hip and pull up garment.
6. Reaching tongs may be helpful to pull garment up or position garment on feet.

Removing

Remove pants or underwear by reversing procedure for donning. Dressing sticks may be helpful to push pants off feet.

*Summarized from Activities of daily living for patients with incoordination, limited range of motion, paraplegia, quadriplegia, and hemiplegia, Cleveland, 1968, Highland View Hospital, Cuyahoga County Hospitals, Division of Occupational Therapy. Mimeographed, unpublished.

SOCKS OR STOCKINGS
Donning

1. Apply socks or stockings while seated on bed.
2. Pull one leg into flexion with one hand.
3. Use other hand to slip sock or stocking over foot and pull it on.

NOTE: Soft stretch socks or stockings are recommended. Panty hose that are slightly large may be useful. Elastic garters or stockings with elastic tops should be avoided. Dressing sticks or a stocking device may be helpful to some clients.

Removing

Remove socks or stockings by flexing leg as described for donning, pushing sock or stocking down over heel. Dressing sticks may be needed to push sock or stocking off heel and toe and to retrieve it.

SLIPS AND SKIRTS
Donning

1. To apply slips and skirts sit on bed, slip garment over head, and let it drop to waist.
2. In semireclining position, roll from hip to hip and pull garment down over hips and thighs.

NOTE: Slips and skirts slightly larger than usually worn are recommended. A-line, wraparound, and full skirts are easier to manage and look better on persons seated in wheelchair than narrow skirts.

Removing

1. In sitting or semireclining position unfasten garment.
2. Roll from hip to hip, pulling garment up to waist level.
3. Pull garment off over head.

SHIRTS
Donning

Shirts, pajama jackets, robes, and dresses opening completely down front may be put on while client is seated in wheelchair. If it is necessary to dress while in bed, following procedure can be used:

1. Balance body by putting palms of hands on mattress on either side of body. If balance is poor, assistance may be needed or bed backrest may be elevated. (If backrest cannot be elevated, one or two pillows may be used to support back.) With backrest elevated both hands are available.
2. If difficulty is encountered in usual methods of applying garment, open garment on lap with collar toward chest. Put arms into sleeves and pull up over elbows. Then hold on to shirttail or back of dress, pull garment over head, adjust and button.

NOTE: Fabrics should be wrinkle-resistant, smooth, and durable. Roomy sleeves and backs and full skirts are more suitable styles than closely fitted garments.

Removing

1. Sitting in wheelchair or bed, open fastening.
2. Remove garment in usual manner.
3. If this is not feasible, grasp collar with one hand while balancing with other hand. Gather material up from collar to hem.
4. Lean forward, duck head, and pull shirt over head.
5. Remove sleeve from supporting arm and then from working arm.

SHOES
Donning

Shoes may be applied by one of the following variations.

Variation I

1. In sitting position on bed pull one knee at a time into flexed position with hands.
2. While supporting leg in flexed position with one hand, use free hand to put on shoe.

Variation II

1. Sit on edge of bed or in wheelchair for back support.
2. Bend one knee up to flexed position, supporting leg with arm, and with free hand slip shoe on.

Variation III

1. Sit on edge of bed or in wheelchair for back support.
2. Cross one leg over other and slip shoe on.
3. Put foot on footrest and push down on knee to push foot into shoe.

Removing

1. Flex or cross leg as described for appropriate variation.
2. For variations I and II remove shoe with one hand while supporting flexed leg with other hand.
3. For variation III remove shoe from crossed leg with one hand while maintaining balance with other hand, if necessary.

Feeding activities. Eating activities should present no special problem for the wheelchair-bound individual with good to normal arm function. Wheelchairs with desk arms and swing-away footrest are recommended so that it is possible to sit close to the table.

Hygiene and grooming. Face and oral hygiene and arm and upper body care should present no problem. Reachers may be helpful to secure towels, washcloths, makeup, deodorant, and shaving supplies from storage areas, if necessary. Tub baths or showers require some special equipment. Transfer techniques for toilet and bathtub will be discussed in Chapter 5. The following are suggestions for facilitating bathing activities:

1. Use a hand-held shower head and keep a finger over the spray to determine sudden temperature changes in water.
2. Use long-handled bath brushes with soap insert for ease in reaching all parts of the body.
3. Use soap bars attached to a cord around the neck.
4. For sponge bath in wheelchair cover the chair with a sheet of plastic.

5. Use shower chairs or bathtub seats.
6. Increase safety during transfers by installing grab bars on wall near bathtub or shower and on bathtub.
7. Fit bathtub or shower bottom with nonskid mat or adhesive material.

Communication and environmental hardware. With the exception of reaching difficulties in some situations, use of the telephone should present no problem. Short-handled reachers may be used to grasp the receiver from the cradle. Dialing could be accomplished with a short, rubber-tipped, ¼-inch dowel stick. Use of writing implements, typewriter, and tape recorder should be easily possible for these clients.

Managing doors may present some difficulties. If the door opens toward the person, opening it can be managed by the following procedure:

1. If doorknob is on right, approach door from right, and turn doorknob with left hand.
2. Open door as far as possible and move wheelchair close enough so it helps keep door open.
3. Holding door open with left hand turn wheelchair with right hand and wheel through door.
4. Start closing door when halfway through.

If the door is very heavy and opens out or away from the person, the following procedure is recommended:

1. Back up to door so knob can be turned with right hand.
2. Open door and back through so big wheels keep it open.
3. Also use left elbow to keep door open.
4. Wheel backward with right hand.[2]

Mobility and transfers. Specific transfer techniques will be discussed in Chapter 5.

Home management activities.[5] When performing homemaking activities from a wheelchair, the major problems are work heights, adequate space for maneuverability, access to storage areas, and transfer of supplies, equipment, and materials from place to place. If funds are available for kitchen remodeling, reducing counters and range to a comfortable height for wheelchair use is recommended. However, such extensive adaptation is often not feasible. Suggestions for home management are as follows:

1. Remove cabinet doors to eliminate the need to maneuver around them for opening and closing. Frequently used items should be stored toward the front of easy-to-reach cabinets above and below the counter surfaces.
2. If entrance and inside doors are not wide enough, use a wheelchair narrower or make doors slightly wider by removing strips along the door jambs.
3. A wheelchair cushion can increase the user's height so that standard counters may be used.

4. Use detachable desk arms and swing-away detachable footrests to allow the wheelchair user to get as close as possible to counters and tables and also to stand at counters, if that is possible (Fig. 4-33).
5. Transport items safely and easily by using a wheelchair lapboard. The lapboard may also serve as a work surface for preparing food and drying dishes. It also protects the lap from injury from hot pans and prevents utensils falling into the lap (Fig. 4-34).
6. Fasten a drop leaf–type board to a bare wall or slide-out board under a counter to give the wheelchair homemaker one work surface that is a comfortable height in a kitchen that is otherwise standard.
7. Fit cabinets with custom- or ready-made lazy Susan devices to eliminate need to reach to rear space (Fig. 4-35.)
8. Ranges should ideally be at a lower level. If this is not possible, place the controls at the front of the range, and hang a mirror angled at the proper degree over the range so that the homemaker can see contents of pots.

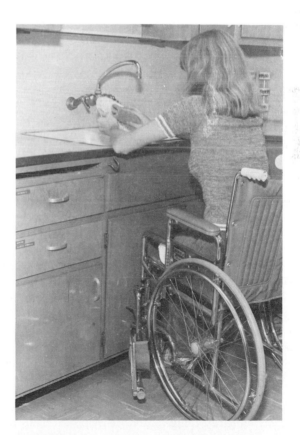

Fig. 4-33. Wheelchair footrests are swung away to allow closer access to sink.

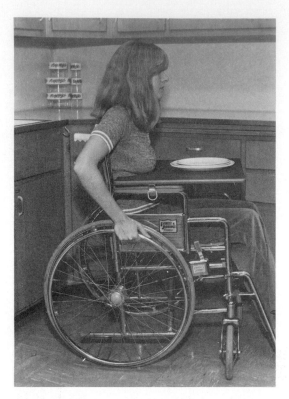

Fig. 4-34. Wheelchair lapboard is used to transport items.

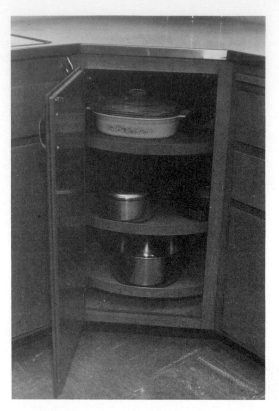

Fig. 4-35. Lazy Susan–type kitchen storage cabinet.

9. Substitute small electric cooking units for the range if it is not safely manageable.
10. Use front-loading washers and dryers.
11. Vacuum carpets with a carpet sweeper or tank-type cleaner that rolls easily and is lightweight or self-propelled. A retractable cord may be helpful to prevent tangling of cord in wheels.

ADL for the wheelchair-bound individual with upper extremity weakness (quadriplegia)

In general, persons with muscle function from spinal cord levels C7 and C8 can follow the methods just described for paraplegia. Individuals with muscle function from C6 can be relatively independent with adaptations and assistive devices, whereas those with muscle function from C4 and C5 will require a considerable amount of special equipment and assistance. Clients with muscle function from C6 may benefit from the use of a wrist-driven flexor hinge splint. Externally powered splints and arm braces or mobile arm supports are recommended for C3, C4, and C5 levels of muscle function.[1]

Dressing activities. The reader is referred to *Self Dressing Techniques for Patients with Spinal Cord Injury* by Margaret Runge[10] for description of specific dressing methods. Assistive devices that can facilitate dressing, depending on the level of muscle function, are dressing sticks, sock aids, trouser pull, ring zipper pull, and buttonhook.

Feeding activities.[1] Eating may be assisted by a variety of devices, again depending on the level of muscle function. Levels C5 and above require mobile arm supports or externally powered splints and braces. A wrist splint and universal cuff may be used together if a flexor hinge splint is not used. The universal cuff holds the eating utensil, and the splint stabilizes the wrist. A nonskid mat and a plate with plate guard may provide adequate stability of the plate for pushing and picking up food (Fig. 4-36).

A regular or swivel spoon-fork combination can be used when there is minimal muscle function (C4 to C5). A long plastic straw with a straw clip to stabilize it in the cup or glass eliminates the need for picking up these drinking vessels. A bilateral or unilateral clip-type holder on a glass or cup makes it possible for many individuals with hand and arm weakness to manage liquids without a straw.

Built-up utensils may be useful for those with some functional grasp or tenodesis grasp. Cutting food may be managed with a quad quip knife if arm strength is adequate to manage the device.

Hygiene and grooming.[1] General suggestions to facilitate hygiene and grooming are as follows:

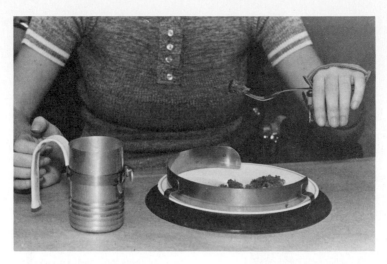

Fig. 4-36. Feeding with aid of universal cuff, plate guard, nonskid mat, and clip-type cup holder to compensate for absent grasp.

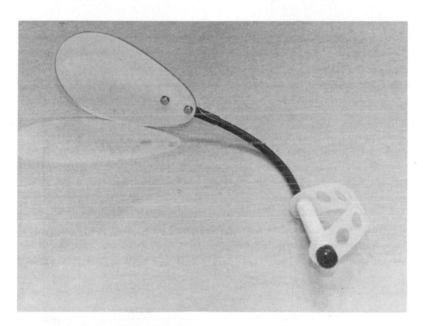

Fig. 4-37. Skin inspection mirror.

1. Use a shower or bathtub seat and transfer board for transfers.
2. Extend reach by using long-handled bath sponges with loop handle or built-up handle.
3. Eliminate need to grasp washcloth by using bath mitts.
4. Hold comb and toothbrush with a universal cuff.
5. Use a clip-type holder for electric razor.
6. Suppository inserters for quadriplegics who can manage bowel care independently with this aid can be used.
7. Use skin inspection mirror with long stem and looped handle for independent skin inspection (Fig. 4-37).

Devices selected and methods must be adapted to the degree of weakness for each individual client.

Communication and environmental hardware. The following are suggestions for facilitating communication:

1. Turn pages with an electric page turner, mouth stick, or head wand if hand and arm function are inadequate.
2. Insert pen, pencil, typing stick, or paintbrush in a universal cuff that has been positioned with the opening on the ulnar side of the palm (Fig. 4-38) for typing, writing, operating a tape recorder, and painting.
3. Dial the telephone with the universal cuff and a

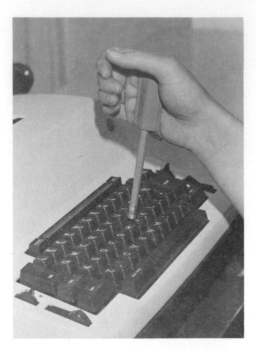

Fig. 4-38. Typing with aid of universal cuff and typing stick.

pencil positioned with eraser down or with mouth stick or head wand if hand and arm function are absent. The receiver may need to be stationed in a telephone arm and positioned for listening. Special adaptations are available to substitute the need to replace the receiver in the cradle.

4. Use electric typewriters, which are easier to use than standard ones.
5. Built-up pencils and pens or special pencil holders are needed for clients with hand weakness.
6. Sophisticated electronic communications devices operated by mouth, suck and blow, and head control are available for clients with no upper extremity function.[11]

Mobility and transfers. Wheelchair transfer techniques for the individual with quadriplegia will be described in Chapter 5. Mobility will depend on degree of weakness. Electric wheelchairs operated by hand or mouth controls have greatly increased the mobility of persons with severe upper and lower extremity weakness. Vans fitted with wheelchair lifts and stabilizing devices have made it possible for such clients to be transported thus to pursue community, vocational, educational, and avocational activities with an assistant.

Adaptations for hand controls have made it possible for many clients with function of at least C6 level to drive independently.

Home management activities. Many individuals with upper extremity weakness who are bound to wheelchair ambulation will be dependent or partially depen-

dent for homemaking activities. Clients with muscle function of C6 or better may be independent for light homemaking, with appropriate devices, adaptations, and safety awareness. Many of the suggestions for wheelchair maneuverability and environmental adaptation outlined for the paraplegic apply here as well. In addition, the client with upper extremity weakness will need to use lightweight equipment and special devices. The *Mealtime Manual for People With Disability and the Aging* compiled by Judith Lannefeld Klinger[5] is an excellent resource for many specific suggestions that apply to the homemaker with weak upper extremities.

REVIEW QUESTIONS
Treatment methods: activities of daily living

1. Define "activities of daily living" (ADL) and list four classifications of tasks that may be considered in ADL.
2. What is the role of occupational therapy in restoring ADL independence?
3. List at least three activities that would be considered self-care skills, three mobility skills, three communication skills, and three home management skills.
4. List three factors that the occupational therapist must consider before commencing ADL performance evaluation and training. Describe how each could limit or effect ADL performance.
5. What is the ultimate goal of the ADL training program?
6. Discuss the concept of maximum independence, as defined in the text.
7. List the general steps in the procedure for ADL evaluation.
8. Describe how the occupational therapist can use the ADL checklist.
9. How does the occupational therapist, with the client, select ADL training objectives after the ADL evaluation?
10. Describe three approaches to teaching ADL skills to a client with perception or memory deficits.
11. List the important factors to include in an ADL progress report.
12. Define three general levels of independence, as defined in the text.
13. Demonstrate the use of at least three assistive devices mentioned in the text.
14. Teach another individual how to don a shirt, using one hand.
15. Teach another individual how to don and remove trousers, as if hemiplegic.
16. Teach another individual how to don and remove trousers, as if the legs were paralyzed.

SECTION FOUR
Sensorimotor approaches to treatment

The normal central nervous system (CNS) functions to produce controlled, well-modulated movement as a result of a balance between the inhibition and facilitation of motor responses. For example, in the normal deep tendon reflex (DTR), the stretch of the muscle excites its muscle spindles, which results in contraction of the muscle stretched. However, the degree of contraction is modulated by the inhibitory influences of the Golgi tendon organs (GTO), resulting in a controlled reflex response. The muscle spindle and GTO receive and mediate responses to proprioceptive stimuli. They act as regulating mechanisms for contraction of extrafusal (voluntary) muscle fibers. They are part of the gamma motor system, which can be thought of as a mini motor system within the major motor system (voluntary muscles). It responds to proprioceptive impulses from stretching and shortening of muscles and regulates voluntary motor activity.[16] The reader is referred to literature in neurophysiology for in-depth study of the gamma system.

In the damaged CNS the inhibition and facilitation of motor responses are out of balance and are not working together to produce smooth, well-modulated, controlled movement. The result can be too much facilitation, producing hypertonic, hyperkinetic, or rigid states of muscle, or too much inhibition, causing hypotonic or hypokinetic states of muscle.

In sensorimotor approaches to treatment it is assumed that specific, controlled sensory input can influence motor responses and that abnormal motor responses can be inhibited and more normal motor responses can be learned by the CNS. All sensorimotor approaches to treatment use proprioceptive stimuli, such as stretching and resistance, to influence thresholds for inhibition and facilitation of movement.[16] Cutaneous stimulation, which has been found to increase stretch receptor sensitivity, may be combined with proprioceptive stimulation to facilitate voluntary contraction of specific muscles.[9] Exteroceptive stimuli, such as brushing to recruit touch receptors and icing to facilitate or inhibit muscle responses, are used. Reflex mechanisms may be used in some approaches. Some of these are the tonic neck and lumbar reflexes, righting and protective reactions, and associated reactions. The sequence in treatment may be based on the recapitulation of ontogenetic development, that is, the development of successive levels of CNS control—spinal, subcortical, then cortical control of movement.[14]

MOVEMENT THERAPY: THE BRUNNSTROM APPROACH TO THE TREATMENT OF HEMIPLEGIA

The material presented here is summarized primarily from *Movement Therapy in Hemiplegia*[4] by Signe Brunnstrom, a physical therapist who developed this treatment approach from her research and extensive work with hemiplegic patients.

The theoretical foundations, treatment goals, and methods are intended as an overview and introduction to some of the procedures that the new practitioner may find helpful. To learn the details of the treatment

approach and additional procedures the reader is referred to the original source for further study.

Theoretical foundations

Following CVA, head injury, or disease producing hemiplegia, the patient progresses through a series of recovery steps or stages in fairly stereotyped fashion (Table 3). The progress through these stages may be rapid or slow, and recovery may be arrested at any stage.

In effect, an "evolution in reverse"[4,12] occurs after neurological disease. Afferent-efferent mechanisms developed in early phylogenesis are retained in man but are inhibited in the developmental process. The basic limb synergies seen in hemiplegic patients are primitive spinal cord patterns[3] of flexion and extension, reminiscent of amphibian patterns of movement, which have been retained through the evolutionary process.[4]

The flexor synergy of the upper limb consists of scapular adduction and elevation, shoulder abduction and external rotation, elbow flexion, forearm supination, wrist flexion, and finger flexion. Elbow flexion is the strongest component, and shoulder abduction and external rotation are the weakest (Fig. 4-39). The extensor synergy consists of scapula abduction and depression, shoulder adduction and internal rotation, elbow extension, forearm pronation, and wrist and finger flexion or extension. Shoulder adduction and internal rotation are the strongest components of the extensor synergy, and elbow extension is the weakest component (Fig. 4-40).

In the lower limb the flexor synergy consists of hip flexion and abduction and external rotation, knee flexion, ankle dorsiflexion and inversion, and toe extension. Hip flexion is the strongest component, and hip abduction and external rotation are the weakest components. The extensor synergy is composed of hip adduction, extension, and internal rotation; knee extension; ankle plantar flexion and inversion; and toe flexion. Hip adduction, knee extension, and ankle plantar flexion are the strong components whereas hip extension and internal rotation are weaker. These patterns are modified in man through the influence of higher centers of nervous system control during development. After CVA, they return to their primitive, stereotyped character. When the influence of higher centers is disturbed or destroyed, primitive and pathological reflexes, such as the tonic neck reflex (TNR), tonic lumbar reflex, and TLR, reappear, and normal reflexes such as the DTR become exaggerated. These reflexes were present at an earlier phylogenetic period and therefore may be considered "normal" when, as in hemiplegia, the CNS has regressed to an earlier developmental stage.[4]

The Brunnstrom approach to the treatment of hemiplegia is based on the use of motor patterns available

Table 3. Motor recovery following cerebral vascular accident[4,16]

Stage	Characteristics		
	Leg	Arm	Hand*
1	Flaccidity	Flaccidity, inability to perform any movements	No hand function
2	Spasticity develops, minimal voluntary movements	Beginning development of spasticity; limb synergies or some of their components begin to appear as associated reactions	Gross grasp is beginning, minimal finger flexion possible
3	Spasticity peaks; flexion and extension synergy present; hip-knee-ankle flexion in sitting and standing	Spasticity increasing; synergy patterns or some of their components can be performed voluntarily	Gross grasp, hook grasp possible; no release
4	Knee flexion past 90° in sitting, with foot sliding backward on floor, dorsiflexion with heel on floor and knee flexed to 90°	Spasticity declining; movement combinations deviating from synergies are now possible	Gross grasp is present; lateral prehension is developing; small amount of finger extension and some thumb movement possible
5	Knee flexion with hip extended in standing; ankle dorsiflexion with hip and knee extended	Synergies are no longer dominant and more movement combinations deviating from synergies can be performed with greater ease	Palmar prehension, spherical and cylindrical grasp, and release are possible
6	Hip abduction in sitting or standing; reciprocal internal and external rotation of hip combined with inversion and eversion of ankle in sitting	Spasticity is gone except when performing rapid movements; isolated joint movements can be performed with ease	All types of prehension, individual finger motion, and full range of voluntary extension possible

*NOTE: Recovery of hand function is variable and may not parallel the six recovery stages of the arm.

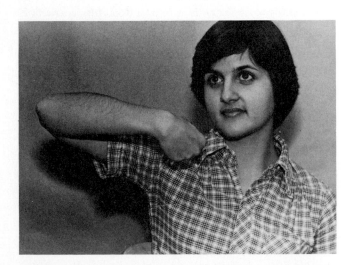

Fig. 4-39. Flexor synergy of upper limb in hemiplegia.

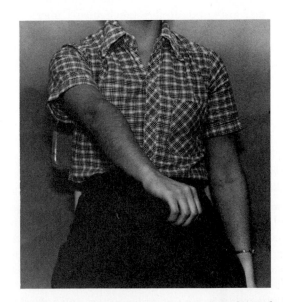

Fig. 4-40. Extensor synergy of upper limb in hemiplegia.

to the patient at any point in the recovery process. It enhances progress through the stages of recovery toward more normal and complex movement patterns. Brunnstrom sees synergies, reflexes, and other "abnormal" movement patterns as a "normal" part of the process the patient must go through before normal voluntary movement can occur. Synergistic movements are used by normal persons all of the time, but they are controlled, occur in a wide variety of patterns, and can be modified or stopped at will. Brunnstrom maintains that the synergies appear to constitute a necessary intermediate stage for further recovery. Gross movement synergies of flexion and extension always precede the restoration of advanced motor functioning following hemiplegia in man.[4] Therefore during the early stages of recovery (stages 1 to 3) Brunnstrom maintains that the patient should be aided to gain control of the limb synergies and that selected afferent stimuli (TNR, TLR, cutaneous and stretch stimuli, positioning and associated reactions) can be advantageous in helping the patient to initiate and gain control of movement. Once the synergies can be performed voluntarily with some ease, they are modified, and simple to complex movement combinations can be performed (stages 4 and 5) that deviate from the stereotyped synergy patterns of flexion and extension.[4]

The advisability of using pathological and primitive reflexes and movement patterns to effect motion is challenged by some experts.[2] It is argued that no pathological responses should be used in training for fear that by repeated use the efferent pathways will become too readily available for use at the expense of normal pathways.[3,4]

Definitions of terms

Some definitions of terms are necessary to comprehend the discussion of treatment principles that follows.

A *limb synergy* of flexion or extension, seen in hemiplegia, is a group of muscles acting as a bound unit in a primitive and stereotyped manner.[4,13] The muscles are neurophysiologically linked and cannot act alone or perform all of their functions. If one muscle in the synergy is activated, each muscle in the synergy responds partially or completely. The patient then cannot perform isolated movements when bound by these synergies.

Associated reactions are movements seen on the affected side in response to voluntary forceful movements in other parts of the body.[4] Resistance to flexion movements of the normal upper extremity usually evokes a flexion synergy or some of its components in the affected upper extremity. By the same token resistance to extension on the sound side evokes extension on the affected side. In the lower extremities the responses are reversed. Resisted flexion of the normal limb evokes extension of the affected limb and vice versa.[13]

Homolateral limb synkinesis appears to be a mutual dependency between the synergies of the affected upper and lower limbs. The same or similar motion occurs in the limb on the same side of the body. For example, efforts at flexion of the affected upper extremity evoke flexion of the lower extremity.[4,13]

The mirroring of movements attempted or performed on the affected side by the unaffected side, perhaps in an effort to facilitate the movement, is called *imitation synkinesis.*[4]

Several specialized reactions can be noted in the hemiplegic hand. These are the proximal traction response, grasp reflex, instinctive grasp reaction, instinctive avoiding reaction, and Souques' finger phenomenon. The *proximal traction response* is elicited by a stretch to the flexor muscles of one joint of the upper limb, which evokes contraction of all flexors of that limb, including the fingers. It may therefore be used to elicit the flexion synergy. To elicit the *grasp reflex* deep pressure is applied to the palm and moved distally over the hand and fingers, mostly on the radial side. The responses are complex but in general there is adduction and flexion of the digits. The *instinctive grasp reaction* is differentiated by Brunnstrom from the grasp reflex. It is a closure of the hand in response to contact of a stationary object with the palm of the hand. The person is unable to release the object-stimulus once the fist has been closed.

A hyperextension reaction of the fingers and thumb in response to forward-upward elevation of the arm is the *instinctive avoiding reaction.* Brunnstrom reported that with the arm in this position, stroking distally over the palm and attempting to reach out and grasp an object resulted in an exaggeration of the reaction. The automatic extension of the fingers when the shoulder is flexed is known as *Souques' finger phenomenon* and can be observed in some but not all hemiplegic patients. Brunnstrom found that although this phenomenon may not be exhibited, the elevated position of the affected arm is a favorable one for the facilitation of finger extension.[4]

General principles of facilitating motor function

The goal of Brunnstrom's movement therapy is to facilitate the patient's progress through the recovery stages that occur after onset of hemiplegia (Table 3). The use of the available afferent-efferent mechanisms of control is the means for attainment of this goal. Some of these mechanisms are summarized here.

Postural and attitudinal reflexes are used as means to increase or decrease tone in specific muscles.[13] For instance, changes in head and body position can influence muscle tone by evoking the tonic reflexes, such as the TNR, tonic lumbar reflex, TLR, and equilibrium and protective reactions. Associated reactions may be used to initiate or elicit synergies in the early stages of recovery by giving resistance to the contralateral muscle group on the normal side. Efforts at flexion synergy of the affected leg may be used to elicit a flexion synergy of the arm through homolateral limb synkinesis.

Stimulation of the skin over a muscle produces contraction of that muscle and facilitation of the synergy to which the muscle belongs. An example is briskly stimulating the triceps muscle during other efforts at performance of the extension synergy, which enhances elbow extension and amplifies the synergy pattern. Muscle contraction is facilitated when muscles are placed in their lengthened position, and the quick stretch of a muscle facilitates its contraction and inhibits its antagonist. Resistance facilitates the contraction of muscles resisted. Synergistic movement may be augmented by the voluntary effort of the patient. Visual stimulation through the use of mirrors, videotape of self, and movement of parts can facilitate motion in some patients as can auditory stimuli in the forms of loud and repetitive commands to perform the desired movement.

The strongest component of one synergy will inhibit its antagonist through reciprocal innervation. It follows that if relaxation of the stronger or spastic muscle can be effected, it may be possible to evoke some activity in the weaker antagonist, which may appear to be functionless because of its inability to overcome the very spastic agonist.[3,13]

General treatment goals and methods for the hemiplegic upper extremity

Prior to the initiation of any intervention strategies the occupational and physical therapists must make a thorough evaluation of the motor, sensory, perceptual, and cognitive functions of the adult hemiplegic. Brunnstrom's Hemiplegia Classification and Progress Record and evaluations of sensation and perception can be found in Chapter 2 of this text. The motor evaluation (Chapter 2) designed by Brunnstrom yields information about stage of recovery, muscle tone, passive motion sense, hand function, sitting and standing balance, leg function, and ambulation. The treatment goals and methods summarized are directed primarily to the rehabilitation of the hemiplegic upper extremity. The point at which the therapist initiates treatment depends on the stage of recovery and muscle tone of the individual client.

One of the early goals in treatment is for the client to achieve good trunk or sitting balance. Most hemiplegic persons demonstrate "listing" to the affected side, which may result in a fall if the appropriate equilibrium responses do not occur. To evoke balance responses the therapist deliberately disturbs the client's erect sitting posture in forward-backward and side-to-

side direction. This may be done while the client sits on a chair, edge of a bed, or mat table. The client is prepared for the procedure with an explanation and is pushed, at first, gently, then more vigorously. The client may support the affected arm by cradling it to protect the shoulder. This prevents him from grasping the supporting surface during the procedure. Later the therapist initiates and assists the client with bending the trunk forward and obliquely forward. The client sits and supports the affected arm as previously described. The therapist holds her hands under the client's elbows. She may use her knees to stabilize the client's knees if balance is poor. In this position the therapist guides the client while inclining the trunk forward and obliquely and attains some passive glenohumeral and scapular motion at the same time.

Trunk rotation is encouraged in a similar manner, with the therapist sitting in front of the client or standing behind and supporting the client's arms as before. Trunk rotation is first performed through a limited range and is gently guided by the therapist. The range is gradually increased. Some neck mobilization may be attained almost automatically during these maneuvers. As the trunk rotates, the client cradles the affected arm and swings the arms rhythmically from side to side to get shoulder abduction and adduction alternately as the trunk rotates. The shoulder components of the flexor and extensor synergies might be evoked during these procedures through the TNR and tonic lumbar reflexes.[4]

A second important early goal in treatment is to maintain or achieve pain-free ROM at the glenohumeral joint. There appears to be a relationship between the shoulder pain, so common in adult hemiplegics, and the stretching of spastic muscles around the shoulder joint. Traditional forced passive exercise procedures may actually produce this stretching and contribute to the development of pain. Such exercise is harmful and contraindicated. Once the client has experienced the pain, his anticipation of it increases the muscular tension that in turn decreases the joint mobility and increases the pain experienced on passive motion. Therefore the shoulder joint should be mobilized without forceful stretching of hypertonic musculature about the shoulder and shoulder girdle.

This is accomplished through guided trunk motion. The client sits erect, cradling the affected arm. The therapist supports the arms under the elbows while the client leans forward. The more the client leans the greater range of shoulder flexion can be obtained. The therapist guides the arms gently and passively into shoulder flexion while the client's attention is focused on the trunk motion. In a similar fashion the therapist can guide the arms into abduction and adduction while the client rotates the trunk from side to side. The TNR and tonic lumbar reflex facilitate relaxation of muscles during this maneuver. When the client is confident that the shoulder can be moved painlessly, active-assisted movements of the arm in relation to the trunk can begin.

First, the client moves both shoulders into elevation and depression and scapula adduction and abduction. These are then combined with glenohumeral movements. The arm is supported by the therapist from behind, with the shoulder between forward flexion and abduction, the elbow flexed less than 90°, and the wrist supported in slight extension. The therapist may ask the client to elevate the shoulders while tapping the upper trapezius. At the same time the therapist is assisting the client to elevate the arm as well. Active shoulder elevation will tend to elicit other components of the flexor synergy that in turn will tend to inhibit the strong adduction component of the extensor synergy (pectoralis major), allowing the therapist to elevate the arm into abduction by small degrees each time the client repeats the active shoulder girdle elevation. The procedure is repeated, and the therapist gives the appropriate verbal commands "pull up, let go." The abduction movement is at an oblique angle between forward flexion and full abduction. Sideward abduction with the arm in the same plane as the trunk is likely to be painful and should be avoided. Alternate pronation and supination of the forearm by the therapist should accompany the elevation and lowering of the arm throughout the procedure. The forearm should be supinated when the shoulder is elevated and pronated when the arm is lowered. Head rotation to the normal side inhibits activity in the pectoralis major muscle through the TNR. When abduction movement above the horizontal has been accomplished without pain, the client can be directed to reach overhead and straighten out the elbow if there has been sufficient recovery to do so. The client is directed to rotate the head to the affected side to facilitate the elbow extension while observing the movement of the arm.

The training procedures for improving arm function are geared to the client's recovery stage. During stages 1 and 2 when the arm is essentially flaccid or some components of the synergy patterns are beginning to appear, the aim is to elicit muscle tone and the synergy patterns on a reflex basis. This is accomplished through a variety of facilitation procedures. Associated reactions and tonic reflexes may be employed to influence tone and evoke reflexive movement. The proximal traction response may be used to activate the flexor synergy. Tapping over the upper and middle trapezius, rhomboids, and biceps may elicit components of the flexor synergy. Tapping over the triceps and stretching of the serratus anterior may activate components of the extensor synergy. Passive movement alternately through each

of the synergy patterns is not only an excellent means for maintaining ROM of several joints but provides the client with proprioceptive and visual feedback for the desired patterns of early movement. Quick stretch to muscles and surface stroking of the skin over them are also used to activate muscles. These methods are not employed in any set order or routine but are selected to suit the particular responses of each individual client. Since the flexor synergy usually appears first, it may be useful to begin trying to elicit the flexor patterns. This should be followed immediately with facilitation of the extensor synergy components, since these tend to be weaker and more difficult to perform in later stages of recovery.[4,12]

When the client has recovered to stages 2 and 3, the synergies or their components are present and may be performed voluntarily. Spasticity is developing and reaches its peak in stage 3. During this period the aim is for the client to achieve voluntary control of the synergy patterns. This is accomplished by repetitious alternating performance of the synergy patterns, first with the assistance and facilitation of the therapist. Facilitation is provided through resistance to voluntary motion, verbal commands, tapping, and cutaneous stimulation. This is followed by voluntary repetition of the synergy patterns without the facilitation and, finally, concentration on the components of the synergies from proximal to distal with, then without, facilitation. Bilateral rowing movements with the therapist holding the client's hands are a useful activity for reciprocal motion of the synergies that should be started during this time.[4,12]

During stages 3 and 4 when the client has voluntary control of the synergies and may begin to be able to use movement combinations that deviate from the synergies, the occupational therapist should help the client to use the newly learned movements for functional and purposeful activities. Some of the activities that can be adapted to use the synergy patterns or gross combined movement patterns are skateboard or powder board exercises (Fig. 4-41), sanding, leather lacing, braid weaving, finger painting, sponging off tabletops, and using a push broom or carpet sweeper. Activities that demand too much cortical control and conscious effort on the part of the client will tend to increase fatigue and muscle tension and should be avoided.

The treatment aim during stages 4 and 5 is to break away from the synergies by mixing components from antagonistic synergies to perform new and increasingly complex patterns of movement. One means for accomplishing this goal is using skateboard or powder board exercises in arcs of movement to get elbow flexion, combined with shoulder horizontal adduction and forearm pronation, and alternating with shoulder horizontal abduction and elbow extension with forearm supina-

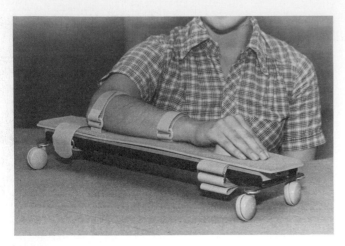

Fig. 4-41. Skateboard exercises for synergy or combined movement patterns in gravity-eliminated plane.

tion. These same movement patterns may be used to perform the therapeutic activities just mentioned. Later the client may be able to perform the more complex figure eight pattern on the skateboard or powder board. At this time the occupational therapist should stress the use of any voluntary movement of the affected limb in performance of ADL. Using the arm for dressing and hygiene skills will translate the movements to purposeful use. It should be borne in mind that the degree to which purposeful, spontaneous use of the arm is possible depends on the sensory status of the limb and not only on the motor recovery achieved.

In the final recovery stages 5 and 6 increasingly complex movement combinations and isolated motions are possible. The aims in treatment are to achieve ease in performance of movement combinations and isolated motion and to increase speed of movement. The activities mentioned earlier can be performed now in their usual manner and can be graded to demand finer and more complex movement patterns. Loom weaving, block printing, gardening, furniture refinishing, leather tooling, rolling out dough, sweeping, dusting, and washing dishes are a few of the activities that may enlist the use of the affected arm purposefully if hand recovery is adequate.

It should be noted that the hemiplegic upper extremity seldom makes a full recovery. If voluntary, spontaneous movement is possible, the client should be trained to use the limb as an assist to the sound arm to the extent possible in bilateral activities.

Methods for retraining hand function are treated separately, since recovery of hand function does not always coincide with arm recovery. Hand retraining commensurate with the recovery status of the client

should be carried out continuously through the treatment program.

The first goal of hand retraining is to achieve mass grasp. The proximal traction response and grasp reflex may be used to elicit early grasp movement on a reflex level. During the proximal traction response maneuver the therapist should maintain the client's wrist in extension and give the command "squeeze."

Because the normal association between wrist extension and grasp is disturbed, another important aim is to achieve wrist fixation for grasp. Wrist extension often accompanies the extensor synergy. Wrist extension can be evoked if the therapist applies resistance to the proximal palm or fist while supporting the arm in the position described earlier for elevation of the arm into abduction. Percussion of the wrist extensors with the elbow in extension and arm elevated and supported by the therapist can activate wrist extension. The proximal portion of the extensors are tapped, and the therapist directs the client to "squeeze" simultaneously. The commands to "squeeze" and "stop squeezing" are given at appropriate points in the facilitation procedures. During the wrist extension and fist closure the therapist carries the elbow forward into extension. During the wrist and finger relaxation the therapist carries the elbow back into flexion. While the client is maintaining fist closure, the therapist may withdraw the wrist support and give the command "hold." The therapist may continue tapping the wrist extensors while the client attempts to hold the posture. The goal is to synchronise the muscles for fist closure with wrist extension.

This procedure should be alternated with a command to "stop squeezing" and the wrist should be allowed to drop and fingers open while the elbow is moved into flexion. These steps are alternated and the wrist extension-fist closure is gradually performed with increasing amounts of elbow flexion so that the client can learn to grasp with wrist stabilization when the arm is in a variety of positions.

A third objective in hand retraining is to achieve active release of grasp. This is difficult, since there is usually a considerable degree of spasticity in the flexor muscles of the hand. A release of tension in the finger flexors, then, is primary to the achievement of any active finger extension. Active grasp should be alternated with manipulations to release tension in the flexors. The therapist sits facing the client and pulls the thumb out of the palm by gripping the thenar eminence. The forearm is supinated. The wrist is allowed to remain in slight flexion. The therapist maintains the grasp around the thumb and alternately pronates and supinates the forearm with emphasis on supination. Pressure on the thumb is decreased during pronation and increased during supination. Cutaneous stimulation is given to the dorsum of the hand and wrist when the forearm is supinated. This manipulation is likely to develop some tension in the finger extensors, and the fingers extend. The client may actually participate in opening the hand when the forearm is supinated. However, strong efforts on the part of the client may evoke flexion instead and should be avoided.

If this manipulation is inadequate, stretch of the finger extensors may be used. With the therapist and client positioned and the hand manipulated as just described, the therapist uses her free hand for distally directed, rapid stroking movements over the proximal phalanges of the affected hand. This causes momentary flexion of the MP joints, which then bounce back into partial extension. The stroking movement is performed so that the proximal, then distal IP joints are included. The movement is performed rapidly and continuously, causing rapid flexion and then bounce back of MP and IP joints. The fingers now become extended, and the finger flexors are relaxed because they are reciprocally inhibited by the stretch reflex response in the extensors. If the flexors are stretched or stroking is performed over the palmar surface of the fingers, the spasticity will return to the finger flexors, and they will act to close the hand.[4] For this reason the fingers should not be pulled into extension.

Active finger extension may be further facilitated by the use of a finger extension exercise glove with rubber bands, which the client uses while the hand is manipulated into supination with the thumb pulled out of the palm as described earlier.

Elevation above the horizontal position evokes the extensor reflexes of the fingers. After flexor spasticity has been decreased by the maneuvers just described, the therapist stands on the affected side and maintains the thumb in abduction and extension and the forearm in pronation. The fingers are kept in extension by pressure over the IP joints and stabilization of the fingertips. The grip on the thumb is released, and the arm is raised above the horizontal position. The therapist strokes distally over the IP joints with the heel of her hand. The fingers will extend or hyperextend, and the therapist gradually discontinues contact with the client's hand. If the client is ready, slight voluntary mental effort can be superimposed on the reflex extension which may bring about additional extension of the fingers.

If the forearm is supinated while the arm is elevated, thumb extension will be enhanced. The hand should be positioned overhead for this maneuver. To facilitate extension of the fourth and fifth fingers the forearm should be pronated as the arm is elevated and friction should be applied over the ulnar side of the dorsum of the forearm.

When reflex extension of the fingers is well-estab-lished, alternate fist opening and closing can begin. The arm is lowered passively, and the elbow is flexed. The forearm and wrist are supported, and the client is asked to "squeeze" then "stop squeezing." As soon as the fingers relax, the manipulations to facilitate finger extension are carried out. These two steps are alternated, and the client's voluntary efforts are superimposed on the reflex activity so that the movements begin to assume a semivoluntary character. Semivoluntary finger extension is influenced by the position of the limb and appears to be linked to gross movements other than the synergy patterns.

Voluntary movements of the thumb appear when semivoluntary mass extension becomes possible. Once the flexor muscles have been relaxed, the hand can be placed in the client's lap, ulnar side down, and the client can attempt to move the thumb away from the first finger, a preliminary for lateral prehension. The therapist may stimulate the tendons of the abductor pollicis and the extensor pollicis brevis by tapping or friction at the point where they pass over the wrist to enhance the client's effort. The client can learn to "twiddle" his thumbs to attain further control of thumb motion. He folds his hands, wrists slightly flexed, and moves the thumbs around each other. Initially the normal thumb may push the other around, but the involved thumb may begin to participate actively. The willed effort, visual input, and sensory feedback from affected and unaffected sides contribute to the development of this movement. During the treatment sessions the client must be comfortable and relaxed. His willed efforts must be slight lest too much effort evoke a flexor rather than the extensor response that is desired. Excessive muscle tension in the limb and entire body must be avoided or finger extension will not occur.

Many adult hemiplegics never achieve good voluntary extension or coordinated fine hand motions. However, if semivoluntary extension can be well-established, voluntary extension usually follows, so that the client can open the hand in all positions.[4]

The accomplishment of palmar prehension and fine hand movements requires the achievement of voluntary opening of the hand, opposition of the thumb to the fingers, and the ability to release objects in contact with the palm of the hand.

THE ROOD APPROACH TO THE TREATMENT OF NEUROMUSCULAR DYSFUNCTION

Margaret S. Rood is an occupational and physical therapist whose treatment approach is based on her extensive study of neurophysiological and developmental literature.[10,15] Her method undergoes continuous change and modification as new information becomes available.[15] Based on her studies Rood designed treatment methods that she tested clinically. However, controlled research on the effectiveness of her approach is limited. The approach is used with apparent success by occupational and physical therapists. There is a need for documentation of the effectiveness of the method. This treatment approach evolved from Rood's work with persons who have cerebral palsy,[10] however, it can be applied to the treatment of persons of any age who have brain damage.[15]

The Rood approach uses cutaneous stimulation to specific areas of the skin to modify muscle tone and facilitate muscle contraction. Fast and slow brushing and quick or prolonged stimulation with ice are often associated with Rood's technique. However, proprioceptive and vestibular stimulation and stimulation of the special senses are used as well.

If mechanical or thermal stimulation is applied to the skin overlying a particular muscle, the gamma efferent innervating stretch receptors in that muscle are activated. The stimulation acts to "tune up" the stretch receptors in the muscle that will result in increased tone and contractile response to stretch. Rood's approach uses cutaneous stimulation to increase stretch receptor activity and proprioceptive stimulation, which facilitates voluntary contraction of the muscles stimulated.

It is possible to reduce spasticity using this approach. Since the gamma efferent system displays reciprocal innervation, stimulation of muscles antagonistic to spastic muscles will result in a decrease of tone in the spastic muscles and an increase of tone in their antagonists, the muscles stimulated.[8]

General principles of the Rood approach

The principles of the Rood approach as stated by Huss[10] are summarized as follows:

1. Because motor output is dependent on sensory input, sensory stimuli are used to activate or inhibit motor responses.
2. Activation of motor responses follows a normal developmental sequence. First there is phasic movement, followed by co-contraction patterns for stability for holding action, then heavy work movement superimposed on the co-contraction as seen in weight bearing, and finally skilled and coordinated movement in a nonweight bearing position with stabilization at the proximal joints.
3. The interaction between somatic, psychic, and autonomic functions within the nervous system makes it possible to use stimuli to influence one or more of these functions directly or indirectly.

This treatment approach may be defined as the activation, facilitation, and inhibition of voluntary and involuntary muscle activity through the reflex arc.[10]

General methods of treatment

Sensory stimulation is provided initially to proprioceptors using vibration, pressure into muscle bellies by rubbing, joint compression, quick stretch to muscles to be facilitated, and vestibular stimulation appropriately applied. If necessary this is followed by exteroceptive stimuli of light touch or rapid brushing. Ice may be used but is applied to the extremities only and with caution. The use of exteroceptive stimuli requires careful follow-up of the patient for several hours, since cutaneous stimuli have a profound effect on the reticular system and adverse effects may result if exteroceptive stimulation is incorrectly applied.

Procedures for overall relaxation that were introduced by Rood are slow stroking, neutral warmth, and slow rolling. Pressure to the muscle insertion can be applied for relaxation of specific muscles. Slow stroking is done over the posterior primary rami adjacent to the vertebral column with firm, light pressure in an alternating pattern. One of the therapist's hands starts in the cervical area and descends to the lower lumbar region. Thus the hands alternate from top to bottom in a stroking movement, and one hand is always in contact with the client. This is done for 3 minutes or less. If there is irregular hair growth pattern, the stroking may be irritating.[10] Neutral warmth is the wrapping of part or all of the client in a cotton towel or blanket until the appropriate relaxation is obtained, usually about 10 to 20 minutes.[15] Slow rolling is done from the supine position to the side and back and is continued until relaxation is observed.

The treatment program is designed to suit the client's muscle tone and developmental level. It may be designed to facilitate, inhibit, or combine facilitation with inhibition of muscle activity to suit the special needs of the individual client. The reader is referred to the original sources[10,14,15] for more detailed information about the developmental patterns of posture and movement as described by Rood.

As muscle tone and activity are normalized, cortical demand for voluntary effort by the client is made. Activities that use motor patterns that have been stimulated are used so that the client's attention is directed to activity and not to specific movements or stabilizing patterns.[10]

Specific techniques and precautions*

Facilitation through cutaneous stimulation. The skin may be stimulated by fast or slow brushing. Fast brushing is accomplished by a battery-driven camel's hair

---

*Summarized from Trombly, C. A., and Scott, A. D.: Occupational therapy for physical dysfunction, Baltimore, 1977, The Williams & Wilkins Co.

brush applied for 3 to 5 seconds on the skin area over each muscle to be stimulated (Fig. 4-42). The dermatome served by the same spinal segment as those muscles that are being facilitated may also be brushed. The brushing should be done for 5 seconds for each area, and if no response is obtained after 30 seconds, the brushing should be repeated three to five times.

Fast brushing of the skin adjacent to the vertebral column facilitates contraction of the tonic muscles of the back. Fast brushing of the skin over the rest of the body facilitates a tonic response of superficial muscles if the corresponding dermatomes are brushed. Precautions to fast brushing include avoiding the pinna of the ear, since this stimulates the vagus nerve and can influence the cardiorespiratory functions, and fast brushing to dermatomes of L1-2, which will result in voiding. Brushing the dermatomes of S2-4 will result in urine retention.

Light touching or stroking of the skin activates the reciprocal action of the phasic or mobilizing muscles that are superficial. For example, light stroking of the dorsal aspects of the finger or toe web spaces or the palms of the hands or soles of the feet elicits a withdrawal of the stimulated limb.

Facilitation through thermal stimulation. Ice is used to facilitate muscle activity. Popsicle maker molds for home use are a convenient way to prepare ice that can be administered easily by the therapist. Ice is thought to have the same effect as brushing and stroking. The ice is held in place firmly for 3 to 5 seconds, and then the water is wiped away (Fig. 4-43). This stimulates postural tonic responses. The skin areas to be stimulated are the same as for fast brushing, except for the areas adjacent to the vertebral column, which should not be iced. If these regions are iced, a sympathetic nervous system response may result.

Quick icing involves wiping the ice very quickly over the skin and evokes a reflex withdrawal similar to that described for the light touch stimulation when ice is applied to the palms or soles or the dorsal webs of the hands or feet. Quick icing is only used in hypotonic conditions when the client is a calm or placid type. The therapist should be aware that quick icing of the upper right quadrant of the abdomen (T7-9 dermatome) will stimulate the diaphragm and that touching the lips with ice results in mouth opening while ice inside the lips and tongue results in mouth closure. These techniques are sometimes used in training for mouth control, feeding, and phonation. Precautions for icing to the pinna of the ear and the L1-2 and S2-3 dermatomes are the same as for brushing.

Facilitation through proprioceptive stimulation. Quick, light stretch of muscle activates a phasic response of the muscle stretched and inhibition of its antagonist.

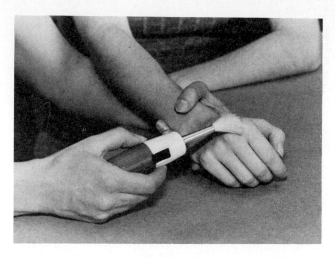

Fig. 4-42. Cutaneous stimulation by battery-operated brush to facilitate contraction of intrinsic muscles of hand.

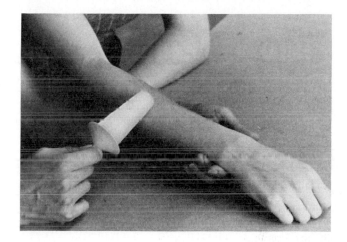

Fig. 4-43. Thermal stimulation with ice water Popsicle.

The effect is immediate. Tapping of the muscle belly or its tendon with the fingertips is another technique that causes stretch of muscle fibers and has the same effect as quick stretch. Pressure on the muscle belly also elicits the stretch reflex response.

Secondary stretch is a maintained stretch of the muscle at the end of the range. Secondary stretch of heavy work muscles (extensors and abductors) facilitates contraction of their antagonists (flexors and adductors).

Joint compression is used to facilitate co-contraction of muscles around a joint that act for its stabilization. The joint compression must be heavy, that is resistance is greater than body weight, and the force is applied through the longitudinal axes of bones that are in approximation with one another. Weight bearing while prone on flexed elbows and prone weight bearing on the hands, quadruped, and standing are positions of heavy joint compression. Weights can be added to the client to increase the resistance for joint compression.

Techniques to inhibit muscle activity. Joint approximation can be used to reduce tone in spastic muscles. Joints are manually approximated or pushed together to reduce spasticity and equalize tone. Slow stroking of the back, rocking, and neutral warmth, described earlier, are methods of inhibiting muscle activity and attaining relaxation.

Pressure on the tendinous insertion of muscle will inhibit it. For example, grasp of a firm handle will apply constant pressure over the long flexor tendons and inhibit the flexor muscles of the hand. A maintained stretch or prolonged maintenance of the muscle in its elongated position will inhibit the muscle's response to the stretch stimulus. A brief maximal contraction of spastic muscles is recommended before placing the limb in the lengthened position. This is thought to activate a large number of GTOs and produce inhibition of the muscle, which will allow it to be placed more easily in its lengthened position.

Conclusion. This is a brief summary of the principles and some of the treatment techniques used in the Rood approach for the treatment of neuromuscular dysfunction. It is intended to orient the reader to the approach rather than to enable him or her to practice it.

The treatment approach needs to be seen in its totality and not as a fragmented series of isolated techniques[12] to be applied appropriately. The therapist needs to have a thorough understanding of kinesiology, neurophysiology, and the development of human motion and its relationship to dysfunction,[12] as well as study and training in this treatment approach to practice it competently.

The reader is referred to the references and supplementary reading list for more details of treatment and its neurophysiological basis.

NEURODEVELOPMENTAL TREATMENT— THE BOBATH APPROACH TO THE TREATMENT OF ADULT HEMIPLEGIA

JAN ZARET DAVIS, O.T.R.

This is an introduction and orientation to the neurodevelopmental treatment approach. It is designed to provide a basic foundation in principles of treatment and describe some general treatment techniques. Those interested in expanding their knowledge in this area are directed to readings from the reference list, particularly to *Adult Hemiplegia: Evaluation and Treatment* by Berta Bobath.[2]

□ Director of Ergotherapie, Klinik Valens, Rehabilitations Zentrum, Valens, Switzerland. Special thanks is given to Pat Davies, M.C.S.B., instructor and clinical specialist at the Bäderklinik in Valens, Switzerland, for her assistance.

Berta Bobath, physical therapist, and her husband Karel Bobath, neuropsychiatrist, have been developing special treatment techniques in England since World War II. This technique, often called neurodevelopmental treatment (NDT), is meant for a wide variety of dysfunctions of the CNS, most commonly for cerebral palsy and acquired adult hemiplegia.[9,15] It is intended to be a 24-hour per day treatment program. Therefore it should be practiced by all those concerned with the client's care. These include the nursing staff, occupational therapists, physical therapists, speech therapists, and family. It is ideal to begin treatment immediately during the acute stage of illness, but treatment can begin at any time.

Rationale for use of neurodevelopmental treatment techniques with adult hemiplegics

The primary goal of NDT is to relearn normal movements. The techniques used are intended for more than just the movements of an arm or leg; they treat the person as a whole, encouraging the use of both sides. The client uses less adaptive equipment (for example, slings, braces, and canes) and is more able to more about freely with normal muscle tone.[2] This creates a better atmosphere for his psychosocial adjustment to family and everyday living. The more normal a person appears to others, with less deformity from spasticity, the better he or she is accepted.

The Bobaths use specific techniques to decrease spasticity and inhibit abnormal patterns of movement. This suppression or inhibition of abnormal patterns (synergies) must be accomplished before normal, selective isolated movement can take place. It is impossible to superimpose normal movement on a person still being influenced by spasticity.[2]

The following are terms often used in describing the NDT techniques of Bobath. Their meanings and uses should become clear as the reader pursues the rest of this section. For more complete definitions and discussion the reader is advised to consult the original source.[2]

Positioning	Reflex inhibiting patterns (RIP)
Rotation of trunk	Normalization of tone
"Placing"	Key points of control
Spasticity	Associated reactions
Inhibition	Associated movements
Weight bearing	Postural reactions
Postural tone	Righting reactions
Scapular mobility	Equilibrium reactions
Reciprocal innervation	Protective extension

Evaluation. The initial phase in treatment is the evaluation. An NDT evaluation includes the assessment of postural tone, motor patterns, sensation, and balance reactions. These are all well-defined and outlined by

Bobath.[2] The occupational therapist must also include an ADL and perceptual evaluation. The client is evaluated by the therapist to see just what he can or cannot do. In evaluation, emphasis is placed on the *quality* of *movement* rather than muscles and joints.[2]

To do an accurate evaluation the therapist should have a good understanding of normal development. This would include normal postural reactions, that is, righting reactions, equilibrium reactions, and protective extension of the arms. It is important to understand what is "normal" and "abnormal" in movement and positioning of the body. Most clients will display at least one abnormal reaction following a CVA. Normal and abnormal movements are listed here for comparison.

Normal	Abnormal
Muscle tone at rest	Flaccidity, spasticity
Voluntary selective movement	Abnormal postural tone
Isolated control	Synergistic movement
Associated movements	Associated reactions
Postural reactions	Lack of or reduced equilibrium reactions

Following the evaluation the therapist uses a variety of techniques to "normalize tone" by reducing spasticity to gain selective movement.

Treatment. Before treatment begins it is important to realize which factors may contribute to or cause spasticity. These are (1) improper positioning, (2) stress—trying too hard, (3) pain, and (4) fear. Fear can be caused by loss of sensation, poor balance reactions, undependable (hemiplegic) side, fear of falling (no protective extension), fear of pain, previous bad experience, aids

taken away after being trained with them, perceptual problems, immobilization for a long period, and lack of trust in therapists.[6] Fear and spasticity are so intertwined that sometimes a vicious cycle appears:

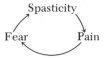

If preventive measures are taken to reduce pain, fear, and other contributing factors, the therapist should have better success with the techniques used to reduce spasticity. It cannot be too strongly emphasized that the establishment of trust and rapport with the client is very important to help him gain confidence through success.

The first rule in the treatment of persons with hemiplegia is *if spasticity begins, stop!* Spasticity should never be encouraged; instead there are several ways of discouraging spasticity in preparation for purposeful movement. These should begin from the time of onset in the *acute* stage. During this first stage the muscle tone is often flaccid, and the client is passive, so all persons attending to the client should follow these suggestions:

1. Position bed so that client must turn toward his affected side[5] (Fig. 4-44).
2. Always approach client from his hemiplegic side, encouraging eye contact.
3. During nursing tasks such as washing, name each body part to increase awareness.
4. Provide sensory stimulation (for example, tactile input to hemiplegic side, and orientation to time and place).

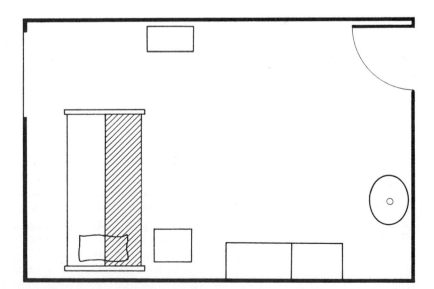

Fig. 4-44. Room arranged so that client must turn to affected side. Shaded area represents affected side of body.

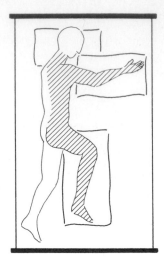

Fig. 4-45. Bed position when lying on unaffected side.

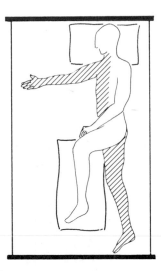

Fig. 4-46. Bed position when lying on affected side.

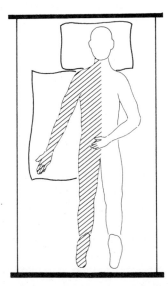

Fig. 4-47. Bed position when lying supine.

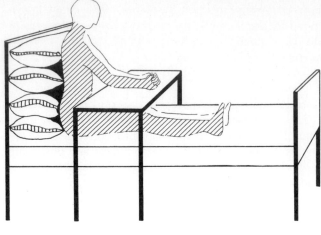

Fig. 4-48. Bed position when sitting upright.

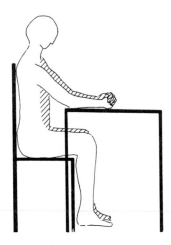

Fig. 4-49. Position when sitting in chair at table. Arms are clasped in front, elbows extended, and shoulders protracted.

5. Position client properly in bed and when sitting[2] (Figs. 4-45 to 4-49).

In each medical setting the roles of occupational therapy and physical therapy may differ slightly. Yet the techniques described are imperative for proper client treatment, and all professional services should be aware of them and be able to apply them appropriately. The general rules of treatment and positioning are followed by a more specific focus on the shoulder, arm, and trunk. The Bobaths strongly stated that the upper and lower extremities must not be separated. Although the role of occupational therapy has traditionally been primarily with the upper extremities, the lower extremities must not be neglected during positioning.

It is typical for persons with hemiplegia to "ignore"

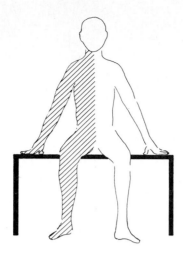

Fig. 4-50. Weight bearing on position of upper limbs in sitting.

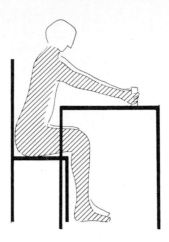

Fig. 4-52. Bilateral activity of upper limbs.

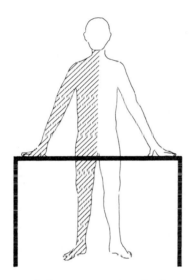

Fig. 4-51. Weight bearing on upper limbs in standing.

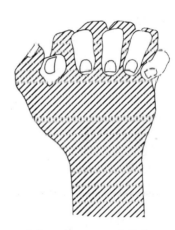

Fig. 4-53. During bilateral activity and when in sitting position hands are clasped as shown. Shaded hand is affected hand.

or neglect the affected side. This is most often due to sensory loss, visual field disturbance, general lack of awareness, and paralysis. To reduce this neglect and provide more normal input to the affected side the following basic working positions are suggested[2,5,6,7]:

1. Weight bearing on the hemiplegic side in sitting and standing (Figs. 4-50 and 4-51). The purposes of weight bearing are to provide proprioceptive input to hemiplegic side, encourage more normal postural tone and balance reactions, decrease fear, reduce spasticity, and prevent contractures of wrist and fingers.
2. Bilateral activities with hands clasped together Figs. 4-52 to 4-54). The purposes of bilateral activities are to increase awareness of hemiplegic side, increase sensory input to hemiplegic side, bring affected arm into visual field, begin "purposeful" movement of hemiplegic arm, discourage flexion synergy by protraction of scapula and extension of the elbow and wrist, develop abduction of fingers and thumb that discourages spasticity of hand; and teach the client reflex inhibiting patterns that he can perform himself.
3. Trunk rotation (Figs. 4-55 and 4-56). The purposes of trunk rotation are to reduce spasticity of trunk, encourage weight bearing on hemiplegic side, increase visual field, begin more normal control of trunk as a whole, and increase normal balance reactions.

The positions just described should be incorporated

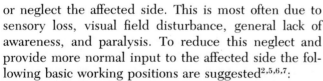

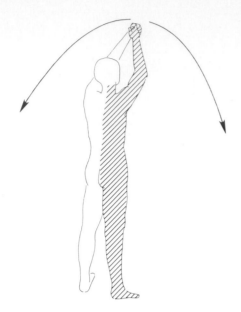

Fig. 4-54. Bilateral exercise of arms.

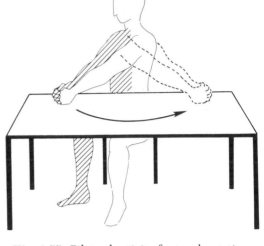

Fig. 4-55. Bilateral activity for trunk rotation.

into all activities in occupational therapy. Each activity can be done in sitting or in standing, depending on the level of the client's progress. At every possible opportunity the client should be treated in a normal chair instead of the wheelchair to obtain maximum benefit.

The shoulder. At all times the affected shoulder should be watched to make sure that the scapula is not pulling back into retraction. This retraction increases spasticity throughout the arm, contributes to shoulder pain, and inhibits normal movement. Protraction of the shoulder can be assisted by gravity and by bilateral activities with the hands clasped together.

When spasticity is too strong for the client to obtain protraction of the shoulder, the therapist must assist. The therapist should use reflex inhibiting patterns to control and reduce spasticity. As Bobath[2] stated, "The main reflex inhibiting pattern counteracting spasticity in trunk and arm is the extension of neck and spine and external rotation of the arm at the shoulder with elbow extended. Further reduction of flexor spasticity can be obtained by adding extension of the wrist with supination and abduction of the thumb" (Fig. 4-57). It is better to use movement patterns rather than static postures to control and reduce spasticity. When the therapist uses static reflex inhibiting postures (controls and holds every part of the body to reduce spasticity), active and more normal movements are impossible.[2]

Rationale for scapula mobilization. In the normal shoulder the scapula glides freely when the arm is fully flexed or abducted. The hemiplegic shoulder is often influenced by spasticity pulling the scapula into retraction. This prevents any gliding movements. Now if the arm is raised higher than 90°, the head of the humerus pushes against the acromion with the supraspinatus muscle and joint capsule pressed in between. This causes intense pain and can also damage the supraspinatus. Therefore the arm must *never* be fully raised before the scapula has been mobilized, and the therapist can feel its gliding movements. Even in a flaccid arm the scapula can be influenced by spasticity of the rhomboids, trapezius, and latissimus, so the therapist should be sure to check for scapula mobility.

Mobilization of the scapula prevents the "frozen shoulder" and usually eliminates the painful shoulder completely. The scapula can be moved into protraction, elevation, and depression, but the therapist should avoid pushing it into retraction.[2,6]

Subluxation. Many professionals are particularly afraid of the subluxed shoulder. Numerous efforts are made to protect it and "prevent" it. Subluxation cannot be "prevented." If the muscles around the shoulder girdle, which are attached to the humerus, are weak enough, the shoulder will be subluxed. Slings do not help subluxation. They only keep the arm in a poor position and may contribute to pain and swelling. Subluxation itself does not cause pain. The pain is caused by the improper *handling* of a subluxed arm. Forcing the head of the humerus back into place can cause trauma and pain. Doing standard ROM procedures on an arm without a gliding scapula can also cause pain. Treatment of the subluxed arm should include proper sitting (Figs. 4-48 and 4-49), weight bearing (Figs. 4-50 and 4-51), and mobilization of the scapula and proper positioning in bed (Figs. 4-45 to 4-47). The goal is to prevent long

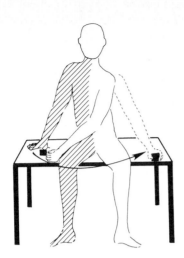

Fig. 4-56. Trunk rotation is practiced while client bears weight on affected arm and transfers objects from one side of bench to other.

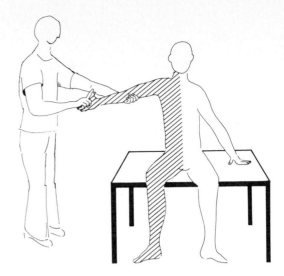

Fig. 4-57. Therapist assists client to obtain reflex-inhibiting pattern for arm.

lasting stretch of the joint capsule and supraspinatus.[6]

The nonfunctional arm. Even if the upper extremity has no potential for functional use, the trunk and arm must be retrained for bilateral activity. At all times the arm should be in front of the body where it can be seen and not hanging down to the side. If emphasis is placed only on the unaffected arm, the client will lose potential for sensory and motor recovery of the affected arm.[2]

Preparing the patient for home

The benefits of the treatment program will be lost if the client is not adequately prepared for returning home. This preparation should include prescribing a home exercise program, family education, and communication with the follow-up therapist if necessary. The hospital or clinic is a very secure setting, and it is very important that both the client and family feel comfortable and confident on their return home. The home exercise program is important to maintain mobilization and movement. The therapist should select exercises that can be done easily and correctly without assistance. If stress is used to complete his exercises, it is likely that the client will form "bad habits" and spasticity will increase.

After the selection of exercises the therapist must train the client in each of them. To encourage consistency the client should follow the same sequence of exercises each day. This should begin long before discharge from occupational therapy so that it is a well-established part of the daily routine.

Each exercise should be written down in the proper sequence. This should include how often they should be done, for example, twice a day; number of repetitions, for example, 10 times each; and diagrams if necessary.

Next the family should be trained so they are also well-acquainted with each exercise. Thus they can guide the home program properly. For best results in family teaching the occupational therapist should demonstrate tasks, explaining the importance; emphasize each major point, for example, position of arm and placement of hands; have the family work with the client under the therapist's guidance; and repeat instructions as often as needed until the family and client are confident enough to do the exercises at home alone. Family education should include a home exercise program and ADL training in areas of dressing, eating, grooming, hygiene, bathing, transfers, and cooking. This program should also include instruction in proper positioning (lying, sitting, and standing) and proper use of equipment. Before discharge from the treatment center the therapist should give the family her name and work telephone number, set up a date for a reevaluation if necessary, and contact the therapist treating the client following discharge from the treatment facility to ensure proper carry over.

General treatment principles[6]

1. Never exercise—*retrain!* The brain knows patterns and movements, not muscles and bones.
2. Start and finish a treatment session with something positive, something the client can do well.
3. Use slow, controlled movements—fast movements can increase spasticity.

4. The client must find the treatment useful, purposeful, and meaningful.
5. Do not magnify pain by dwelling on it.
6. If the client thinks there has been no progress, it may be due to memory loss.
7. Proper sequence of activities leads to success.
8. After spasticity is inhibited, follow with a purposeful movement—put it to use! Do not inhibit spasticity unless you plan to use the limb.
9. Do not ask a client who is influenced by spasticity to relax—he cannot.
10. Encourage the client to look at his arm.
11. Tell the client when he has done a movement correctly so he can *feel* it.
12. It is of great importance to train proprioceptive, tactile, and spatial sensation.
13. Discourage stressful or excessive efforts of the sound arm, which increase associated reactions of the affected arm.
14. Ask for "automatic movements" to reduce stress. The client then will think about the activity rather than the arm.
15. If spasticity starts, *stop!*
16. The client often has to relearn movements, even on his "good" side.

Popular misconceptions about adult hemiplegia[6]

1. Shoulder subluxation causes pain.
2. A person with hemiplegia has a normal side.
3. Slings prevent shoulder subluxation.
4. The harder the client tries, the better he will get.
5. Strength is more important than control.
6. Hemianopsia is the primary reason for neglect of the hemiplegic side.
7. Hemiplegia of long standing cannot be changed.
8. Return of sensation is totally dependent on the lesion.
9. Walking is enough of a rehabilitation goal.
10. If the affected arm has no functional use, forget it.
11. An arm with an intravenous drain in place is an immobilized arm.

Summary

The NDT approach was developed by Karel and Berta Bobath. It may be effectively used with a wide variety of CNS dysfunctions but is most widely known for its application in treatment of cerebral palsy and adult hemiplegia.

The NDT approach is based on normal neuromotor development and function. Its primary goal is to enhance the relearning of normal movement patterns. Special techniques of positioning and motion are used to inhibit spasticity, abnormal patterns of movement, and abnormal reflex activity.

Emphasis is on treating the client as a whole rather than using an isolated approach to treatment of the arm, leg, or trunk. Quality of movement, control, and coordination are developed through the treatment techniques rather than muscle strength and joint motion per se.

Sensory reeducation and involvement of the family in the rehabilitation program are important elements in this approach to treatment.

REVIEW QUESTIONS
Treatment methods: sensorimotor approaches to treatment

1. What is the fundamental hypothesis that underlies all sensorimotor approaches to treatment of CNS dysfunction?

Brunnstrom approach

1. List the stages of recovery of arm function after CVA, as described by Brunnstrom.
2. List the motions in the flexor and extensor synergies of the arm, and draw stick figures to illustrate the positions.
3. What is the strongest component of the flexor synergy of the arm?
4. What is the weakest component of the extensor synergy of the arm?
5. What is the basis of the Brunnstrom approach to the treatment of hemiplegia?
6. For what purposes does Brunnstrom recommend the use of primitive reflexes and associated reactions in the early recovery stages after onset of hemiplegia?
7. Define or describe the following terms: limb synergy, associated reactions, imitation synkinesis, proximal traction response, grasp reflex, Souque's finger phenomenon.
8. Describe or demonstrate the procedure that Brunnstrom recommended to maintain or achieve pain-free ROM at the glenohumeral joint.
9. What is the aim of treatment for functional recovery of the arm during stages 1 and 2? Stages 2 and 3? Stages 3 and 4?
10. List two treatment methods that could be used to achieve each of these aims.
11. Describe three activities besides those listed in the text that may be used in occupational therapy to enhance voluntary control of the flexor and extensor synergies.
12. What is the effect of the proximal traction response on muscle function?
13. Describe or demonstrate the procedure that Brunnstrom recommends to establish wrist fixation in association with grasp.
14. Describe the procedure that may be used to relax spastic finger flexion and facilitate finger extension.

Rood approach

1. What types of sensory stimuli are used *primarily* in the Rood approach?
2. What is the effect of mechanical or thermal stimulation of the skin on underlying muscle?
3. How does Rood use cutaneous and proprioceptive stimulation to reduce tone in spastic muscles?
4. Describe the sequence and type of motor responses that Rood recommends and the rationale for this.
5. List four types of sensory stimulation used in the Rood approach to facilitate or inhibit muscle activity.
6. Describe three procedures that will result in overall relaxation of muscle tone.
7. What are the precautions for fast brushing?
8. Describe how ice is used to facilitate muscle activity.
9. What are the precautions for the use of ice?
10. Describe three methods to elicit the stretch reflex. What is the effect on the muscles stretched?
11. What is the purpose and effect of joint compression?
12. List three techniques that could be used to inhibit muscle tone.

The neurodevelopmental (Bobath) approach

1. What is the fundamental or primary goal of the NDT approach?
2. List three advantages of this approach stated in the text.
3. What are the elements of an NDT evaluation?
4. List four factors that can cause or increase spasticity.
5. Describe the vicious cycle that may occur that contributes to the maintenance of spasticity.
6. What are some of the factors that contribute to the neglect of the hemiplegic side?
7. Describe the positions that Bobath recommends to reduce this neglect in sitting and standing.
8. What are the purposes of trunk rotation? Bilateral activities?
9. Describe recommended positioning and mobilization procedures used to prevent shoulder pain and severe spasticity around the shoulder and shoulder girdle.
10. How is subluxation treated in the NDT approach?
11. What is the role of the occupational therapist in preparing the client to go home?
12. Why does Bobath stress scapula protraction in positioning and movement of the hemiplegic arm?
13. According to the NDT approach how should the hemiplegic arm be positioned when the client is seated? What is the rationale for this position?

REFERENCES

Introduction and section one

1. Anonymous: Muscle reeducation, Downey, Calif., 1963, Rancho Los Amigos Hospital. Mimeographed.
2. Anonymous: Progressive resistive and static exercise: principles and techniques, Downey, Calif., Rancho Los Amigos Hospital. Mimeographed.
3. Ayres, A.J.: Occupational therapy for motor disorders resulting from impairment of the central nervous system, Rehabil. Lit. **21:** 302, 1960.
4. Cynkin, S.: Occupational therapy: toward health through activities, Boston, 1979, Little, Brown & Co.
5. Huddleston, O.L.: Therapeutic exercises, Philadelphia, 1961, F.A. Davis Co.
6. Kottke, F.J.: Therapeutic exercise. In Krusen, F.H., Kottke, F.J., and Ellwood, P.M., editors: Handbook of physical medicine and rehabilitation, Philadelphia, 1965, W.B. Saunders Co.
7. Kraus, H.: Therapeutic exercise, Springfield, Ill., 1963, Charles C Thomas, Publisher.
8. Reynolds, M.: Therapeutic exercise, lecture, San Jose, Calif., 1971, Department of Occupational Therapy, San Jose State College.
9. Willard, H.S., and Spackman, C.S., editors: Occupational therapy, ed. 4, Philadelphia, 1971, J.B. Lippincott Co.

Section two

1. Cynkin, S.: Occupational therapy: toward health through activities, Boston, 1979, Little, Brown & Co.
2. Hopkins, H.L., Smith, H.D., and Tiffany, E.G.: The activity process. In Hopkins, H.L., and Smith, H.D., editors: Willard and Spackman's occupational therapy, ed. 5, Philadelphia, 1978, J.B. Lippincott Co.
3. Llorens, L.: Activity analysis for sensory integration (CPM) dysfunction, 1978. Mimeographed.
4. Occupational Therapy Newspaper, Rockville, Md., June 1979, American Occupational Therapy Association.
5. Trombly, C.A., and Scott, A.D.: Occupational therapy for physical dysfunction, Baltimore, 1977, The Williams & Wilkins Co.
6. Willard, H.S., and Spackman, C.S., editors: Occupational therapy, ed. 4, Philadelphia, 1971, J.B. Lippincott Co.

Section three

1. Anonymous: Activities of daily living for patients with incoordination, limited range of motion, paraplegia, quadriplegia, and hemiplegia, Cleveland, 1968, Highland View Hospital, Cuyahoga County Hospitals, Division of Occupational Therapy. Mimeographed, unpublished.
2. Buchwald, E.: Physical rehabilitation for daily living, New York, 1952, McGraw-Hill, Inc.
3. Holser, P., Jones, M., and Ilanit, T.: A study of the upper extremity control brace, Am. J. Occup. Ther. 16:170, 1962.
4. Hopkins, H.L.: Treatment process and procedures. In Hopkins, H.L., and Smith, H.D., editors: Willard and Spackman's occupational therapy, ed. 5, Philadelphia, 1978, J.B. Lippincott Co.
5. Klinger, J.L.: Mealtime manual for people with disabilities and the aging, Camden, N.J., 1978, Campbell Soup Co.
6. Malick, M.H., and Sherry, B.: Activities of daily living and homemaking. In Hopkins, H.L., and Smith, H.D., editors: Willard and Spackman's occupational therapy, ed. 5, Philadelphia, 1978, J.B. Lippincott Co.
7. Malick, M.H., and Sherry, B.: Life work tasks. In Hopkins, H.L., and Smith, H.D., editors: Willard and Spackman's occupational therapy, ed. 5, Philadelphia, 1978, J.B. Lippincott Co.
8. Melvin, J.L.: Rheumatic disease: occupational therapy and rehabilitation, Philadelphia, 1977, F.A. Davis Co.
9. The Professional Manual Subcommittee of the Education Committee, Allied Health Professional Section of the Arthritis Foundation: Arthritis manual for allied health professionals, New York, 1973, The Arthritis Foundation.
10. Runge, M.: Self-dressing techniques for patients with spinal cord injury, Am. J. Occup. Ther. 21:367, 1967.
11. Trombly, C.A., and Scott, A.D.: Occupational therapy for physical dysfunction, Baltimore, 1977, The Williams & Wilkins Co.

Section four

1. Benaron, C.: Occupational therapy in treatment of hemiplegia, Br. J. Occup. Ther. 1978.
2. Bobath, B.: Adult hemiplegia: evaluation and treatment, London, 1977, Heinemann Ltd.
3. Brunnstrom, S.: Motor behavior in adult hemiplegic patients, Am. J. Occup. Ther. 15:6, 1961.
4. Brunnstrom, S.: Movement therapy in hemiplegia, New York, 1970, Harper & Row, Publishers, Inc.
5. Cash, J.: Neurology for physiotherapists, London, 1977, Faber & Faber Ltd.
6. Davies, P.: Treatment techniques for adult hemiplegia, study course, Bäderklinik, Valens, Switzerland, 1979.
7. Eggers, O.: Ergotherapie bei hemiplegie, Basel, 1979, Sekrerariat des Verbandes Schweizerischer Ergotherapeuten.
8. Harris, F.A.: Facilitation techniques in therapeutic exercise. In Basmajian, J.V., editor: Therapeutic exercise, ed. 3, Baltimore, 1978, The Williams & Wilkins Co.
9. Hopkins, H.L., and Smith, H.D., editors: Willard and Spackman's occupational therapy, ed. 5, Philadelphia, 1978, J.B. Lippincott Co.
10. Huss, J.: Sensorimotor approaches. In Hopkins, H.L., and Smith, H.D., editors: Willard and Spackman's occupational therapy, ed. 5, Philadelphia, 1978, J.B. Lippincott Co.
11. Luria, A.R.: The working brain, New York, 1973, Penguin Books.
12. Perry, C.: Principles and techniques of the Brunnstrom approach to the treatment of hemiplegia, Am. J. Phys. Med. 46:789, 1967.
13. Sawner, K.: Brunnstrom approach to treatment of adult patients with hemiplegia: rationale for facilitation procedures, Buffalo, 1969, State University of New York. Mimeographed.

14. Stockmeyer, S.A.: An interpretation of the approach of Rood to the treatment of neuromuscular dysfunction, Am. J. Phys. Med. **46**:900, 1967.
15. Trombly, C.A., and Scott, A.D.: Occupational therapy for physical dysfunction, Baltimore, 1977, The Williams & Wilkins Co.
16. Willard, H.L., and Spackman, C.S., editors: Occupational therapy, ed. 4, Philadelphia, 1971, J.B. Lippincott Co.

SUPPLEMENTARY READING (Section three only)

American Heart Association: Up and around. Pamphlet.
Bonner, C.D., editor: The team approach to hemiplegia, Springfield, Ill., 1969, Charles C Thomas, Publisher.
Collins, A.D.: Adapted plate for use in microwave oven, Am. J. Occup. Ther. **32**:586, 1978.
Fastow, K.: Adapted fitted bed sheets, Am. J. Occup. Ther. **31**:393, 1977.
Ford, J., and Duckworth, B.: Physical management for the quadriplegic patient, Philadelphia, 1974, F.A. Davis Co.
Holmlund, B.A., and Kavanaugh, R.N.: Communication aids for the handicapped, Am. J. Occup. Ther. **21**:357, 1967.
Leff, R.B.: Teaching stroke patients to dial the telephone, Am. J. Occup. Ther. **30**:313, 1976.
Lowman, E.W.: Arthritis, Boston, 1959, Little, Brown & Co.
Marker, M.A.: Adapted living aids for the bilateral shoulder disarticulation, Am. J. Occup. Ther. **31**:584, 1977.
May, E.E., Waggoner, N.R., and Boettke, E.: Homemaking for the handicapped, New York, 1966, Dodd, Mead & Co.
Moore, J.W.: Adapted knife for rheumatoid arthritics, Am. J. Occup. Ther. **32**:112, 1978.
Sammons, F.: Be OK self-help aids, Professional & Institutional Catalog, 1979, Box 32, Brookfield, Ill. 60513.
White, L.W., and Dallas, M.J.: Clothing adaptations: the occupational therapist and clothing designer collaborate, Am. J. Occup. Ther. **31**:90, 1977.
Wittmeyer, M.B., and Stolov, W.C.: Educating wheelchair patients on home architectural barriers, Am. J. Occup. Ther. **32**:557, 1978.

Chapter 5

Wheelchairs and special equipment

LORRAINE WILLIAMS PEDRETTI and GREGORY STONE, M.Ed., B.F.A., C.O.T.A.

WHEELCHAIRS

The wheelchair (Fig. 5-1) provides a comfortable and efficient mode of ambulation for those persons whose physical dysfunction makes walking impossible or impracticable. Others who ordinarily walk with supportive devices such as canes or crutches may find a wheelchair helpful when daily activities require speed or physical endurance that would be overtaxing. A wheelchair, for such persons, can enrich life experiences by making activities, such as trips to shopping centers, theaters, and amusement parks and sight-seeing vacations, possible.

In a sense the wheelchair becomes an extension of the self or the body. The user must learn to manage the wheelchair skillfully, safely, and efficiently, learn to measure space and judge speed and distance with the wheelchair, adapt to viewing the world from a different eye level, and cope with the symbolic meaning of the device to himself and the society.

Occupational and physical therapists are usually responsible for measuring the client for a wheelchair, recommending the wheelchair style and accessories that are most appropriate for the client in his life-style and teaching wheelchair safety and mobility.

Wheelchair size

To effect the best comfort and use efficiency the wheelchair should fit the person who will use it. An ill-fitting wheelchair can produce discomfort and undue fatigue and can contribute to the development of postural deformities.[12] Therefore the occupational or physical therapist should measure the client, as a preparatory step to completing a wheelchair prescription.

When properly fitted the wheelchair should conform to the following specifications[12]:

1. The seat width should be 2 inches wider than the widest point across the client's hips or thighs. This is to prevent pressure of the body against the sides of the chair. If braces are worn, the measurement across the hips should include the braces.
2. The seat depth should be 2 or 3 inches less than the distance from the rear of the buttocks to the inside of the bent knee. The purposes are to distribute weight evenly along the thighs, thus relieving pressure on the buttocks, and to prevent pressure in the popliteal area.
3. The seat height and footrest adjustments are determined by measuring from the rear of the bent knee to the bottom of the heel. The correct adjustments will result in a clearance of 1 inch of height and 1⅛ inches of depth under the thighs, while the step plates clear the floor by at least 2 inches for safety. If a wheelchair cushion is to be used, this must be considered when measuring for seat height and footrest adjustments. Special seat heights are available for unusually tall persons.
4. The wheelchair armrest helps in maintenance of posture and balance and provides a comfortable support for the arms. The armrest height should be approximately 1 inch greater than the distance from the seat level to the bottom of the flexed elbow. When the armrest is properly fitted, the client's shoulders should not be elevated nor should he lean to meet the armrests. If a cushion is to be used, this must be considered when measuring for arm height.
5. The height of the standard seat back is 4 inches less than the distance from the seat level to the posterior aspect of the axilla when the shoulder is flexed to 90°. The seat back should provide support to the client's back, help to maintain posture, and permit free arm movement without irritation. If full trunk support is required, semireclining or reclining seat backs or a headrest extension is available.

□ Gregory Stone, Lecturer, Department of Occupational Therapy, San Jose State University, San Jose, Calif.

It is possible to fit most wheelchair users with one of the manufacturers' standard sizes. However, custom modifications are possible at some additional expense to accommodate individual needs.[12]

Wheelchair selection

Besides proper fit of the wheelchair several other factors should be considered before the wheelchair prescription is completed and the wheelchair is ordered. The diagnosis, prognosis, age, life-style of the client, and environments in which the wheelchair is to be used are also important considerations. These factors influence selection of the type of frame, wheels, and special accessories.

The universal frame with the large wheels in the rear and 8-inch front casters is the most frequently recommended frame for the majority of wheelchair users. It is designed for indoor and outdoor use and is easily modified.[11]

The client with a bilateral lower extremity amputation may benefit from the amputee frame. On this type the large wheels are set further back than on the universal frame to improve balance. Since the client's weight is centered more to the rear of the chair, this frame type prevents tipping over backward.[11]

The traveler frame has the large wheel in front and the casters in the rear. It is primarily for indoor use and has many disadvantages in maneuverability, as compared to the universal frame. It may be more useful for individuals with limited ROM, however.[9,11]

Wheelchair construction is designed in standard, heavy-duty or lightweight models, depending on weight, endurance, strength, and activities of the wheelchair user.

Propelling a wheelchair may be accomplished in a variety of ways, depending on the physical capacities of the user. The standard drive has the hand rims attached directly to the large wheels. These are operated by pushing-pulling motions of the arms and by grasp. This is the most common type of propulsion and assumes sufficient grasp, arm strength, and physical endurance to propel the chair and body weight for daily living.[11]

When grasp strength is inadequate but there is sufficient arm strength and motion, a hand rim with projections may be ordered. The chair is operated by pushing the heel of the hand against the hand rim projections to push the large wheels. This type of operation is often used by quadriplegics with good arm function but inadequate grasp strength.

The one-arm drive has both hand rims on the same side of the chair. The outer rim, which is slightly smaller than the inner one, operates the opposite wheel. The

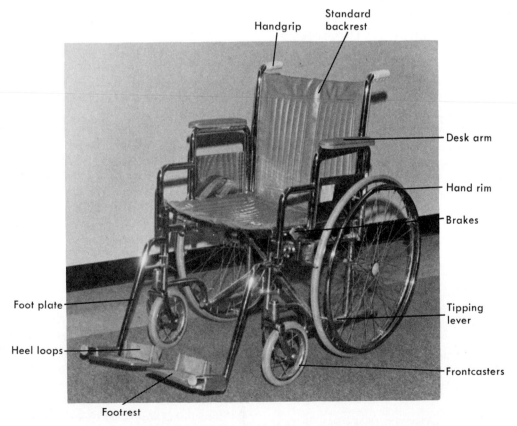

Fig. 5-1. Standard adult wheelchair with detachable desk arms and detachable swing-away footrests.

inner one is attached directly to the wheel on the same side.[11] This propulsion system is used by individuals with only one functional upper extremity and lower extremity involvement such as in triplegia. It may be used by individuals with hemiplegia in some instances. However, they can benefit from a hand-and-foot method of wheelchair propulsion, using a standard wheelchair (Fig. 5-2).

For those with severe disability and minimal use of the arms the power drive or electric wheelchair is the choice if some independence is to be achieved. The usual system has a control box that can be located near either hand, with a single stick lever projecting from it. The wheelchair is operated by pushing the lever in a variety of directions to effect the desired movement. If upper extremity function is insufficient for this control system, the controls can be adapted for operation by head, chin, mouth, elbow, foot, or toe.[11]

There are many wheelchair accessories available. Some of the major accessories and their benefits are discussed here.

Armrests come in standard, offset, desk, and detachable styles. The standard armrest is a continuous part of the frame and is not detachable. It limits proximity to table, counter, and desk surfaces and prohibits side transfers. Offset armrests give extra width for those wearing casts or braces without increasing the overall width of the chair. Desk armrests have a "step" in the front to permit fitting under desk or table surfaces. Detachable armrests permit side transfers.[11]

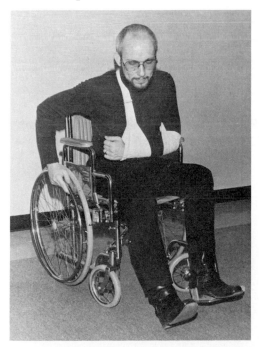

Fig. 5-2. Persons with hemiplegia can propel standard wheelchair by using unaffected arm and leg.

Footrests may be standard swinging detachable or swinging detachable and elevating. The standard footrests are fixed to the wheelchair frame and do not move. They prohibit getting close to counters and may make some types of transfers more difficult. The swinging detachable footrests can be moved to the side of the chair or removed entirely from the chair. They allow a closer approach to bed, bathtub, or counters, and when removed, reduce the overall wheelchair length and weight, for easy loading into a car. They lock into place when on the chair, with a pin- or lever-type locking device. They are recommended for most wheelchair users. Elevating footrests are recommended to aid circulation or when disability necessitates periodic rest. They are usually used when the wheelchair has a reclining backrest.[11] The footrest step plates may have heel loops or toe loops. The heel loops prevent the foot from slipping backward off the step plate. The toe loops help to control involuntary motion and maintain the position of the foot on the step plate.[11]

Backrests are standard or reclining. These may be fully reclining or semireclining. A headrest extension can be added to any backrest to give greater trunk support. The backrest may be obtained in detachable or zip-open styles that allow for a rear transfer.

Wheelchair tires are usually solid. Pneumatic tires are available as well, primarily for rough and uneven surfaces.[11] They are more difficult to use indoors than the solid tires. Some wheelchair users who are active in the outdoors choose to have two wheelchairs to meet their needs.

Before the wheelchair is selected, the therapist(s) should make a home evaluation to ascertain wheelchair accessibility and maneuverability. Deep pile carpets, doorsills, stairs, arrangement of furniture and appliances, floor plan, and entrance can influence wheelchair use in the living place. Modifications to the home, as well as to the wheelchair, may need to be considered. In some instances a change of living place is necessary to accommodate the wheelchair.

If a ramp needs to be installed to allow the wheelchair user to enter and exit, it should be 1 foot of length for every inch of stair height of the home entrance. At this incline the wheelchair user can usually manage the ramp safely and independently.

The life-style of the wheelchair candidate should also be considered. Is he going to be active in sports and outdoor activities? If so heavy-duty construction and pneumatic tires should be considered. Is he going to be involved primarily in indoor work and leisure? If so the universal construction should be adequate. Does he have limited arm strength or endurance? Then the lightweight construction may be the best choice.

These are some of the important considerations before wheelchair prescription and selection. The process should be carefully guided by the professionals working with the client and his family to obtain a wheelchair that fits properly, provides comfort and increased mobility, and is adequate for the client's life-style.

Wheelchair safety

Elements of safety for the wheelchair user and an assistant are as follows:

1. Brakes should be locked during all transfers.
2. Step plates should never be stood on and should be up during transfers.
3. In most transfers it is an advantage to have footrests swung away if possible.
4. If an assistant is pushing the chair, she should be sure that the client's elbows are not protruding from the armrests and hands are *not* on the hand rims. If approaching from behind to assist in moving the wheelchair the assistant should inform the client of this intent and check the position of the feet and arms before proceeding.
5. If the assistant wishes to push the client up a ramp, she should move in a normal, forward direction.
6. If the assistant wishes to push the client down a ramp, she may move down the ramp backwards while the client maintains some control of the large wheels to prevent rapid backward motion. This approach is useful if the grade is relatively steep. Ramps with only a slight grade can be managed in a forward direction if the assistant maintains grasp and pull on the hand grips, and the client again maintains some control of the big wheels to prevent rapid forward motion.
7. An assistant can manage ascending curbs by approaching them forward, tipping the wheelchair back, and using the tipping levers, thus lifting the front casters onto the curb and pushing forward. The large wheels then are in contact with the curb and will roll on with ease as the chair is lifted slightly onto the curb.
8. To descend the curb using a forward approach the wheelchair is tilted backward, and the large wheels are rolled off the curb in a controlled manner, while the front casters are tilted up. When the large wheels are off the curb, the assistant can slowly reduce the tilt of the wheelchair until the casters are once again on the street surface. The curb may be descended using a backward approach. The assistant can move herself and the chair around as the curb is approached. She can tilt the chair back slightly and guide the large wheels off the curb, tilt the chair back to clear the casters, move backward, lower the casters to the street surface, and then turn around.

With good strength and coordination, many clients can be trained to manage curbs independently by doing "wheelies," which require forcefully pulling back on the hand rims to elevate the casters. Clients should be trained to do this under safe and controlled conditions.

Transfer techniques

The major and most obvious purpose of transfers is to move a client from one surface to another. Transfer techniques for moving the client specifically from wheelchair to bed, chair, toilet, or bathtub are included in this section. Assuming that a client has some physical incapacity, it will be necessary for the therapist to assist in or supervise a transfer. Many therapists question which transfer to employ or feel perplexed when a particular one does not succeed with the client. It is important to remember that each client, therapist, and situation is different. The techniques outlined here are not all-inclusive but are basic ones. Each must be adapted for the particular client and his needs.

Preliminary concepts. It is important for the therapist to be aware of the following concepts when selecting and carrying out transfer techniques:

1. The therapist should be aware of the client's assets and deficits, especially his physical and cognitive abilities.
2. The therapist should know her own assets and limitations and whether she can communicate clear, sequential instructions to the client.
3. The therapist should be aware of and employ correct moving and lifting techniques.[13] The following are adapted from the guidelines of the Sister Kenny Institute*:
   a. Maintain broad base of support by standing with feet apart (shoulder's width), knees flexed, and one foot slightly forward. Head and trunk should remain upright.
   b. Maintain center of gravity by carrying, supporting, or lifting others as close to the body as possible.
   c. Lift with the legs, not the back.
   d. Avoid spine rotation; move the feet to turn.
   e. Know personal limitations: do *not* lift alone if in doubt.
4. The therapist should be acutely aware of the safety aspects of transfers.
   a. Maintain all equipment in proper order and state of repair.
   b. Stabilize or lock all surfaces, including wheelchairs, beds, or chairs.

---

*Yates, J., and Lundberg, A.: Moving and lifting patients: principles and techniques, Minneapolis, 1970, Sister Kenny Institute.

c. Employ a transfer belt securely fastened around the client's waist.

d. Clear the work area by removing wheelchair footrests and legrests when possible and armrests when appropriate.

5. The therapist should employ the following basic principles applicable to most transfers:

a. Stabilize surfaces (for *safety*).

b. Equalize heights of surfaces as much as possible.

c. Unless otherwise necessary position wheelchair to bed, chair, or toilet at optimal angle of approximately 60°.

d. Support the client using a transfer belt. If necessary to hold onto the client, support him around his back with an open hand.

e. Avoid grasping the client's arm, as, in general, this offers poor support.

f. Always explain the transfer procedure to the client so that both client and therapist are working toward the same goal.

It is important for the therapist to be familiar with as many types of transfers as possible so that she can resolve each situation as it arises. Some excellent resources regarding transfers, which go beyond the scope of this text, include Sister Kenny Institute publications on transfers and the following texts:

Ford, J.R., and Duckworth, B.: Physical management for the quadriplegic patient, Philadelphia, 1974, F.A. Davis Co.

Hale, G., editor: The source book for the disabled, London, 1979, Paddington Press Ltd.

Kamenetz, H.L.: The wheelchair book, Springfield, Ill., 1969, Charles C Thomas, Publisher.

Directions for some transfer techniques that are most commonly employed in practice are outlined later. The standing-pivot transfers and the seated-sliding transfers to bed, chair, toilet, and bathtub are included. Many classifications of transfers exist, based on the amount of therapist participation. Classifications can range from dependent, where the client is unable to participate and the therapist moves the client, to independent, where the client moves himself while the therapist merely supervises or observes. In general, progression of therapist participation should begin with active assistance, then gradually the assistance is withdrawn if and when the client's abilities and performance improve.

Standing-pivot transfers. The standing-pivot transfer requires that the client is able to come to standing and pivot on one or both feet. It is most commonly used with those clients who have hemiplegia, hemiparesis, or general loss of strength or balance.

Wheelchair-to-bed assisted transfer (Fig. 5-3). The

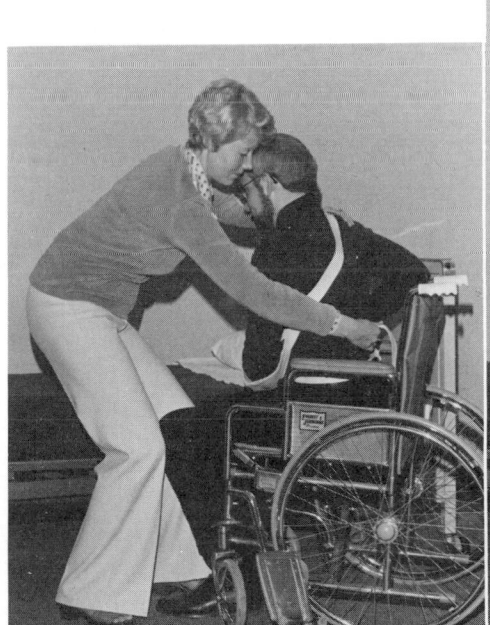 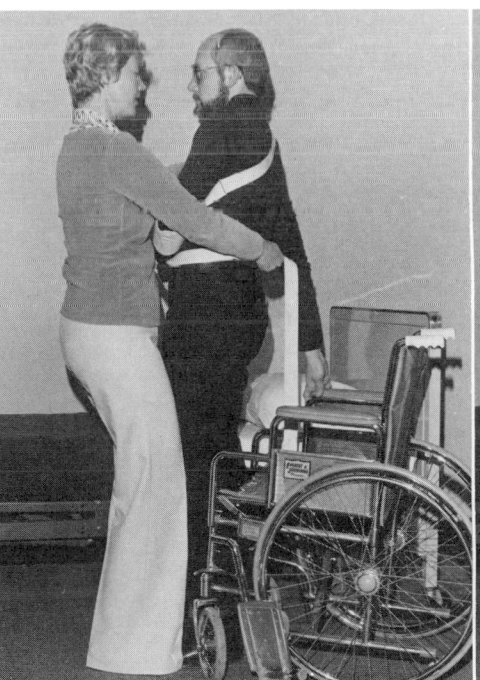 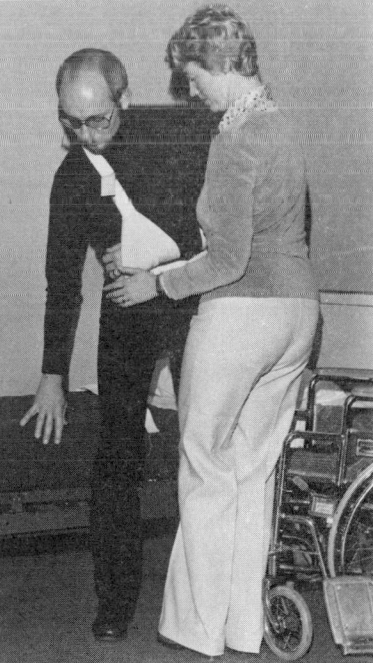

A   B   C

Fig. 5-3. A, Wheelchair and client are prepared for transfer, and therapist is positioned to assist client to stand. **B,** Client is standing and therapist assists him to pivot to prepare to sit down on bed. **C,** Client has completed pivot, reaches for bed, and sits as therapist assists.

procedure for accomplishing the wheelchair-to-bed assisted transfer with client and therapist is as follows:

1. The therapist positions the wheelchair at an approximately 60° angle next to the bed, which should be on the client's stronger side.
2. The therapist sets the brakes and removes the footrests.
3. The therapist positions the client's feet (with shoes on) securely on the floor 6 to 10 inches apart, directly below and slightly behind knees.
4. The therapist applies the transfer belt.
5. The therapist should be sure the client knows the transfer procedure.
6. The therapist positions herself as shown, stabilizing the client's foot and knee with her own.
7. The therapist asks the client to lean forward so that the shoulders are above the knees.
8. The therapist grasps the transfer belt at the client's back and lifts by extending her knees and hips, *not* her back!
9. At the same time the client pushes on the armrest(s) and straightens the lower extremity or extremities.
10. The client comes to a complete standing position.
11. The client pivots on the unaffected foot, as the therapist pivots and repositions her rear foot.
12. The client reaches for the bed and sits as the therapist flexes her knees and hips to lower him, avoiding the use of her back for this maneuver.
13. The therapist then ensures that the client is firmly and safely seated on the bed and assists him to recline.
14. The therapist removes the transfer belt.

Bed-to-wheelchair transfer (Fig. 5-4). The bed-to-wheelchair transfer procedure is essentially the same as the wheelchair-to-bed assisted transfer, except for the following points:

1. The client is positioned on the edge of the bed, sitting with feet securely on the floor. The therapist should be aware of the bed's instability and the possibility of the client slipping from its edge.
2. It is more difficult for the client to come to a standing position, since there is no armrest, and it is difficult to push off from the soft bed.
3. After coming to a standing position and pivoting the client reaches for the armrest to assist in sitting.
4. After the client is sitting, the therapist removes the transfer belt, fastens the seat belt (if used), and repositions the footrests.

Wheelchair-to-chair and return transfer (Fig. 5-5). The wheelchair-to-chair and return transfer is similar to the transfer to bed, as described earlier, except for the following differences:

1. The therapist and the client should be aware that the chair may be light and less stable than a bed.
2. When lowering to the chair the client reaches for the *seat* of the chair. He avoids reaching for the armrest or back of the chair, since this may cause the chair to tip over.
3. When moving from the chair to the wheelchair the client pushes with arm(s) from the seat of the chair as he comes to standing.
4. Standing from a chair is often more difficult if the chair is low or seat cushions are soft.

Wheelchair-to-toilet and return transfer (Fig. 5-6). In general, the wheelchair-to-toilet and return transfer is a very difficult transfer for both the therapist and the client, because of the confined space of most bathrooms, compounded by the client's usual and justified fear of transferring to the slick and small surface area of a toilet seat. Problems that may arise include the following:

1. It may be necessary to position the wheelchair at a greater angle than 60°, often even facing the toilet, requiring up to a 180° pivot.
2. It may not be possible to position the wheelchair so that a hemiplegic client moves *toward* the strong side.
3. The confined quarters may force both the therapist and the client to assume foot positions of less than optimal stability.
4. The client may have to reach for and sit on the toilet seat, but therapist and client should be aware of the instability of the hinged seat.

Some comments should be made concerning removal of lower clothing for toilet use. There are advantages and disadvantages of removing clothing before the transfer or after being seated on the toilet. *Before* the transfer waist closures may be loosened so that trousers and underwear can be lowered when coming to standing. Skirts or dresses may be rolled up or tucked into the belt. This can present problems, since it is often difficult to lower clothing when standing or clothing dropped to knees-ankles may encumber the pivot. *After* the transfer clothes may be removed when seated on the toilet. This, however, requires leaning and hip-hiking (often difficult for the client), and the clothes may get wet in the bowl. No simple solutions are available, except for therapist and client to discover the best and safest method for them.

Independent pivot transfer (Fig. 5-7). All of the transfers just discussed may be accomplished by the client independently; the obvious difference here is that the client does *all* of the tasks. An independent transfer from one surface to another requires the client to perform the following steps:

1. Position wheelchair and set brakes.
2. Flip up or remove footrests.

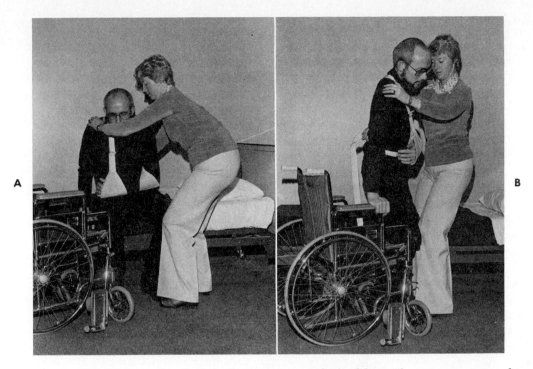

Fig. 5-4. A, Client is seated on bed, ready to move toward wheelchair. Therapist is positioned to assist. **B,** Client has stood and pivoted, reaches for wheelchair armrest, and lowers himself into wheelchair.

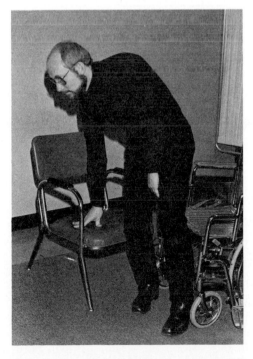

Fig. 5-5. Client, in midtransfer, reaches for seat of chair, pivots, and lowers himself to sitting.

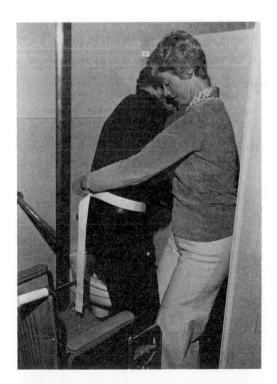

Fig. 5-6. Standing pivot transfer to toilet.

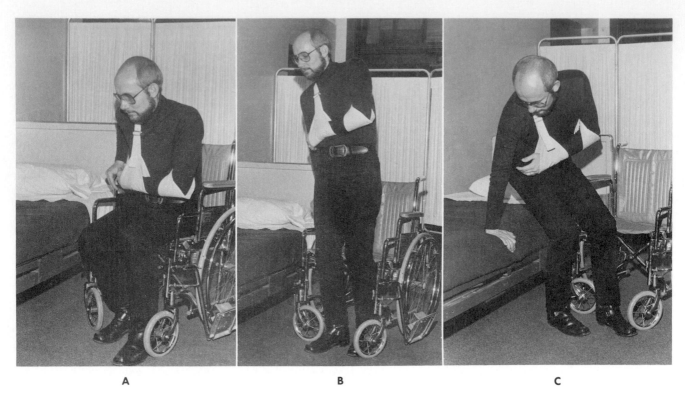

A   B   C

Fig. 5-7. A, Client is properly positioned and leaning on armrest, ready to stand. **B,** Client comes to standing and begins to pivot. **C,** Client reaches for bed and lowers himself to sitting.

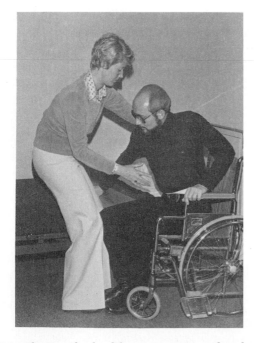

Fig. 5-8. Client and wheelchair are positioned and transfer board has been placed under buttocks and on edge of bed.

3. Scoot forward in chair.
4. Position feet directly below and slightly behind knees at 6 to 10 inches apart.
5. Lean forward so that shoulders are over the knees.
6. Push down with the arm(s) on the armrest(s), while extending the knees and hips.
7. Come to a complete standing position and pivot.
8. Reach for the stable area of a bed, chair, or toilet, and sit.
9. Unlock the wheelchair and reposition (if necessary) to be ready for the return transfer.

Seated-sliding transfers. Seated-sliding transfers are best suited for those individuals who cannot bear weight on the lower extremities or who are too unstable to accomplish a standing transfer. The transfers require the ability to use the upper extremities and are most often employed with persons who have lower extremity amputations or paraplegia or those who have quadriplegia with adequate upper extremity function.

In the previous section on standing-pivot transfers each was first discussed as a therapist assisted the transfer. Subsequently the independent transfer was outlined. In this section the techniques will be discussed from the point of view of the therapist *supervising* the transfer. Active assistance will be assumed to be min-

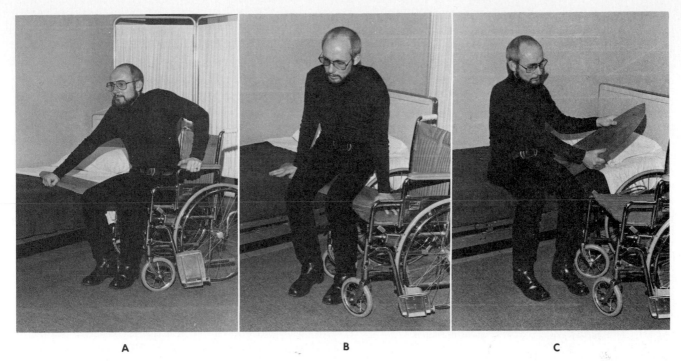

A   B   C

Fig. 5-9. **A,** Client moves across board toward bed. **B,** Client is on middle of transfer board, lifting his weight from surface. **C,** Client reaches bed and removes transfer board.

imal. Initial assistance might include helping the client to move his body by lifting on his transfer belt or ensuring that the client does not fall or injure himself.

It is assumed that all proper lifting, moving, and *safety* techniques are employed. In general, use of additional equipment is discouraged so that the client may learn to perform as independently as possible. With these transfers, however, instruction often begins with the use of a sliding board that is eventually eliminated if and when the client has become stronger and more stable and confident in his transfer abilities. NOTE: The client might initially manifest poor balance and decreased strength, which will require more assistance from the therapist. In general, the therapist should position herself in front of the client to offer both physical and psychological support by holding on to the client's transfer belt (Fig. 5-8).

Wheelchair-to-bed and return transfer with sliding board (Fig. 5-9). The wheelchair-to-bed transfer with a sliding board can be accomplished by using the following procedure:

1. The client positions the locked wheelchair next to the bed at a 60° to 90° angle.
2. The client removes the armrest of the wheelchair that is nearest the bed.
3. The client slips the transfer board under buttocks, as shown, and bridges the board securely across to the bed.

4. The client then lifts his body by pushing down with one hand on the sliding board and the other hand on the seat or arm of the wheelchair.
5. Then by lifting his buttocks from the surface the client moves on the board toward the bed in a series of small shoves or moves.
6. When secure on the bed surface the client removes the sliding board and lifts his legs onto the bed.

To return the following procedure is used:

1. The client sits on the edge of the bed with his feet on the floor for stability (if the bed is low enough).
2. The sliding board is positioned under his buttocks and bridged to the wheelchair.
3. Again, in a series of small moves, the client lifts his body weight and edges to the wheelchair seat.

NOTE: In moving from the wheelchair to the bed or return there is a tendency for the weaker, less stable client to pitch forward or backward. Also, this transfer is made more difficult if surfaces are of unequal heights.

Wheelchair-to-bed and return transfer without sliding board (Fig. 5-10). There are two recommended techniques if the client is stronger and more stable and does not require the use of a sliding board.

The first technique, similar to the transfer just discussed, is as follows:

1. The client positions the locked wheelchair at a 60° to 90° angle next to the bed with the armrest nearest the bed removed.

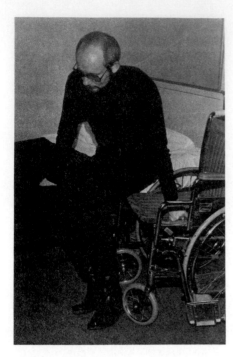

Fig. 5-10. Client has pushed up and is shifting from wheelchair to bed without transfer board.

2. The client positions himself in the wheelchair as close to the bed as possible.
3. The client places one hand on the seat or armrest of the chair (seat preferred for stability) and the other hand approximately 12 to 18 inches onto the bed surface.
4. The client pushes his body weight up from the seat and swings his buttocks onto the bed.
5. The process is reversed to return.

The second technique is a forward-backward approach, whereby the locked wheelchair is positioned directly facing and touching the edge of the bed. This technique, more easily used to move from the bed to the wheelchair, is as follows (Fig. 5-11):

1. The client sits on the bed with his back toward the wheelchair.
2. The client places a hand on each armrest.
3. The client pushes his body up and over into the seat of the wheelchair.

Wheelchair-to-chair and return transfer. The wheelchair-to-chair and return process is very similar to the wheelchair-to-bed transfer. In general, it is best accomplished when the client can transfer without using a sliding board, since a chair allows less room for maneuverability. This transfer is also further complicated because a chair is less stable or secure than a bed. The steps are as in the first seated-sliding transfer described earlier. This transfer is easier than a bed transfer if the

chair used is a hard, straight back type and is of equal height to the wheelchair.

Wheelchair-to-toilet transfer (Fig. 5-12). The wheelchair-to-toilet transfer is also like the first wheelchair-to-bed transfer described earlier if the wheelchair can be positioned next to or at an acute angle to the toilet. In some instances a second method is employed, whereby the wheelchair is positioned facing the toilet as closely as possible. Then by performing a forward-backward transfer the client slides directly on and off the toilet, facing the rear or tank end of the bowl.

Wheelchair-to-bathtub, standing or seated, transfers (Fig. 5-13). The bathtub transfer is more dangerous than others because the bathtub is considered one of the most hazardous areas of the home. It is *not* recommended that a client transfer directly from the wheelchair to the floor of the bathtub but rather from the wheelchair to either a commercially produced bathtub chair or a well-secured straight back chair placed in the bathtub. Therefore whether a standing or sliding transfer is employed, the technique is basically similar to a wheelchair-to-chair transfer. However, the transfer is further complicated by the confined space, the slick bathtub surfaces, and the bathtub wall between the wheelchair and the bathtub seat.

If a standing pivot transfer is employed, it is recommended that the locked wheelchair be placed at a 60° angle to the bathtub if possible. The client should stand, pivot, sit on the bathtub chair, and *then* place the lower extremities into the bathtub.

If a seated transfer is used, the wheelchair is placed next to the bathtub with the armrest removed. The client should then slide to the bathtub chair (with or without a sliding board). In some instances more capable clients may transfer to the edge of the bathtub and then to the bathtub chair or even the bathtub floor. This obviously requires greater strength and balance and good judgment on the part of the client.

In general, the client may exit by first placing his feet securely outside of the bathtub on a nonskid floor surface *and then* performing a standing or seated transfer back to the wheelchair.

Dependent standing transfer (Fig. 5-14). The dependent standing transfer is more specifically designed for use with the individual who has virtually no functional ability. Its purpose is to move the client from surface to surface. The transfer is used with the highly involved quadriplegic client. The requirements are that the client be cooperative and willing to follow the instructions. The therapist should be keenly aware of correct leverage and lifting techniques, as well as her own physical abilities and limitations.

If performed incorrectly this is a potentially dangerous

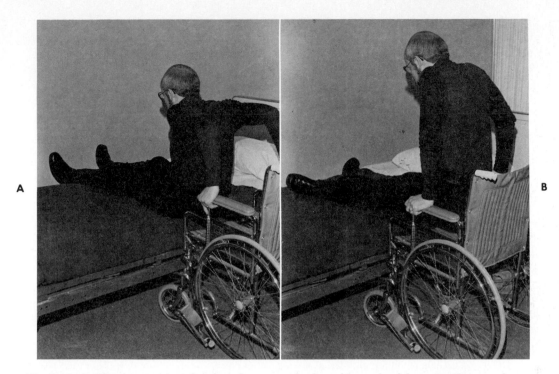

Fig. 5-11. A, Client is positioned and ready to move backward into wheelchair. **B,** Client pushes up and pulls himself back into wheelchair.

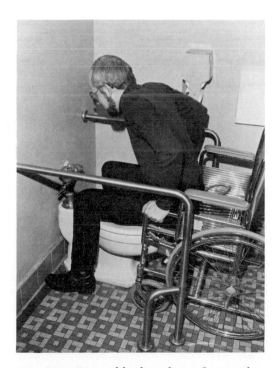

Fig. 5-12. Forward-backward transfer to toilet.

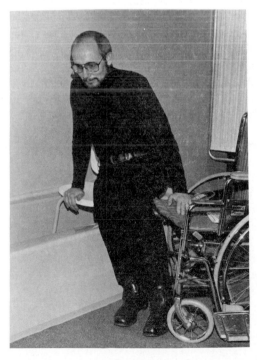

Fig. 5-13. Seated transfer from wheelchair to bathtub chair. Legs are lifted into bathtub following transfer.

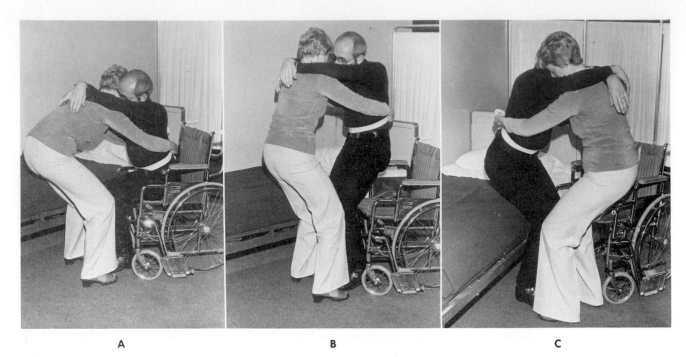

| A | B | C |

Fig. 5-14. A, Wheelchair, client, and therapist are positioned and ready to move. **B,** Therapist assists client to semistanding position and pivots with him toward bed. **C,** Therapist lowers client to bed and assists him to recline.

transfer for both the therapist and the client. Therefore this should be first practiced with able individuals and *initially* employed with the client only if standby assistants are available. The procedure is as follows:

1. The therapist positions the locked wheelchair at a 60° angle to the bed.
2. The therapist positions the client's feet together directly under his knees.
3. The therapist then stabilizes the client's feet by placing her feet laterally to each of the client's feet.
4. The therapist then stabilizes the client's knees by placing her knees toward the anterior-lateral aspect of the client's knees.
5. The therapist assists the client to lean forward over his knees with his arms draped securely over her shoulders.
6. The therapist grasps the transfer belt with both hands toward the midline of the back, positioning herself and the client as close together as possible.
7. The therapist then rocks gently forward and backward with the client to gain momentum.
8. On the count of three, as the client rocks forward, the therapist extends her knees and hips while lifting the belt to bring the client up from the seat, taking care *not* to lift with her back. The therapist stabilizes the client's feet and knees with her feet and knees.
9. At this point one of two actions takes place. Either

the therapist comes to a standing position with the client, pivots in place, and flexes her knees and hips to lower the client to the bed or, without coming to a full stand but using the previously gained momentum, the therapist pivots the client from the wheelchair to the bed in a semiseated position.
10. The therapist secures the client on the bed, assists him to recline, and lifts his feet onto the bed.

This transfer can be adapted to move a client from one surface to another. It is recommended that transfers to other surfaces be attempted only when the therapist and the client feel secure with this first procedure.

THE BICYCLE JIGSAW[1,10]

The bicycle jigsaw is a traditional piece of occupational therapy equipment. The one illustrated is a popular model known as the Oliver Rehabilitation Machine[10] (Fig. 5-15). It has been used for many years. The first bicycle jigsaws used were actual prepower devices employed by carpenters. Later models for therapeutic purposes were devised to allow for a variety of gradations of the activity.

This piece of equipment is one of a few that can provide graded activity for improving lower extremity function. It can be used for strengthening and increasing ROM of the lower extremities, increasing cardiovascular function, and improving physical endurance, coordina-

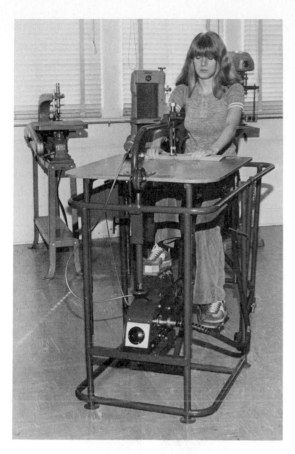

Fig. 5-15. Oliver Rehabilitation Machine or bicycle jigsaw.

tion, and reciprocal movements. In spite of these benefits and a wide variety of possible therapeutic uses, it appears to have fallen into disuse in many treatment facilities. Occupational therapists often claim to treat the "whole" person, yet it sometimes appears that the client is severed at the waist, and the lower extremities are the province of the physical therapist.

It is proposed here that the bicycle jigsaw can be a valuable and useful piece of therapeutic equipment if its uses and functions are understood.

Candidates for use

All clients with disabilities producing lower extremity muscle weakness, incoordination, and loss of joint motion, such as quadriparesis, paraparesis, hemiparesis, multiple sclerosis, and fractures, may benefit from the bicycle jigsaw. Clients with above- and below-knee amputations may use the equipment with special adaptations described by Jones.[7] The bicycle jigsaw is contraindicated for persons with severe spastic paralysis; flexion contractures of the hips and knees, which are severe and irreversible; inflammatory arthritis; osteoarthritis; and severe incoordination.

Goals of treatment

The bicycle jigsaw can be used to achieve or enhance achievement of the following goals:
1. Increase ROM at hips, knees, and ankles.
2. Increase strength of lower extremity musculature, especially hip and knee extensors.
3. Increase physical endurance.
4. Establish reciprocal walking pattern.
5. Stimulate good circulation and healing of injured or residual parts.
6. Improve eye-hand-leg coordination.
7. Increase cardiovascular function.

Use of the Oliver Rehabilitation Machine[1,10]

Adjustments of equipment. The height of the seat above the pedal shaft is adjusted by cranking the handle directly under the seat near the floor. This may be done with the client sitting on the seat. There are numbered calibrations on the shaft supporting the seat. The average height for adults is number 6. The seat is raised to decrease range of hip and knee flexion and increase range of hip and knee extension. The seat is lowered to decrease hip and knee extension and increase hip and knee flexion.

The pedal radius is adjusted by loosening the pedal with a socket wrench and an allen wrench simultaneously. The pedal is moved to the desired level on the shaft and fixed in place by tightening with wrenches. There are numbered calibrations from 1 to 7 (6 to 13 inches) in diameter on the pedal shaft. The average radius is number 4. The pedal is above number 4 to increase ROM at hip and knees and below number 4 to decrease ROM at hip and knees.

The toe and heel supports of the pedal footboards are adjusted by turning thumbscrews under the footboards and sliding support backward or forward. These are adjusted for size of foot and to lend maximum support. If the toe and heel supports are positioned forward, the foot will tend to be positioned in plantar flexion as the pedal rotates around. If the toe and heel supports are positioned backward, this will tend to position the foot in dorsiflexion as the pedal rotates around. Increasing pedal radius increases the leverage and results in easier pedaling.

The distance of the seat to the tabletop is adjusted by pushing the seat cradle forward or backward. The pin is placed through the holes in the seat cradle and the locating bars on the worktable unit. There are numbered calibrations on the locating bars. The average position is number 2. The seat unit is pushed forward or backward for working comfort or to increase or decrease ROM in combination with seat height and pedal radius adjustments.

The brake is adjusted by turning the knob at the side

Date	Seat cradle location	Seat height	Pedal crank no.	Table height	Gear position
Duration of treatment	Speed to be maintained	Brake position	Mileage at start of session	Mileage at end of session	Saw head or drill head

Fig. 5-16. Form for recording progress and settings on bicycle jigsaw.

or front of the gearbox assembly. The higher numbers increase resistance to pedaling, whereas the lower numbers decrease resistance to pedaling. Calibrations allow for recording progress and keeping record of the desired setting for the client.

Gears can be shifted to numbers 1, 2, or 3 by pressing down on the small lever at the right side of the worktable unit. The lowest position is the lowest gear and reduces resistance to pedaling. The highest position is the highest gear and increases resistance to pedaling. Resistance may also be controlled by the type of wood or material used for sawing.

The position of the back of the seat is adjusted forward or backward by turning the handle under the back of the seat. The seat is usually set all the way back. The forward position of the seat back increases hip flexion. Adjustments are made for comfort and correct posture of the client. The seat back height is adjusted by turning the handle to the right of the seat back and sliding the back up or down on its shaft.

Speedometer and odometer dials are at the right of the saw assembly support. These measure miles per hour and the total miles pedaled. They are useful as motivating devices and a means of recording day-to-day progress of physical endurance. They provide a guide for maintaining rhythmic pedaling to the client.

Table height is adjusted by turning the screw handles on the forward vertical table posts and cranking the jack at the back of the jigsaw just above the gear box. The vertical post on the left is calibrated from numbers 1 to 13, and the average position is number 5 or 6. The purpose of adjusting the table height is for working comfort and good visibility.

Procedure for use. To transfer the client to the seat the seat cradle unit is removed from the worktable unit. The client is wheeled up to the worktable unit so he is facing the saw. The client then stands or is assisted to stand up in front of the saw and holds onto the cutout handles on the tabletop. The seat cradle is then brought up to the back of the client, with the seat lowered to the height of the groin. The client is instructed to or assisted to lower himself onto the seat, still holding onto the tabletop handles. The seat cradle is moved forward on the locating bars, and the pins are secured in the first or second notch. Feet are secured on the pedals and the seat cradle is pushed forward to correct the working position. The pins are repositioned.

The foot pedals are prepositioned for the correct radius. The feet are placed on the pedals and the toe and heel supports are adjusted to accommodate the client's foot. The feet are strapped in position. The seat is set at the correct height by raising it, so that the knee joint is at a 165° to 170° angle when the leg is extended with the pedal in the lowest position. The backrest is raised or lowered so that it fits in the lumbar curve for the correct support and comfort.

The gears are adjusted to the client's need and power. Treatment usually begins with the lowest gear and is

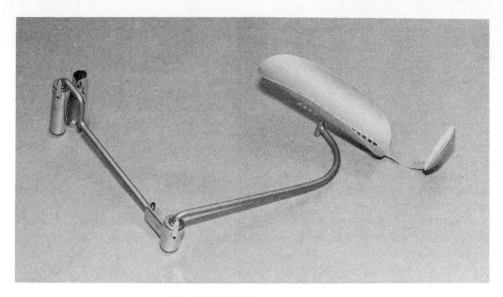

Fig. 5-17. Mobile arm support.

graded to the highest. The worktable is adjusted in height so that it is level with the client's elbows.

To start pedaling the client begins with one pedal raised to a position 30° in front of the vertical, for the best mechanical advantage to overcome the initial inertia of the machine. The therapist may have to assist manually if the client cannot overcome the initial inertia of the machine. The client then pedals, maintaining a uniform rate of speed by referring to the speedometer. An average rate is 10 to 15 miles per hour. Quick pedaling is best for mobilization of joints, and slow, strong pedaling is best for increasing strength. Fig. 5-16 is a suggested form for recording progress and settings on the bicycle jigsaw.

Common substitution patterns used on the bicycle jigsaw include (1) rocking the pelvic girdle to assist pedaling, which may mean that the seat is too high; (2) pushing the knee with the hand to substitute for quadriceps action; (3) using the momentum of the machine to carry the legs along; (4) pedaling with one leg, carrying the weaker leg along passively; (5) abducting and externally rotating the hip to substitute for weak or absent hip flexion; and (6) bending forward at the hip to use extensor power of the gluteus maximi.

THE MOBILE ARM SUPPORT[3a, 4]

The mobile arm support (MAS), referred to as a feeder, is usually mounted on the wheelchair backrest upright (Fig. 5-17). It is adjusted so that gravity is used to assist weak muscles. Various adjustments are possible, and these are individualized to suit the needs of the particular client. The MAS provides assistance for shoulder and elbow movement by using gravity to aid lost muscle power. It provides a large, usable range of arm motion over the tabletop that would otherwise not be available to the client. It helps support, assist, and strengthen weakened musculature and enables clients to perform simple ADL and recreational and avocational activities that they could not perform without them.[3]

Candidates for use of the mobile arm support

Generally those clients with disabilities that result in muscle weakness but intact coordination, such as poliomyelitis, spinal cord injuries, and muscular dystrophy, are candidates for MAS. When there is moderate to severe muscle weakness in the upper extremities (muscle grades 0 to F at the elbow and grades 0 to F at the shoulder) and limited endurance for sustained movement, the MAS could increase function.[3a]

The client must have a source of muscle power to initiate movement of the MAS. This may be at the neck, trunk, shoulder, or leg. There must be adequate, pain-free ROM as follows: (1) shoulder flexion to 90°, abduction to 90°, external rotation to 30°, and internal rotation to 80°; (2) elbow flexion from 25° to 140°; (3) full forearm pronation from midposition and supination to midposition; and (4) hip flexion from 0° to 100°.

The client must have sufficient coordination to cope with and control movement of the freely swinging arms of the MAS. Involuntary movement precludes effective use. There must be sufficient motivation to use the MAS and enough frustration tolerance to persevere at the training program until use is mastered. Sitting tolerance and balance must be adequate to engage in the training program, and later, make use of the MAS worthwhile.[4]

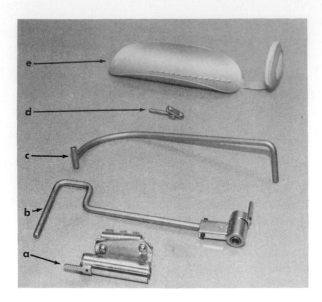

Fig. 5-18. Parts of mobile arm support. *a*, Bracket assembly. *b*, Proximal swivel arm. *c*, Distal swivel arm. *d*, Rocket arm assembly. *e*, Forearm trough.

Parts and their functions[3]

The parts of the MAS are shown in Fig. 5-18. The *bracket assembly* holds the MAS to the chair. It supports the proximal arm and controls the height of the MAS. It can be adjusted to assist horizontal movement at the shoulder and elbow. It may be adapted for use in the reclining position, but the upright position is most desirable.[4] The *proximal swivel arm* permits shoulder motions and contains the distal ball bearings. It may be adjusted to produce a second inclined plane to allow gravity to assist elbow motion. The *distal swivel arm* permits forearm motion in the horizontal plane. It supports the rocker arm assembly and forearm trough. Attached to the forearm trough is the *rocker arm assembly*. It is positioned in the distal swivel arm and permits vertical (hand-to-mouth) motions. It swivels to produce added horizontal motion. The *forearm trough* supports the forearm. It offers stable elbow support but may limit elbow extension. The elbow dial can be bent to produce adjustments for comfort and vertical motions. The elbow dial is sometimes removed.[3]

How the MAS works

The client must use a source of muscle power to get the device swinging back and forth for horizontal motions and use available muscle power to perform vertical motions. Gravity can be used to assist movement in the direction of weakest motion by adjusting parts of the MAS. The ball bearing bracket assembly tilts to allow gravity to assist either shoulder flexion and adduction or shoulder extension and abduction. The position of the rocker arm assembly may be adjusted under the forearm trough to assist internal or external rotation for vertical motions.

Adjustment and checkout of the MAS[2]

To adjust the MAS the therapist must find the best position for the client in the wheelchair, choose the correct bracket assembly for the arm being fitted, since the right and left are not interchangeable, and set the height of the bracket to position the whole MAS at the proper height for the client. The forearm trough is then fitted to the client. It is balanced for maximum range and force in vertical motion. The bracket is adjusted for maximum range and force in horizontal motion at the glenohumeral joint. The therapist must then tilt the distal bearing, if necessary, to produce the maximum range and force in horizontal motion at the elbow joint. She should then reevaluate range and force of combined horizontal motions of the glenohumeral and elbow joints and reevaluate the vertical motion of the trough. Some clients may require special attachments such as straps to stabilize the forearm in the trough.

The following questions can serve as a guide for the therapist to determine the correctness of fit and adjustments of the MAS.[2]

1. Are the client's hips set back in the chair?
2. Is the spine in good vertical alignment?
3. Does the client have lateral trunk stability?
4. Is the chair seat adequate for comfort and stability?
5. Is the client able to sit upright?
6. If the client wears hand splints, does he have them on?
7. Does the client meet requirements for passive ROM?
8. Are all the screws tight?
9. Is the bracket tight on the wheelchair?
10. Are all arms and joints freely movable?
11. Is the proximal arm all the way down in the bracket?
12. Is the bracket at the proper height so that the shoulders are not forced into elevation?
13. Does the elbow dial clear the lapboard when the trough is in the "up" position?
14. When the trough is in the "up" position, is the client's hand as close to his mouth as possible?
15. Can the client obtain maximum active reach?
16. Is the trough short enough to allow wrist flexion?
17. Are the trough edges rolled so that they do not contact the forearm?
18. Is the elbow secure and comfortable in the elbow support?
19. Is the trough balanced correctly?

20. In vertical motion is the dial free of the distal arm?
21. Can the client control motion of the proximal arm from either extreme?
22. Can the client control motion of the distal arm from either extreme?
23. Can the client control vertical motion of the trough from either extreme?
24. Have stops been applied to limit range, if necessary?
25. What is the client's maximum reach in front of his body (measured from the bracket)?
26. What is the distance between the two extremes of the horizontal arc?
27. What is the client's vertical range (in degrees)?
28. What is the maximum weight the client can lift from the lapboard to the face?
29. What is the distance from the hand to the mouth when the trough is in the "up" position?

Training in use of the MAS

The therapist should be sure that supports are fitting well and adjusted correctly before attempting to instruct the client in their use. If two MASs are used, the client should practice with one at a time until each is mastered. Bilateral use of MASs requires considerable practice. Early use includes training in vertical motions (external and internal rotation of the shoulder). External rotation is accomplished by depressing the shoulder to elevate the hand, shifting the body weight to the side of the MAS, rolling the shoulder back, tilting or turning the head toward the side of the device, or leaning backward. Internal rotation is accomplished by gravity, elevating the shoulder on the same side as the mobile arm support, shifting the body weight to the opposite side from the device, rolling the shoulder forward, tilting and turning the head to the opposite side from the MAS, or leaning forward. Work is started on horizontal adduction and abduction with the trough balanced at midposition. Then the client can proceed to practice these motions with the trough at various heights between wheelchair tray and head. Practice progresses to include elbow flexion and extension with the trough at various heights. Activities that are designed to offer practice in the use of MASs are typing on an electric typewriter, turning book pages, dialing the phone, playing the chord organ, and playing games, such as checkers, chess, cards, and puzzles.

The MAS offers the client with significant upper extremity weakness the necessary assistance to make maximum use of minimal muscle power. Once assembled, fitted, and adjusted it enables the client to perform a variety of self-care and avocational activities that promote self-esteem, a sense of independence, and pleasure in doing. The reader is referred to the supplementary readings for more comprehensive discussion of MASs and their use.

REVIEW QUESTIONS

1. If the wheelchair is properly fitted, what is the correct seat width?
2. What is the danger of having a wheelchair seat that is too deep?
3. What is the minimum distance for safety from the floor to the bottom of the wheelchair step plate?
4. List three types of wheelchair frames and the general uses of each.
5. Describe three types of wheelchair propulsion systems and when each would be used.
6. What are the advantages of detachable desk arms and swing-away footrests?
7. Discuss the factors for consideration before wheelchair selection.
8. Name and discuss the rationale for at least three general wheelchair safety principles.
9. Describe or demonstrate how to descend a curb in a wheelchair with the help of an assistant.
10. Describe or demonstrate how to descend a ramp in a wheelchair with the help of an assistant.
11. List four safety principles for correct moving and lifting technique during wheelchair transfers.
12. Describe or demonstrate the basic standing-pivot transfer from wheelchair to bed and wheelchair to toilet.
13. Describe or demonstrate the wheelchair-to-bed transfer, using a sliding board.
14. Name three conditions in which the bicycle jigsaw would not be beneficial and tell why in each instance.
15. List two primary goals of treatment when using the bicycle jigsaw as a treatment method.
16. List two adjustments on the bicycle jigsaw that will increase ROM at the hip and knee.
17. List two adjustments on the bicycle jigsaw that can increase or decrease resistance to pedaling.
18. Describe three substitution patterns therapists should watch for when the client is using the bicycle jigsaw.
19. Describe the procedure for transferring a wheelchair client to the bicycle jigsaw.
20. What kinds of clients are good candidates for use of the MAS (in terms of disability or muscle grades)?
21. What kinds of clients are poor candidates for use of the MAS? Why?
22. List the five criteria a client must meet to use the MAS successfully.
23. Describe how the MAS works (refer to parts and their functions, how the device is activated, and how it is adjusted so that gravity assists movement).
24. What kinds of activities can be performed with the MAS that could not be performed without it?
25. List the three major steps in training the client to use MAS.
26. List two ways external rotation motion can be accomplished.
27. List two ways internal rotation motion can be accomplished.
28. What are some activities that are good for practicing use of the MAS?

REFERENCES

1. Anonymous: Bicycle saw, Minneapolis, Sister Kenny Rehabilitation Institute. Mimeographed.
2. Anonymous: How to fit and adjust a ball bearing feeder, Downey, Calif., 1962, Rancho Los Amigos Hospital. Mimeographed.

3. Anonymous: Mobile arms supports, ball bearing, suspension, and friction feeders, parts and their function, Downey, Calif., 1962, Rancho Los Amigos Hospital. Mimeographed.

3a. Anonymous: The uses and limitations of mobile arm supports, Downey, Calif., 1962, Rancho Los Amigos Hospital. Mimeographed.

4. Dicus, R.G.: Mobile arm supports, part 1, film, Downey, Calif., 1970, Rancho Los Amigos Hospital, S.R.S. Service Dept. (Available at the Instructional Resources Center, San Jose State University.)

5. Ford, J.R., and Duckworth, B.: Physical management for the quadriplegic patient, Philadelphia, 1974, F.A. Davis Co.

6. Hale, G., editor: The source book for the disabled, London, 1979, Paddington Press Ltd.

7. Jones, M.S.: An approach to occupational therapy, London, 1964, Butterworth & Co. Ltd.

8. Kamenetz, H.L.: The wheelchair book, Springfield, Ill., 1969, Charles C Thomas, Publisher.

9. Modification and accessory analysis form, Los Angeles, Calif., 1972, Everest and Jennings, Inc.

10. Oliver, E.R.: The Oliver Rehabilitation Machine, Nottingham, England, Nottingham Handcraft Company.

11. Wheelchair features and benefits, Los Angeles, Calif., 1969, Everest and Jennings, Inc.

12. Wheelchair prescription: measuring the patient, Los Angeles, Calif., 1968, Everest and Jennings, Inc.

13. Yates, J., and Lundberg, A.: Moving and lifting patients: principles and techniques, Minneapolis, 1970, Sister Kenny Institute.

SUPPLEMENTARY READING

Flaherty, P., and Jurkovich, S.: Transfers for patients with acute and chronic conditions, Minneapolis, 1970, Sister Kenny Institute.

Thenn, J.E.: Mobile arm support, installation, and use, Brookfield, Ill., 1975, Fred Sammons, Inc.

Trombly, C.A., and Scott, A.D.: Occupational therapy for physical dysfunction, Baltimore, 1979. The Williams & Wilkins Co.

Chapter 6

Hand splinting

The purposes of this chapter are to introduce the reader to the elementary principles of hand splinting and to enable him or her to construct and evaluate two hand splints through the use of a self-instruction program. The reader is referred to other sources[3,4] for in-depth study of hand splinting.

It is important for the occupational therapist to understand the principles of hand splinting and to be able to construct some types of hand splints. The occupational therapist is usually the professional who works most closely with hand rehabilitation. Therefore she is depended on to analyze hand dysfunction, make suggestions for splinting needs, evaluate splint performance, and train the client in the use of the splint.[1,6] The occupational therapist may determine when the goals of splinting have been achieved, recommend changes in the splint, or see that its use is discontinued.[3]

Temporary splints made of high- and low-temperature thermoplastic materials are often made by the occupational therapist. These splints are usually used in treating temporary conditions of muscle weakness and joint limitation. They may be used to prevent or correct deformity, substitute for lost muscle power, and assist weak muscles in normal patterns of motion.

Splints required for long-term use to treat permanent conditions are often made of metal and should be referred to a certified orthotist for design and construction.[2]

NORMAL HAND FUNCTION

The occupational therapist must understand normal hand function and hand-to-upper extremity relationships to perform splint design and construction accurately and effectively.

The normal hand has many assets, several of which cannot be replaced or helped with splints. The normal hand is capable of mobility and stability at all joints. Splinting can provide one or the other but usually not both. The normal hand has strength and skill in a wide variety of grasp and prehension patterns. Splinting may assist in only one or two patterns such as palmar prehension or grasp. The normal hand has considerable dexterity and can move in a quick, accurate manner. The use of a splint may aid in the ultimate recovery of dexterity, but while the splint is being worn, dexterity is hindered or limited. Sensation is a major asset of the normal hand. The normal hand has the ability to sense pain and temperature and interpret qualities of objects, such as size, weight, and texture. Splinting can do nothing to aid sensation and actually limits sensation during wear.

The normal hand has unique padding on the palm and fingertips that contributes to the effectiveness of grasp and pinch. Splinting may limit or hinder the function of this unique padding. The hand is supplied with complex blood-vascular and lymphatic systems. Effective splinting and splint use can aid good circulation, whereas poor splinting can limit circulation. Finally the hand has cosmetic significance in that, after the face, it is a primary organ of expression. After splinting a more cosmetically acceptable hand may be achieved, but during splinting the hand is less cosmetically appealing.[1]

The joints of the upper extremity must have adequate ROM to ensure normal hand function. This will allow the hand to reach the object or perform the activity. Joints of the hand and arm must have stability and the ability to be fixed or to co-contract at any point in their ranges of motion. The hand and arm must have enough muscle power for the reaching, placing, performing, or holding that is required by the task to be done.[3]

Wide ranges of shoulder motions are critical to placing the hand at some distance from the body, such as extending over the head and reaching behind and out to the side of the body. A lesser degree of shoulder motion is essential for hand-to-mouth and hand-to-body activities such as toileting and combing hair.[3]

To perform hand-to-face activities the elbow must have full range of flexion. Full extension is required if activities at some distance from the body are to be accomplished such as putting on socks or reaching to high shelves. Pronation and supination are essential for placing the hand at the correct angle for holding or activity performance.

Lesser ranges of motion at the wrist are required for basic hand function. More important is the wrist's sta-

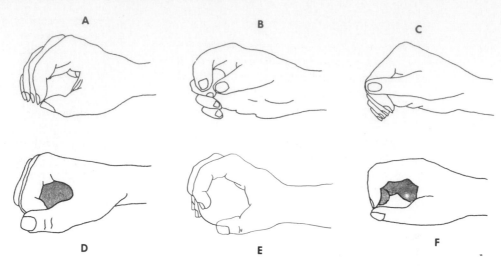

Fig. 6-1. Basic types of prehension and grasp. **A,** Fingertip prehension. **B,** Palmar prehension. **C,** Lateral prehension. **D,** Cylindrical grasp. **E,** Spherical grasp. **F,** Hook grasp.

bility. For the hand to function maximally it should be possible to stabilize the wrist at any point in its ROM and make fine adjustments in the degree of wrist motion. This ability to stabilize and make fine adjustments in the wrist contributes to the fine coordination possible in the hand. Wrist extension is most important, since finger flexion and grasp are best performed with the wrist in extension. If the wrist is flexed, grasp will be limited and the arches of the hand will tend to flatten.

Prehension and grasp are the primary functions of the hand. Hand movements are complex and occur in smooth sequence and combinations. However, it is possible to reduce these movements to several basic types of prehension and grasp.[3]

Types of prehension and grasp (Fig. 6-1)

Fingertip prehension (Fig. 6-1, *A*). Fingertip prehension, contact of the thumb pad with that of the index or middle fingers, is used to pick up small objects, such as pins, nails, and buttons, and to fasten buttons and snaps and hold a needle for sewing. It requires very fine coordination.

Palmar prehension (Fig. 6-1, *B*). Palmar prehension, also called "three-jaw chuck grip" or "palmar tripod pinch,"[3] is the contact of the thumb pad with the middle and index fingers. It is the most common type of prehension and requires a high level of coordination. It is used to pick up and hold small square, cylindrical, or spherical objects, such as a marble, pen, or small cube, and is the prehension pattern used for holding a pen or eating utensil.

Lateral prehension (Fig. 6-1, *C*). During lateral prehension the thumb pad is in contact with the lateral surface of the index finger at the middle or distal phalanx. For this to be a functional prehension pattern the thumb and index finger must have good stability, and the first dorsal interosseous muscle must have good to normal strength. The fourth and fifth fingers must act as a support to the index and middle fingers. Lateral prehension is used for turning a key or thumbscrew, carrying a plate or teacup, and winding a watch. It is a stronger type of prehension than fingertip or palmar prehension and requires less coordination to perform.

Cylindrical grasp (Fig. 6-1, *D*). The cylindrical grasp is the position the normal hand assumes when holding objects, such as a tumbler, rail, hammer, or pot handle. The object is stabilized against the palm by the fingers, which close or flex around it. Intrinsic and thenar muscle strength are essential to the power of this grasp. It is one of the earliest grasp patterns, occurring reflexly in infants and developing later into voluntary gross grasp.[3]

Spherical grasp (Fig. 6-1, *E*). The spherical grasp, also called "ball grasp," is the position the normal hand assumes when grasping a small rubber ball such as a tennis ball. The five fingers are flexed around the object and hold it against the palm, which is in an arched position. It is used to hold balls, apples, oranges, and round doorknobs. Its power depends on the stability of the wrist and finger joints and the strength of the intrinsic and extrinsic muscles of the hand.

Hook grasp (Fig. 6-1, *F*). The hook grasp is the position the normal hand assumes when carrying a briefcase or similar bag handle. The grip can be accomplished entirely by the fingers. The thumb remains outside the fingers and is relatively passive. It acts simply to close the hook, but its presence and power are not essential to hook function. The hook grasp requires strength and stability of the IP joints, primarily. The MP joints and the wrist remain in the neutral position and need not be completely stabilized. This type of grasp is used to carry heavy objects, such as pails, suitcases, and shopping bags, and may also be used to pull open drawers and cabinets with hardware that require four fingers to hook to pull them.

Arches of the hand (Fig. 6-2)

There are three arches of the hand that must be considered when making splints. There are the metacarpal and carpal transverse arches and the longitudinal arch.

Metacarpal transverse arch. The metacarpal transverse arch lies across the distal metacarpal heads at a slightly oblique angle. The second and third metacarpal bones are relatively stable elements in the arch, whereas the fourth and fifth metacarpal bones are the more mobile elements. The normal arch increases as the hand is used functionally. The dexterity and function of the fingers are dependent on the mobility and flexibility of this arch. Grasp function will be impaired if the mobility of the metacarpal bones is limited and if the transverse arch is flattened or prevented from increasing during functional use. These conditions can be caused by poor positioning of the hand in the splint, poorly constructed or ill-fitting splints, intrinsic paralysis, edema, and scarring and contracture of the dorsal skin of the hand.[3]

The arch should be considered in splinting, since the splint should be designed to maintain the normal arch of the hand and allow the arch to increase during hand use. If the metacarpal transverse arch is flattened, the thumb will be unable to oppose the fingers and thus hand function will be considerably impaired.

Carpal transverse arch. The carpal transverse arch is located at the wrist. It is troughlike and is formed by the annular ligaments and carpal bones. It provides the mechanical advantage to the finger flexor tendons by acting as the fulcrum.

Longitudinal arch. The longitudinal arch follows the long lines of the carpal and metacarpal bones at a slightly oblique angle and primarily involves the third finger. The relationship of this arch to the metacarpal transverse arch accounts for the dual obliquity of the hand. The carpal and metacarpal bones are the fixed units, and the fingers through their flexion and extension abilities are the mobile units. This flexibility allows for a wide range of prehension patterns. The function of the longitudinal arch can be disturbed by intrinsic paralysis, poor hand positioning, edema, scarring of the dorsal skin, and adhesions of extensor tendons or bony obstructions.[3]

Creases of the hand (Fig. 6-3)

The palmar skin is tough and not very pliable or mobile. These qualities allow for stability and fixation of

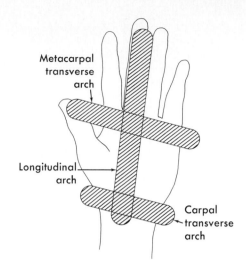

Fig. 6-2. Arches of hand.

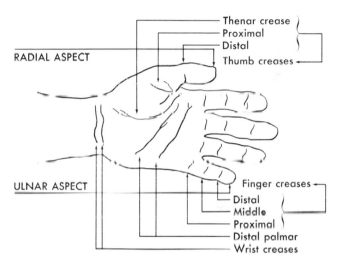

Fig. 6-3. Palmar creases of hand. (Reproduced with author's permission from Malick, M.H.: Manual on static hand splinting, Pittsburgh, Harmarville Rehabilitation Center.)

the palmar skin during motion and grasp. The palm has several skin creases that can act as guides in individual design and fitting of splints.

Splints should not obstruct the distal palmar crease if full MP flexion is to be allowed. The thenar crease must not be obstructed if opposition is to occur or if the hand is to be in the position of function. The wrist creases are good points for locating the wrist strap if the splint is to remain in a good position and not slide forward.[3]

Position of function (Fig. 6-4)

The functional position of the hand is a position similar to that which the hand assumes when grasping a

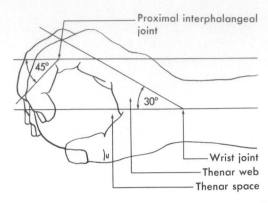

Fig. 6-4. Position of function, lateral view, right hand. (Reproduced with author's permission from Malick, M.H.: Manual on static hand splinting, Pittsburgh, Harmarville Rehabilitation Center.)

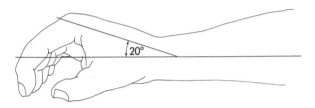

Fig. 6-5. Position of rest. (Reproduced with author's permission from Malick, M.H.: Manual on static hand splinting, Pittsburgh, Harmarville Rehabilitation Center.)

ball. The wrist is in 20° to 30° of extension. The transverse metacarpal arch is rounded. The thumb is in abduction and is in opposition to the pads of the four fingers. The metacarpal joints are flexed to about 30° and the PIP joints are flexed to about 45°.[3]

The functional position of the hand may be described as the midposition of the ROM of every joint. In this position there is equal tension of all musculature, and the muscles are in the best mechanical position for efficient function.

The functional position is an important concept, since it is usually desirable to splint the hand in a position as near the functional position as possible.[1] Placing the hand in the functional position alone will improve its performance and decrease the possibility of developing deformity in many instances.

Position of rest (Fig. 6-5)

The position of rest is slightly more relaxed than the position of function. It is similar to the position the normal hand assumes when resting passively on a tabletop. The wrist is in 10° to 20° of extension. All finger joints are slightly flexed. The thumb is in partial opposition and abduction, and the thumb pad faces the pad

of the index finger. The metacarpal, carpal, and longitudinal arches are maintained when the hand is in the position of rest.[3] The hand is often splinted in this position in a static resting splint if joint rest or prevention of deformity is desirable in conditions such as peripheral nerve injuries and rheumatoid arthritis.

PRINCIPLES OF HAND SPLINTING
Types of splints

There are two types of hand splints—static and dynamic. *Static splints* have no moving parts. Except in special circumstances they should hold the involved part in a functional position or as close to a functional position as is physically possible. The antideformity splint for the burned hand is an exception to this rule. Its position is determined by the importance of preventing thumb web space contracture and shortening of the collateral ligaments at the MP joints.

All splints should be designed to meet the client's physiological and functional needs. The splint must achieve the desired purposes while not creating dysfunction. All static splints must be removed periodically for exercise of the affected part, and the client should be encouraged to use the part as frequently as possible while wearing the splint.[3]

Static splints may be used for three major purposes. The first purpose is for protection of weak muscles. A static splint can protect weak muscles from overstretching and therefore prevent their antagonists from contracture. Prevention of overstretching muscles weak because of temporary paralysis is important to ensure good function when nerve and muscle recovery occurs.

The second major purpose of static splints is for support. A joint may be supported or immobilized for resting purposes, as in rheumatoid arthritis, or for healing purposes, as in tendon lacerations and skin grafting. The function of the hand can often be improved if the wrist is supported in extension. Therefore a simple static wrist cock-up splint can improve finger function for grasp and prehension.

The third major purpose of static splinting is for prevention or correction of deformity. The splint may be designed to force the involved joint into correct or near correct alignment, such as the protective ulnar drift splint used in rheumatoid arthritis.[5]

The *dynamic hand splint* has a static base and one or more moving parts. Thus the same splint may incorporate both static and dynamic elements. Some parts may be supported in their best anatomical position for function, whereas other parts are assisted in movement by the dynamic feature of the splint. The splint is designed to apply a relatively constant force on a part as it moves. It provides mobility to the joints with control on the direction and degree of motion. The splint is designed

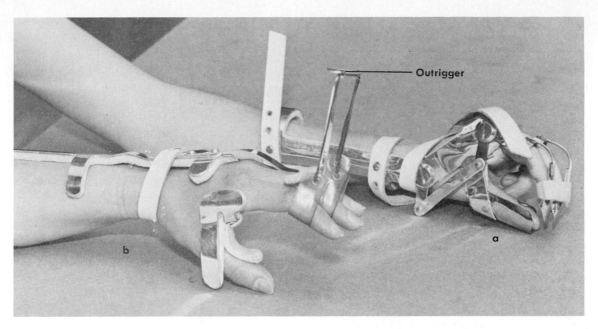

Fig. 6-6. *a*, Wrist driven flexor hinge splint. Wrist extension effects palmar prehension; flexing or dropping wrist effects release. *b*, MP extensor assist. Finger extension is assisted by tension of rubber bands attached to outrigger.

to assist weak muscles or substitute for lost muscle power.[4]

Movement in dynamic splints may be effected by another part of the body or available muscle group, as in the wrist-driven flexor hinge splint (Fig. 6-6, *A*); by springs, pulleys, and rubber bands, as in the wrist cock-up splint with outrigger and MP extensor assist (Fig. 6-6, *B*); or by an external power source such as electricity or gas.[4,6]

General guidelines for splint design and fitting

The wrist is the key joint of the upper extremity in relation to hand function. Wrist stability is essential to optimum function of hand muscles, and wrist extension is critical to forceful grasp and prehension patterns. When the wrist is flexed due to pain, paralysis, or deformity, the long extensor tendons stretch, the metacarpal transverse arch flattens, and the thumb drifts into the plane of the palm of the hand. To prevent this nonfunctional position and potential deformity from developing, the wrist should be splinted in slight extension. There are exceptions, of course, depending on the particular dysfunction, limitations already present at the wrist, degree of paralysis, and goals of hand splinting. Individual variations in wrist positioning will depend on these factors and should be determined by the therapist in concert with the supervising physician.

The MP joints are the key joints of the fingers. Their ability to flex and be stabilized at any point in their range of flexion is critical to grasp and prehension. When the

MP joints are hyperextended, the IP joints flex due to the stretch placed on the long flexor tendons of the fingers in this position. If the MP joints are allowed to remain in hyperextension for a prolonged period, claw-hand deformity may ultimately develop. In the extended or hyperextended position the MP joints will become limited in their ROM or immobilized because of shortening and thickening of the collateral ligaments. These ligaments are at their shortened length when the MP joints are extended.[1] If the collateral ligaments develop contractures due to poor positioning, MP flexion may be difficult or impossible even if recovery of muscle function occurs. If splinted the MP joints should be positioned between 30° and 80° of flexion, depending on the particular dysfunction and the goals of splinting.

The thumb is the most valuable element of the hand. One or two other fingers and the thumb will make a more functional hand than four fingers and no thumb. Thumb opposition is critical to all of the prehension patterns. It acts as a flexible force in strong grasp patterns. It must be possible for the thumb to rotate at the CMC joint if true opposition of thumb pad to finger pads is to take place. Hand splints are often used to stabilize and position the thumb properly for some grasp and prehension patterns.[1] In some instances splints may be used to assist thumb extension, abduction, or opposition.[4]

The normal hand can perform a wide variety of prehension and grasp patterns, which have already been reviewed. The finer prehension patterns require minimal strength and flexibility in the hand, whereas grasp patterns require more strength and flexibility in the hand. The grasp and prehension patterns that may be provided by hand splinting are determined by the muscles that are functioning, potential and present deformities, and how the hand is to be used.[1]

Pronation and supination are valuable in positioning the hand at the desired angle for function. Full pronation is required if the hand is to perform adequately. Supination to midposition is sufficient for adequate function.

The carpal and metacarpal transverse arches are critical to hand function. Motion and opposition of the thumb and little finger, ability to grasp round or large objects, convergence of the fingers during flexion, and strength or pressing with the palm are dependent on these arches.[1] The arches must be maintained if the hand is splinted. Flattening of the MP transverse arch will place the hand in a nonfunctional position and will severely limit the types of grasp and prehension possible.

Purposes of splints

A hand splint may be prescribed and fitted for more than one purpose. If there is limited joint motion, the splint may be a positioning or corrective device, and more function may not be achieved until the ROM is improved. In such instances performance of hand skills may be greater without the splint, although not necessarily in the most desirable patterns of motion. A splint may be a positioning device to enhance function during the day and a corrective device at night.

The ultimate and idealistic goal of hand splinting is to assist in the development of as near a normal hand as possible. The following are some specific goals of hand splinting:

1. Prevent deformity due to joint tightness, or muscle contracture. Contracture of muscles whose antagonists are weak or paralyzed can be prevented by placing the muscle at its resting length in the functional position and facilitating motion through the splint or passively.
2. Protect weak muscles from overstretching so that maximum efficiency will be obtained when the muscle regains its function. This goal is related to number 1.
3. Prevent increased muscle imbalance by providing assistance to the weaker muscle group, for example, using rubber bands, to pull the part through the full ROM. This will enable weak muscles to work and allows active ROM.
4. Strengthen weak muscles by providing assistive motion first. Assistance is gradually decreased as muscle function improves. The goal

is related to number 3. The MP extensor assist or opponens assist are examples of splints with these purposes.
5. Correct or prevent deformity by maintaining the ROM gained in forced stretching exercise or maintaining corrected alignment of joints.
6. Provide temporary support for a painful part while permitting motion of uninvolved segments. An example is the wrist cock-up splint to support an arthritic wrist while allowing some hand function.
7. Prepare the hand for future surgery to approximate the position or motions to be gained by surgery and provide the needed ROM and strength, if possible.
8. Place the hand in the correct or appropriate position after burn, surgery, trauma, or skin grafting.
9. Aid in the development of a useful tenodesis tightness in the long finger flexors for the wrist-driven flexor hinge splint.
10. Transfer power from one joint to another for increased function. An example is the wrist-driven flexor hinge splint, where wrist extension effects palmar prehension and wrist flexion effects release through the splint. Later with the controlled development of some finger flexor tightness many clients can discard this splint and use the tenodesis action of the hand for some prehensile function.
11. Substitute for permanently paralyzed muscles through the use of external power such as electricity or the carbon dioxide muscle. Example of this type of splint is the battery-driven flexor hinge splint and the Rancho electric arm.[6]
12. Encourage use of normal movement patterns, prevent substitutions, and facilitate muscle reeducation. These purposes may be achieved by placing the part in a functional position and providing as near a normal range as possible. Return of function will be facilitated by use of the hand in coordinated movement patterns. Proper position and motion will aid returning muscles to work to their maximum but will have no effect on reinnervation of the muscle itself.[1]

Limitations of hand splints

Motion and sensation are intimately related in hand and upper extremity function. Sensory information and feedback from the parts are essential to normal motion. A person with severely limited sensation will have limited motor function even if muscles are normal or near normal. Splinting cannot aid in the restoration of sensation. Splints reduce the amount of sensory information being received from the part. The possibility of the development of pressure points and the resultant skin breakdown from splints is greater in the person with sensory deficits. Such clients must be taught how to compensate for and guard the affected part through the use of vision. The therapist and the client must be responsible for vigilant precautions against the adverse effects of splinting.

A splint cannot provide both mobility and stability of a joint, as in the normal hand, at the same time. Therefore a choice for one or the other must be made in relation to the dysfunction, purposes of splinting, potential deformities, and use of the hand.

The cosmetic appearance of the hand can be improved by splinting. However, during splint wear or use the hand may be less cosmetically appealing. This may influence the client's acceptance and use of the device.[1]

Precautions of splinting

Of greatest importance is the prevention of the adverse effects of immobilization. Prolonged immobility from splinting or positioning can produce limitations in joint ROM and, ultimately, joint stiffness and immobility. All static splints must be removed about every 2 hours, and active or passive exercise must be performed at splinted joints unless contraindicated by surgery, infection, or trauma.

Joints that do not require splinting should not be limited or immobilized by the splint. All joints proximal and distal to the splinted joint(s) should be used actively or exercised passively if active motion is not possible.

To ensure that proper fit and comfort have been achieved, the splint should be removed after short periods of wear (½ to 1 hour), and the part should be checked for indentations of the skin, redness, edema, pain, and changes in the degree of joint mobility.

The splint should be evaluated for function. Is it achieving the desired goals? Is it making no difference? Is it increasing dysfunction or deformity?[1,3]

Criteria for assessing splints

Certain general criteria can be outlined to estimate the practicality of splint construction by the occupational therapist. Static splints should be fitted soon after injury, surgery, or disease. They should be simple in design, easily adjustable, lightweight, cosmetically pleasing, and comfortable and should offer adequate support to achieve the objectives of the splint. It should be possible to fabricate the splint in a reasonable period. The splint should be inexpensive when materials and the therapist's time for construction are considered.[3] The splint should be neat, durable, and easy to clean.

For function the splint should follow the natural contours of the hand and arm as closely as possible without causing pressure areas. If the splint is to be lined or padded, this must be allowed for when first molding the splint by padding the client's arm.

The arches of the hand must be maintained, and the normal padding of the fingers and the hypothenar and thenar eminences must not be flattened. Joints should be positioned in correct anatomical alignment, and the hand should be positioned in or as nearly as possible to the position of function unless contraindicated.[1,6] In dynamic splints the joints of the splint should be lined up with the normal axes of anatomical joints. The therapist should be aware of and check the splints for shifts in position, which therefore change their function and support of the part.

If the splint is used for progressive increase of joint motion, three points of pressure should be used (Fig. 6-7).[1]

INDEPENDENT SPLINT CONSTRUCTION: A SELF-INSTRUCTION PROGRAM

This self-instruction program was designed to enable the reader to construct two simple static splints frequently fabricated by occupational therapists. These are the volar wrist cock-up splint and the resting splint. The wrist cock-up splint may be used to immobilize the wrist in a functional position while allowing finger function. It is used for rheumatoid arthritis, if rest or stabilization of the wrist is desirable, and also to protect the wrist and finger extensors from overstretching when there is muscle weakness producing the wrist-drop position.

The resting splint is worn for similar purposes but immobilizes the thumb and fingers as well as the wrist in the position of rest or function. It may be modified

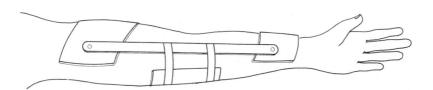

Fig. 6-7. Three-point elbow extension splint illustrates points of pressure proximal and distal to elbow joint and over it to increase or maintain extension.

to the antideformity position required for splinting the hand with dorsal burns. In this position the wrist is at neutral, the MP joints are flexed to approximately 80°, and the IP joints are in full extension. The thumb is midway between radial and palmar abduction to maintain full stretch on the thumb web space.

The resting splint is sometimes used to prevent contractures of the hand with flexor spasticity. When the client wears the splint, no hand function is possible. Therefore it is often worn when the client is at rest or asleep or is worn on one side at a time if bilateral splinting is required.

Steps in making a hand splint independently

Study the preceding sections of this chapter and review the illustrations of grasp, prehension, hand creases, position of function, and position of rest. Then begin construction of the splint using the following steps:
1. Decide which type of splint is to be constructed.
2. Make a pattern for the splint according to the directions.
3. Follow the directions for splint construction.

Supplies needed. For making the splint pattern the following supplies will be needed:
1. Strip of paper towel 18 to 20 inches long
2. Twelve-inch flexible ruler
3. Soft pencil or felt tip pen
4. Scissors

For molding the splint the items listed here will be required:
1. Piece of low-temperature thermoplastic material, such as Orthoplast or Kay-Splint, 8 × 12 inches*
2. Marking crayon or stylus
3. Large scissors*
4. Heat gun*
5. Shallow pan filled with water ¾-inch deep, candy thermometer, and range or hot plate as heat source or thermostatically controlled rectangular, electric frying pan*
6. Tongs*
7. Pot holder or oven mitts*
8. Two Ace bandages or stockinette tubing*
9. Edger for smoothing splint edges*

For applying straps two or three prefabricated, self-adhesive Velcro straps with D rings* and a pair of scissors are needed.

Making a pattern for a splint. The following are instructions for making a pattern for two basic types of hand splints. The reader is directed to choose *one* and construct a splint, making the pattern for the splint selected and constructing the splint on another person.

---

*These items are available from Fred Sammons, Inc., Box 32, Brookfield, Ill. 60513.

1. Position the affected hand and forearm palm down on a long piece of paper towel. The fingers should be adducted and the wrist should be in a neutral position with the thumb against the index metacarpal and finger.
2. Draw a line around the hand, forearm, and thumb, keeping the pencil perpendicular to paper at all times.
3. With the hand still in place mark the wrist joint and the MP joints of the fingers on the radial and ulnar sides of the hand. Mark the MP joint of the thumb. Mark the ulna styloid and the olecranon of the elbow (Fig. 6-8). Later when you are ready draw the splint pattern around this hand tracing.

Resting splint pattern[2] (Fig. 6-9)
1. On the tracing of the hand, beginning at the MP joint of the index finger, draw a line ¼ inch around hand tracing, ending at the wrist on the ulnar side (line a). Extend the line on the radial side straight down to the CMC joint of the thumb and extend it another ½ inch (line b).
2. Measure the width of the thumb and add ¼ inch to this measurement. Mark this distance inward from line b at MP joint of index finger. Draw a line from this mark toward the wrist (line c). This line should be parallel to line b and equal in length to the length of the thumb from the tip of the MP joint plus ½ inch. Taper this line inward slightly at the top and round the bottom.
3. From the mark that designates the olecranon of the elbow, measure 2½ to 3 inches toward the hand and draw a line across the forearm at this point, indicating the length of the splint trough (line d). Extend this line 1 inch on either side of the forearm tracing.
4. Beginning approximately ½ inch away on the ulnar side and 1 inch away on the radial side of the wrist, draw two lines extending to meet line d on each side of the forearm (line e).
5. Cut pattern out and fit to hand, adding or trimming as necessary for proper fit. Cut along line c for the thumb support. Round out all sharp edges.

Proper fit
1. Hand section should not extend more than ¼ inch around hand or thumb.
2. Narrowest point at wrist should be about the width of the wrist.
3. Sides of trough should extend halfway up the sides of the forearm at all points.

Wrist cock-up splint pattern[2] (Fig. 6-10)
1. Draw a line connecting the MP joint marks across the palm of the drawing (line a). Draw a line ¼ inch below this line, beginning ¾ inch lateral to radial side and extending ¾ inch beyond ulnar side of the hand (line b).
2. Draw a line ½ inch down from the radial side of line b (line 1) and another line on the ulnar side of line b, extending past the ulna styloid and parallel to the ulnar side of the arm (line 2).

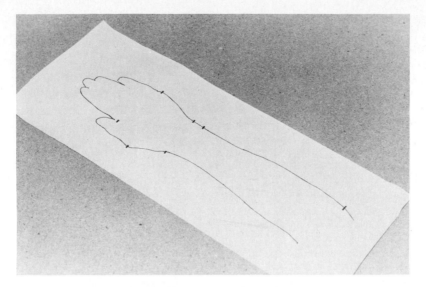

Fig. 6-8. Tracing of subject's arm marked to indicate location of joints.

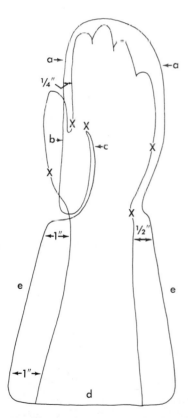

Fig. 6-9. Resting splint pattern.

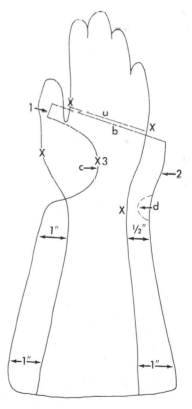

Fig. 6-10. Cock-up splint pattern.

3. To mark the thenar eminence measure the thumb from the tip to the MP joint and subtract ½ inch. Using this measurement make an X in toward the palm from the MP joint of the thumb (3).
4. Draw a curved line (line c) from line 1, arching through the X (3) end at the wrist.
5. Repeat steps 3, 4, and 5 of the resting splint pattern.
6. Ulna styloid should not be under the splint trough. Cut a notch in the splint to accommodate the ulna styloid if it is a potential pressure point (d).

Proper fit

1. Ulnar side of the splint at hand should extend halfway up the side of the hand.
2. Top of the splint should not prevent full flexion of MP joints (splint should fall just below distal palmar crease).
3. Radial side of top of splint should curve around the hand ½ to ¾ inch on the radial side.
4. Opposition and abduction of the thumb should have full ROM (move thumb into this position and check pattern).
5. Narrowest point at wrist should be slightly wider than the width of the wrist.
6. Sides of trough should extend halfway up the sides of the forearm at all points except at the wrist, where they should be slightly beneath the halfway line.

DIRECTIONS FOR USING LOW-TEMPERATURE THERMOPLASTICS IN THE CONSTRUCTION OF HAND SPLINTS[7]

1. Low-temperature thermoplastic materials soften when exposed to heat. Sources of heat used to soften them are hot water, ovens, or heat guns. Use hot water in a shallow flat pan or the heat gun as sources of heat. These materials soften at 130° to 160° F. If heated too hot or reheated more than two times, they may tend to shrink, stretch, or change their molding characteristics. Read directions for material in use carefully before proceeding.
2. Trace the pattern on the thermoplastic before it is heated, using the marking crayon or stylus (Fig. 6-11).
3. Place the thermoplastic, with the tracing on it, in a shallow pan of water or in the electric frying pan that has been heated to the temperature recommended by the manu-

facturer. Be sure the water is not boiling! Use a candy thermometer to monitor water temperature if a pan is used on the range or hot plate.
4. Within 2 or 3 minutes the material will have softened and can be removed from the hot water with tongs for cutting.
5. Low-temperature thermoplastics do not retain the heat and usually can be handled easily while cutting. With ordinary household shears cut the pattern out of the material, rounding all sharp corners. Since the material sets in 5 to 10 minutes after it has been removed from the heat, it may be necessary to place it back in the hot water for 1 or 2 minutes before molding (Fig. 6-12).
6. It is usually possible to mold the material directly over the skin without harm. However, to prevent risk of burn

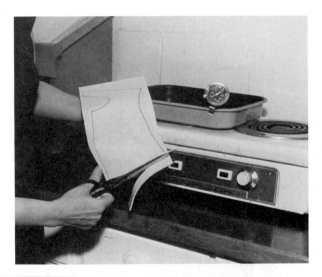

Fig. 6-12. Cutting splint out of thermoplastic.

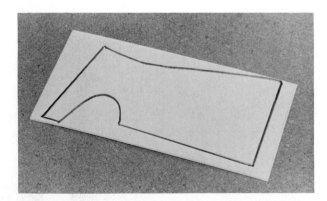

Fig. 6-11. Splint pattern traced on thermoplastic.

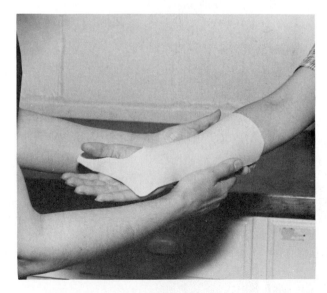

Fig. 6-13. Molding thermoplastic on forearm.

or for hypersensitivity to heat the part may be wrapped with one layer of Ace bandage or a piece of stockinette tubing may be applied to the arm where the splint will be molded.

7. Place the softened material over the arm. Support the arm in the desired position. Mold the thermoplastic around the forearm (Fig. 6-13).
8. If it is not possible to hold the thermoplastic in position on the forearm while molding the hand section (and later when the splint sets), wrap an Ace bandage *loosely* on the subject's arm to mold the material in place. Be careful *not* to wrap too tightly or twist the splint on the forearm while wrapping.
9. While holding the forearm section in place (the subject may help do this), press a thumb into the concavity of the palm to be sure to get the contour of the arch of the hand into the splint. Be sure the subject's wrist is extended between 10° and 30° when this is done (Fig. 6-14).
10. Have the subject abduct and oppose the thumb to the little finger to get a fold in the thermoplastic that will mark the medial border of the thenar eminence (Fig. 6-15).
11. Then with the thumb moved out of the way roll this edge over. Mold the radial extension through the thumb web space and flat against the dorsum of the hand (Fig. 6-16).
12. Also have the subject flex the MP joints and roll over the distal end of the splint. These rolls give the splint strength, provide a smooth edge against the skin, and should be formed to allow for full flexion of MP joints and full opposition of the thumb (Fig. 6-17).
13. If necessary, resoften the proximal end of the splint and roll over this end ⅛ to ¼ inch as well.

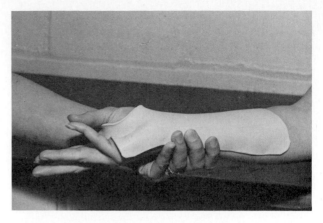

Fig. 6-15. Subject opposing thumb to little finger to attain medial fold on thenar eminence.

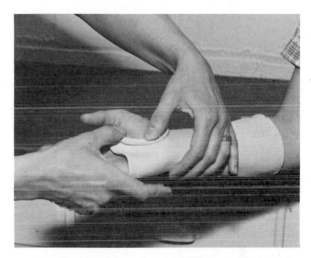

Fig. 6-16. Therapist rolls over thenar edge of splint.

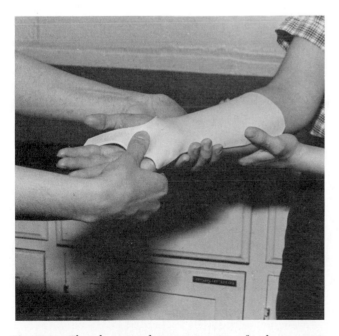

Fig. 6-14. Thumb pressed into concavity of palm to attain metacarpal palmar arch.

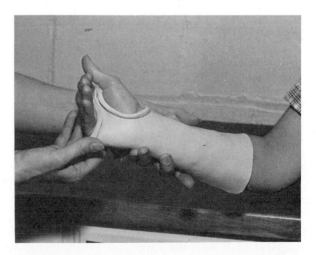

Fig. 6-17. Subject flexes MP joints, and therapist rolls over distal edge of splint.

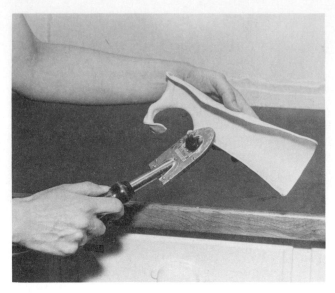

Fig. 6-18. Edger is used to smooth edges of splint.

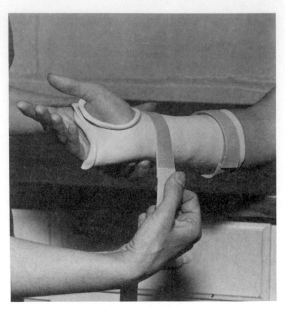

Fig. 6-19. Self-adhesive Velcro straps are applied to splint.

NOTE: If the thermoplastic sets before the desired contours are formed, it is possible to reheat all or part of the splint and remold as desired. If reheating is necessary after the basic contours of the splint are formed, remove the splint, which is set, from the subject's arm and spot heat at the desired area only by dipping the small area in the hot water; using the spot heater tip on the heat gun; or pouring small amounts of very hot tap water over the desired area with a cup, repeatedly, until the area is softened. When the desired pliability is reobtained, replace the splint on the subject's arm and remold. This same procedure can be followed if it is necessary to trim some material from the splint.

14. After the splint has been molded to the exact form desired, smooth any rough edges of the splint with the edger. Heat the edger to "medium" and touch it lightly to the splint, using gentle strokes (Fig. 6-18).

NOTE: Too much heat or pressure will cause the thermoplastic to melt along the edges, and its appearance gets worse instead of improving.

Attaching straps to the splints

1. Using two Velcro self-adhesive straps place one strap on the splint at the proximal end and the other strap over the wrist, but not on top of the ulna styloid, which is a potential pressure point.
2. A third strap may be placed on the splint around the hand just proximal to the MP joints (Fig. 6-19).

Evaluation of splint construction. Finished splints may be evaluated for molding technique, function, fit, and appearance. Both the wrist cock-up and the resting splints should be evaluated for molding technique and fit by the following criteria:

1. Is the splint smoothly molded?
2. Is the trough twisted, or is it well-aligned to the forearm?
3. Are all of the corners rounded?
4. Are the straps correctly placed to afford stability and avoid pressure points?
5. Do the sides of the trough extend about halfway around the forearm at all points?
6. Does the splint fit loosely enough to prevent pressure areas along edges and over bony prominences?
7. Is there evidence of pressure (redness, soreness, or edema) after 1 to 2 hours of wear?

Appearance of both the wrist cock-up and the resting splints may be evaluated according to the following criteria:

1. Is the thermoplastic material clean and free of bumps, dents, cuts, and ridges?
2. Are the straps clean and attached straight?
3. Does the splint have a neat appearance that would be acceptable for wear?

For function the resting splint may be evaluated by the following criteria:

1. Are the arches of the hand maintained?
2. Is the hand splinted in a resting position, that is, with the wrist in 10° to 30° extension, MP joints in 20° to 30° flexion, IP joints in 10° to 15° flexion, and thumb in palmar abduction and opposition, aligned with index finger?

The cock-up splint may be evaluated for function by the following criteria:

1. Are the arches of the hand maintained?
2. Does the splint allow full ROM at the MP joints?
3. Does the splint allow full, normal opposition to the little finger?
4. Is the wrist positioned in 10° to 30° of extension?
5. Can the subject use the hand for grasp and release while wrist stability is maintained?

REVIEW QUESTIONS

1. What is the role of the occupational therapist in hand splinting?
2. List five assets of the normal hand.
3. Describe the relationship of shoulder, elbow, and wrist function to hand use.
4. Which type of prehension is used to pick up a straight pin?
5. Which type of prehension is used to turn a key in a lock?
6. Which type of grasp is used to hold a tumbler?
7. What is the role and importance of the metacarpal transverse arch in hand function?
8. What happens to hand function if this arch is flattened?
9. In which position are the muscles of the hand at the best mechanical advantage to function efficiently?
10. Name two major classifications of splints. Give one example of each.
11. How are the adverse effects of immobilization by splinting best prevented?
12. What is the optimum position for splinting the wrist?
13. What effect does wrist flexion have on hand function?
14. Why is it important to splint the MP joints in some flexion if these joints are to be splinted?
15. What is the optimum position for splinting the thumb?
16. Describe six purposes of splinting.
17. List and describe three limitations of splints.
18. What are the factors that influence the practicability of splint construction by the occupational therapist?
19. List six general rules for achieving optimum fit and function of the splint.
20. Describe the purposes of the resting and wrist cock-up splints.

REFERENCES

1. Anonymous: Principles of hand splinting, Downey, Calif., 1962, Occupational Therapy Department, Rancho Los Amigos Hospital. Mimeographed, unpublished.
2. Anonymous: Splinting manual, Jamaica Plain, Mass., 1972, Occupational Therapy Department, Lemuel Shattuck Hospital. Mimeographed, unpublished.
3. Malick, M.: Manual on static hand splinting, vol. 1, rev. ed., Pittsburgh, 1972, The Harmarville Rehabilitation Center.
4. Malick, M.: Manual on dynamic hand splinting with thermoplastic materials, Pittsburgh, 1974, The Harmarville Rehabilitation Center.
5. Melvin, J.L.: Rheumatic disease: occupational therapy and rehabilitation, Philadelphia, 1977, F.A. Davis Co.
6. Trombly, C.A., and Scott, A.D.: Occupational therapy for physical dysfunction, Baltimore, 1977, The Williams & Wilkins Co.
7. Von Prince, K.: Orthoplast splint construction, San Jose, Calif., 1971, special study, Department of Occupational Therapy, San Jose State College. Mimeographed, unpublished.

SUPPLEMENTARY READING

Buckner, G.: A dynamic finger splint, Am. J. Occup. Ther. **27**:39, 1973.
Butts, D., and Goldberg, M.J.: Congenital absence of the radius: the occupational therapist and a new orthosis, Am. J. Occup. Ther. **31**:95, 1977.
Doubilet, L., and Polkow, L.S.: Theory and design of a finger abduction splint for the spastic hand, Am. J. Occup. Ther. **31**:2, 1977.
Fishwick, G.M., and Tobin, D.: Splinting the burned hand with primary excision and early grafting, Am. J. Occup. Ther. **32**:182, 1978.
Frankhauser, J.N.: Self-ranging foot splint, Am. J. Occup. Ther. **31**:316, 1977.
Gorham, J.A.: A mouth splint for burn microstomia, Am. J. Occup. Ther. **31**:105, 1977.
Kuntavanish, A.A.: Dynamic facial palsy splint, Am. J. Occup. Ther. **28**:433, 1974.
McKenzie, M.W.: The ratchet hand splint, Am. J. Occup. Ther. **27**:477, 1973.
Millender, L.H., and Philips, C.: Uses of proximal interphalangeal joint gutter splint, Am. J. Occup. Ther. **27**:8, 1973.
Petersen, P.: A conformer for the reduction of facial burn contractures: a preliminary report, Am. J. Occup. Ther. **31**:101, 1977.
Pomerantz, P., and Gurves, M.: Ptosis splint, Am. J. Occup. Ther. **28**:821, 1974.
Rivers, E., State, R.G., and Solem, L.D.: The transparent face mask, Am. J. Occup. Ther. **33**:108, 1979.
Solie, G.A.: Short opponens hand orthosis, Am. J. Occup. Ther. **32**:588, 1978.
Torres, J.: Little finger splint, Am. J. Occup. Ther. **29**:230, 1975.
Vigliotta, C.L.: Traction splint for maximum interphalangeal joint flexion, Am. J. Occup. Ther. **32**:175, 1978.

Chapter 7

Amputations and prosthetics

Limb loss can result from disease, injury, or congenital causes. Congenital amputees or those whose amputations occurred very early in life grow and develop sensorimotor skills and self-images without the amputated part. The individual who incurs amputation of a part in adolescence or adulthood is confronted with the task of adjusting to the loss of a part that was well-integrated into the body scheme and self-image.

These two types of amputees present somewhat different problems for the rehabilitation worker.[4] This chapter will be limited to discussion of the adult with acquired above-elbow (AE), below-elbow (BE), or lower extremity (LE) amputations.

Physical therapy is usually responsible for the preprosthetic preparation and prosthetic training of the LE amputee. Occupational therapy may be useful to the LE amputee for functional use training, standing and walking tolerance, and prevocational explorations. The preprosthetic and prosthetic training of the upper extremity (UE) amputee, on the other hand, is usually the primary responsibility of the occupational therapist. Psychosocial adjustment, controls and use training, wearing tolerance, and prevocational assessment are important aspects of the occupational therapy program.[4]

Etiology

Amputations may result from trauma, peripheral vascular disease, thrombosis, embolism, and cancer.[2,4] The most common reason for UE amputations in adults is trauma, and LE amputations are most frequently the result of peripheral vascular disease.[2]

Surgical management

The surgeon attempts to preserve as much tissue as possible during the amputation procedure. During and after surgery it is a primary goal to form the stump in a way to maintain maximum function of the remaining tissue and obtain a result that will allow maximum use of the prosthesis. Blood vessels and nerves are cut and allowed to retract so that they do not cause pain in the stump when the prosthesis is used. In any amputation the muscles involved in the function of the amputated part are affected by the loss.

A closed or open surgical procedure may be performed. The open method allows drainage and minimizes the possibility of infection. The closed method reduces the period of hospitalization but also reduces free drainage and increases the risk of infection. In either case the stump that results must be strong and resilient. It must be possible to fit the prosthesis socket to the stump snugly and comfortably, since the amputee will be exerting much pressure on the stump when using the prosthesis.[4]

Special considerations and problems

There are several factors and potential problems that can affect the outcome of the amputee's rehabilitation. Stump length, skin coverage, stump edema, hypersensitivity, rate of healing, infections, and allergic reactions to the prosthesis are some of the physical problems that can affect the fitting and use of the prosthesis.

The loss of feedback sensation from the amputated part is one of the major problems that confronts the amputee. The amputee must rely on visual and proprioceptive sensory feedback to control the use and function of the prosthesis. Sensation in the stump is functionally lost when the prosthesis is applied. An ill-fitting socket or a stump that is not well formed at the distal end can cause pain and discomfort when the prosthesis is worn. Besides the loss of normal sensation the amputee must become accustomed to new sensations as well. The pressure of the stump inside the socket and the feeling of the harnessing system must be accommodated.[4] Neuromas and phantom sensation or pain are two problems that may interfere with use of the prosthesis. The neuroma is nerve tissue growing into scar tissue that causes pain in the area when it is pressed or moved. It is treated by surgical excision or ultrasound therapy. The stump socket may be fabricated to accommodate the neuroma.[6]

Phantom sensation is a common experience among amputees. It is the sensation of the presence of the amputated part or a distal portion of it. The phantom sensation may be present for life or may eventually disappear. Phantom sensation does not usually interfere with good prosthetic usage. A much less common phenomenon that can prohibit good use of the prosthesis is phantom pain. In this condition the amputated limb is not only perceived as present but is painful as well.[6]

Surgical revision of the stump is sometimes necessary to alleviate the discomfort. Phantom sensations occur most frequently in crush injuries and are usually felt as distal parts, that is, a hand or foot, rather than the entire extremity. Supportive counseling and early use of the stump with a temporary or permanent prosthesis are effective measures for dealing with phantom sensations.[4] The therapist can allay the client's fears about these phenomena by offering information, support, and reassurance, unless she considers these fears an indication of some mental imbalance. It is best not to dwell on discussion of phantom sensation but rather to focus on prosthetic training and the advantages of using a prosthesis. The appearance of phantom pain or overconcern with phantom sensation may require the intervention of a psychiatric specialist who may work with the client or provide advice to the occupational therapist.[6]

Psychological adjustment

Amputation is likely to be accompanied by a profound psychological shock. Reactions are less severe in clients who have been well prepared for amputation surgery and more severe in persons who have experienced sudden traumatic injury that causes or necessitates amputation. The amputee may manifest depression, hostility, denial, or feelings of futility. Older persons may demonstrate postoperative confusion whereas younger persons may have a sense of mutilation or emasculation. The amputee will need a lot of reassurance during the preoperative, postoperative, and rehabilitative phases of care.[2]

Loss of a body part necessitates a revision of the body image. The amputee must accept the new body image. Such adjustment will have a beneficial effect on prosthetic training, since the amputee must integrate the prosthesis into the body scheme, and it must become part of the self before it can be used most effectively. Difficulties with acceptance of body scheme change may cause difficulties in prosthetic training.[4]

Levels of amputation and functional losses in the upper extremity (Fig. 7-1)

The higher the level of amputation the greater the functional loss of the part, and the more the amputee must depend on the prosthesis for function and cosmesis. The higher level amputations require more complex and extensive prostheses and prosthetic training. The more complex prostheses can be more difficult to operate and use effectively.[4]

The shoulder forequarter and shoulder disarticula-

tion (SD) amputations will result in the loss of all arm and hand functions. The short AE amputation will result in the loss of all hand, wrist and elbow functions and rotation of the shoulder. The long AE and elbow disarticulation amputations will result in loss of hand, wrist, and elbow functions, but good shoulder function will remain. The short BE amputation will result in loss of hand and wrist function, forearm pronation and supination, and reduction in the force of elbow flexion. Shoulder function will be intact and good. The long BE amputation will result in loss of hand and wrist function and most of the forearm pronation and supination. Elbow function and force of elbow flexion will be good. The wrist disarticulation will result in complete loss of hand and wrist function and about a 50% loss of pronation and supination. Amputations below the wrist across the metacarpal bones are called transmetacarpal or partial hand amputations. Functions of all the joints of the

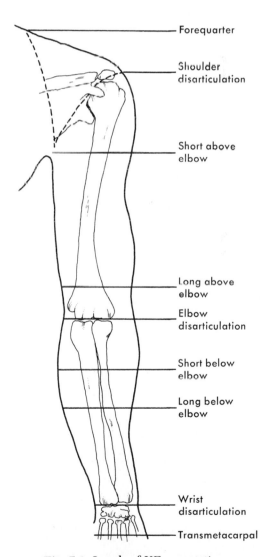

Fig. 7-1. Levels of UE amputation.

arm are intact, and there may be some hand function available, depending on whether the thumb was amputated or left intact.

Many types of prostheses are available for each level of amputation. Each prosthesis is individually prescribed according to the client's needs and life-style and is individually fitted and custom-made.[4]

Accessories and component parts of the UE prosthesis (Fig. 7-2)

Stump sock. A stump sock of knit wool, cotton, or Orlon-Lycra is usually worn by the amputee. It absorbs perspiration and protects from potential discomfort or irritation that could result from direct contact of the skin with the socket of the prosthesis. It accommodates

volume change in the stump and aids with fit and comfort of the stump in the socket.[4,7]

Harness. The purposes of the harness are to suspend the prosthesis and to provide the anchor point for the control cables. The figure eight Dacron harness is a commonly used design, although others are available. Extra straps may be added to the figure eight as needed.[3,4,6] The higher the level of amputation the more complex the harnessing system. The amount of muscle power and ROM loss may necessitate variations in the harness design.

Cable and components. The cable is made of stainless steel and is contained in a flexible stainless steel housing. It is fastened to the prosthesis by a retainer unit made of a base plate and a retainer butterfly or a housing crossbar and a leather loop. A ball or ball swivel fitting at one end of the cable attaches it to the terminal device (TD) while a T bar or hanger fittings at the other end attach it to the harness.[3,6]

Upper-arm cuff. The upper-arm cuff is used on the BE prosthesis to increase stability and control of the prosthesis and provide an anchor point through which the cable passes to the TD. It prevents the control cable from floating freely and incorporates the elbow hinges to hold the forearm socket to the harness.

Socket. The forearm socket for the BE amputee is made of plastic resins and may be single or double wall. The socket must be anchored stably on the stump to allow the wearer full power and control of the prosthesis. The BE stump socket may be constructed to allow any remaining pronation and supination to be used. The single wall socket is used when the outside diameter of the distal end of the stump is sufficient to permit tapering to the wrist unit. The double wall socket is used when the stump is too short or slender to achieve the desired contour or tapering. The inner wall conforms to the stump and the outer wall gives the required length and contour for the forearm replacement. A rota-

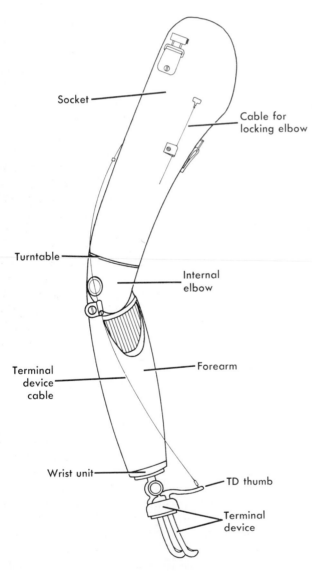

Socket

Cable for locking elbow

Turntable

Internal elbow

Terminal device cable

Forearm

Wrist unit

TD thumb

Terminal device

Fig. 7-2. Component parts of standard AE prosthesis. (Adapted from Santschi, W., editor: Manual for upper extremity prosthetics, ed. 2, Los Angeles, 1958, University of California Press.)

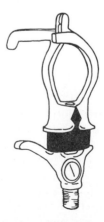

Fig. 7-3. "Farmer's hook," Dorrance model 7, heavy-duty stainless steel.

tion unit that fastens to the inner socket and rotates inside the outer shell may be used to increase the remaining pronation and supination. This unit is driven by the forearm stump and has a step-up ratio of 2:1.[4,6]

The AE stump socket is a double wall unit. There is a locking elbow unit laminated onto the socket. The elbow unit provides elbow flexion, extension, and locking at various points in the ROM by the control cable system. The socket must fit snugly and firmly but allow full ROM at the shoulder.[4,6]

Elbow unit. The elbow unit on the AE prosthesis allows the maximum ROM possible, locking of the elbow in 11 different locking positions at 45° of motion, and prepositioning of the prosthesis for arm rotation by a manual control friction turntable unit.

The BE prosthesis has flexible metal or leather hinges that allow amputees with longer stumps to use the available normal pronation and supination.

A rigid metal hinge with a step-up mechanism is available for the short BE stump. It allows the amputee to achieve a range of elbow flexion that would otherwise not be possible. The forearm socket and TD flex 2° for every 1° of flexion of the stump through this mechanism.

The forearm socket on the AE prosthesis provides the connection between the wrist and elbow units. It contains the wrist unit and TD and is fabricated to fit the arm length requirements of the individual amputee. The forearm lift loop, which allows the amputee to flex the prosthesis forearm, is fastened to this forearm socket.[6]

Wrist units. The wrist unit joins the TD to the forearm socket. There are three basic types of wrist units. These are the friction, locking, and oval types. The wrist unit allows prepositioning of the TD to accommodate the task to be performed. It serves as a disconnect unit so that TDs may be interchanged. The locking unit allows wrist flexion by manual operation or with the aid of another object such as the edge of a table. It is usually used by the bilateral amputee for facilitating activities close to the body. The friction unit requires prepositioning of the TD manually or with the aid of another object. There is a rubber washer in the unit that creates the friction sufficient to hold the TD, as it was prepositioned, against moderate loads.[4,6,7]

The oval unit is used with the wrist disarticulation prosthesis. It minimizes the length of the components so that the prosthesis will match the length of the sound arm more closely.

The wrist unit is usually selected for its ability to meet the use needs of the amputee in daily living and vocational activities.[4]

TD. Two types of TDs that are available are the hook and the cosmetic hand. These may be either voluntary-opening or voluntary-closing in design.

The voluntary-opening TD opens when the amputee exerts tension on the control cable, which connects to the "thumb" of the TD. When tension is released, rubber bands, springs, or coils close the fingers of the TD. The voluntary-opening type is the most frequently prescribed.[6]

The voluntary-closing TD is also activated when tension is applied to the control cable. The tension effects locking and maintaining the grasp force on the object in the desired position.

The hook TD may be made of aluminum or steel. It may have canted or lyre-shaped fingers and usually has a neoprene lining for the protection of the objects grasped. It is the most functional and most frequently prescribed and used TD. Several types of hooks are available to meet the individual needs of the amputee. The farmer's and carpenter's hooks allow for ease in handling tools, and narrow-opening hooks may be used for handling fine objects (Fig. 7-3). On the hook TD, the number of rubber bands controls the amount of grasp pressure. Training usually begins with one rubber band, and the number increases to three to four rubber bands as training progresses.

The cosmetic TD, designed to duplicate the amputee's hand as nearly as possible, is available in addition to the hook. One type of cosmetic hand that is used primarily for its appearance is the flesh-colored glove, which covers a partial hand. It may be used to hold light objects or position objects by pushing or pulling. Another type of cosmetic hand is the functional hand, which may be attached to the wrist unit and activated by the same control cable that operates the hook. It comes in voluntary-opening and voluntary-closing types. The thumb of the functional hand is prepositioned manually in either of two positions to accommodate small or large objects. The fingers are controlled at the MP joints by the prosthesis control cable, and palmar prehension between the thumb and these two fingers is possible through the control system. A natural-looking plastic glove fits over the mechanical hand.[4]

THE UE PROSTHETIC TRAINING PROGRAM
Preprosthetic training

During the period between the amputation and the fitting of the prosthesis the amputee is engaged in a training program designed to promote stump shrinkage, desensitize the stump, maintain ROM of proximal joints, and increase the strength of the stump and proximal muscles. In addition aiding in adjustment to the loss and achieving independence in self-care are important aspects of the training program.[5]

During the preprosthetic period the amputee should be encouraged to use the sound arm to perform ADL. If the dominant arm was amputated, special training may be required for the nondominant limb to assume the dominant role. Practice in writing and activities

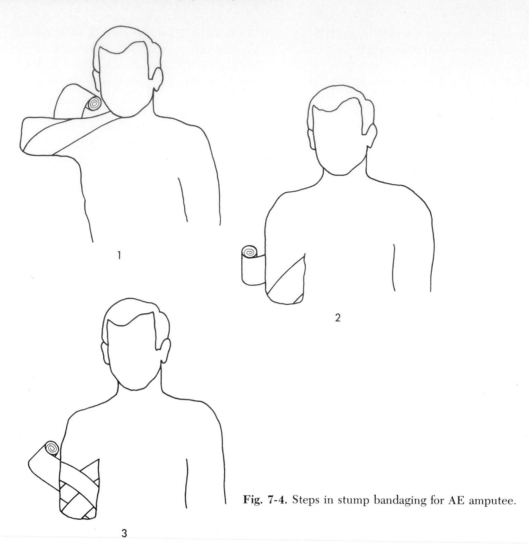

Fig. 7-4. Steps in stump bandaging for AE amputee.

requiring dexterity and coordination may be helpful in the retraining process.[4,6] Most amputees change dominance to the sound extremity automatically.

During the preprosthetic period the client may be counseled about the acceptance of the amputation and about the prosthesis and its benefits. It is important for the therapist to be aware of what the amputation and the prosthesis may mean to the client. It is also important to consider whether the client's primary need is function or cosmesis in selecting the prosthesis and presenting it to the amputee.

With medical approval stump exercises may be commenced. These are designed to encourage use of the stump, maintain ROM of joints proximal to the amputation site, and strengthen muscles of the arm and shoulder. Many of these muscles will ultimately be used to operate the prosthesis, so strength and endurance are the desired results of training.

The loss of weight of the amputated part will cause a shift in the body's center of gravity. Early exercise programs geared toward correcting faulty body mechanics can help to prevent muscular atrophy, scoliosis, and compensatory curves, which can result from this shift in the center of gravity.

The client is encouraged to move and use the stump as much as possible during the healing period. After complete healing the stump is massaged. This increases circulation, aids with desensitization, reduces swelling, and discourages adhesions from scar tissue. It helps the patient overcome fear of handling the stump.

Stump shrinkage and shaping are effected with Ace bandaging of the stump several times a day. The bandage is applied from the distal to the proximal end of the stump. The bandage must be applied smoothly, evenly, and not too tightly[4,6] (Fig. 7-4).

Small utensils may be strapped to the stump to encourage its functional use. A temporary prosthesis fashioned of plaster or leather may be applied to the stump. This enhances early use of the stump for function and helps to accustom the amputee to prosthesis wear and use. Bilateral activities should be encouraged during the preprosthetic period. The early use of a temporary pros-

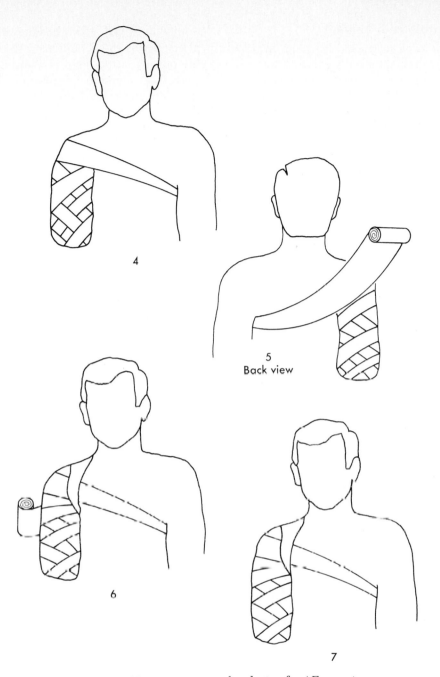

Fig. 7-4, cont'd. Steps in stump bandaging for AE amputee.

thesis may aid in psychological adjustment and increase the possibility of the acceptance and use of the prosthesis by the amputee.

Checkout of the prosthesis

When the prosthesis is received, it is checked by the members of the rehabilitation team to ensure that it is functioning efficiently, is mechanically sound, and meets prescription requirements. The prosthesis is checked for fit and function against the mechanical stan-

dards outlined by Wellerson[6] and Trombly and Scott[5] that were developed from actual tests on prostheses worn by amputees. Ranges of motion with the prosthesis on and off are compared. Control system function and efficiency, TD opening in various positions, degree of slippage of the socket on the stump under various degrees of load or tension, compression fit and comfort, and force required to flex the forearm are several of the factors that are measured against prescribed standards during the initial checkout.[6]

Common considerations in training

The amputee should be instructed in stump hygiene and care of the stump sock in the early phase of the prosthetic training program. The stump and armpits should be washed daily and blotted dry. Underarm deodorant or deodorant powder should be applied every day. At least six stump socks of cotton, wool, or Orlon-Lycra should be obtained. A clean stump sock should be worn every day. The socks should be washed daily and squeezed out, not wrung, gently. The sock is placed on a flat surface to dry and spread gently to its original dimension and contours. A T shirt for men and an underblouse for women are recommended for wear under the harness. These will absorb perspiration and protect the skin from irritation in the axillae and across the back. Stump socks and undergarments may need to be changed twice a day in very warm weather.[6,7]

The amputee should learn the names and functions of the parts of the prosthesis. This is important so that the amputee can communicate with the therapist, physician, or prosthetist, using terminology understood by all. It is especially important if the amputee is having difficulties with the prosthesis or if it is in need of repairs. The amputee then is trained in donning and removing the prosthesis with ease.[6,7]

Training the unilateral BE amputee

Donning and removing the prosthesis. The amputee dons the stump sock with the sound arm. To apply the prosthesis the amputee places it on a table or bed and pushes the stump between the control cable and Y strap from the medial side into the socket. The harness is placed across the shoulder on the amputated side, and the opposite axilla loop is allowed to dangle down the back. The sound hand reaches around the back and slips into the axilla loop. The amputee then slips into the harness as if putting on a coat. The shoulders are shrugged to shift the harness forward and into the correct position.

To remove the prosthesis the amputee slips the axila shoulder strap off on the sound side with the TD and then slips the shoulder strap off on the amputated side. The harness is then slipped off like a coat.[6]

TD control. Scapula abduction and glenohumeral flexion on the amputated side are the motions necessary to operate the TD. The therapist takes the movable finger on the TD and opens it, holding it to show the amputee that the control cable in back is slack. She then pulls the prosthesis forward, so that the amputee's shoulder is in a flexed position and releases the TD, asking the amputee to maintain the tension on the control cable (Fig. 7-5). This will hold the TD open. The amputee is then asked to gradually move the shoulder back into extension, releasing the tension on the control cable and allowing the TD to close. The therapist will then hold her hand at the back of the amputee's stump and passively move the humerus into flexion (Fig. 7-6).[7] The therapist returns the stump to the neutral position at the amputee's side. During this procedure the amputee watches the TD operate and gains a sense of the tension on the prosthesis control cable. The amputee then repeats the motions without the therapist's assistance

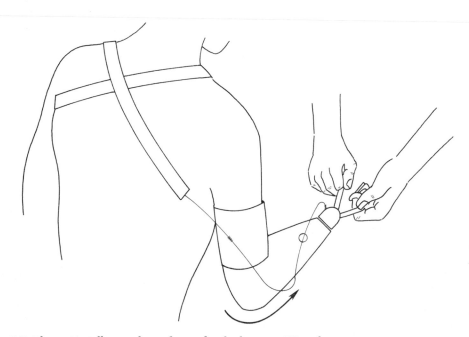

Fig. 7-5. Therapist pulls prosthesis forward, which opens TD, asks amputee to maintain tension on control cable, and then releases her hands.

and verbalizes the actions that occurred during operation.

This same procedure is repeated, except that scapula abduction is used as the control motion. The therapist stands in front of the amputee and passively draws the shoulders together, rounding his back. The amputee feels and observes the effect of the motion on the TD and repeats the motion actively. This procedure is again repeated, using scapula depression as the control motion. The therapist instructs the amputee to hold the humerus at his side with the elbow extended. The therapist places her hand directly under the TD and asks the amputee to push down and push her hand away. The amputee again feels and observes the effect on the TD and repeats the movements, verbalizing the actions that are occurring.

If forearm stump is more than 50% of the normal forearm length, pronation and supination should be practiced. The therapist stands behind the amputee and asks him to flex the elbow to 90°. The therapist holds the amputee's elbow adducted to the side of the body, and the amputee pronates and supinates the forearm stump, observing the effect on the TD. The amputee then repeats the motion without assistance. The therapist then instructs the amputee to repeat all of these motions in one continuous sequence in both sitting and standing positions until they are smooth and natural.[6]

The amputee will then be instructed to open and close the TD in a variety of ranges of elbow and shoulder motion. TD opening and closing should be accomplished easily with the elbow extended, and at 30°, 45°, 90°, and full elbow flexion, as well as with the arm overhead, down at the side, out to the side, and leaning over to the floor level.[7]

Training the unilateral AE amputee

Elbow controls. After learning to don and remove the prosthesis as just described, the AE amputee is instructed in elbow controls. Learning to flex the mechanical elbow is the first step in the training process. The therapist places one hand on the amputee's shoulder and the other on the forearm. She passively flexes the prosthesis into full elbow flexion for the amputee, noting that the control cable is slackened by this maneuver (Fig. 7-7). The therapist then flexes the amputee's shoulder forward and asks the amputee to hold this position while she releases her hands (Fig. 7-8). The amputee gains a sense of the control cable tension across the scapula from this maneuver. The amputee is then asked to relax the stump to the side of the body once again, slowly allowing the forearm to extend (Fig. 7-9). This procedure is repeated by asking the amputee to flex the humerus and abduct the scapula to accomplish elbow flexion and relax the stump back slowly into shoulder extension to achieve elbow extension. This is repeated until the amputee gains enough control of cable tension to accomplish elbow flexion and extension smoothly and with ease.[7] The therapist should be aware of the possible need for adjustment of the prosthesis and should consult with the prosthetist if this need becomes apparent.

The therapist then teaches elbow locking by placing her hand on the amputee's shoulder and the other hand on the TD. She passively pushes the humerus into hyperextension with the elbow flexed thus locking the elbow (Fig. 7-10). She brings the arm back to the neutral position and removes her hands from the prosthesis, demonstrating that the elbow mechanism is locked. She

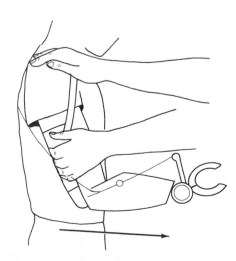

Fig. 7-6. Therapist moves stump forward to attain cable tension and TD opening.

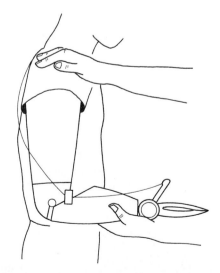

Fig. 7-7. Therapist passively flexes elbow to cause slackening of control cable.

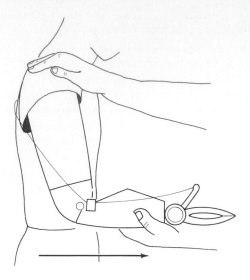

Fig. 7-8. Forearm is moved forward, which causes tension on control cable, to maintain elbow flexion.

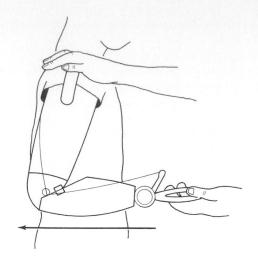

Fig. 7-10. Therapist pushes humerus into hyperextension to lock elbow.

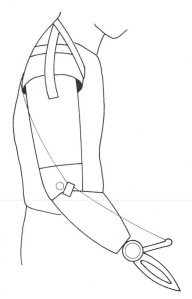

Fig. 7-9. Amputee relaxes stump to allow controlled extension of forearm.

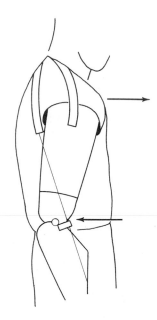

Fig. 7-11. Shoulder is rolled forward, scapula abducted, and humerus hyperextended to lock or unlock elbow at various points in ROM.

repeats this maneuver, demonstrating that the elbow is now unlocked. The amputee is then asked to lock the elbow by moving the humerus into hyperextension and rolling the shoulder forward, using scapular depression and abduction at the same time to lock the elbow. This control motion may be difficult to master. It requires practice and the development of a "proprioceptive memory." The same motions are used to unlock the elbow mechanism. The amputee is then asked to practice locking and unlocking the elbow in various ranges of elbow flexion and extension until full flexion and extension are obtained[7] (Fig. 7-11).

TD control. Once elbow controls have been mastered, TD control training can begin. With the elbow locked the same motions of shoulder flexion and scapula abduction that were used to flex the forearm can now be used to control the TD. The amputee is instructed to lock the elbow, first at 90°, and perform the control motions to open the TD. The sequence of elbow flexion, elbow locking, TD operation, elbow unlock, and elbow extension is repeated at various points in the range of elbow motion from full extension to full flexion.[5,7]

Once elbow controls are achieved, the therapist should show the amputee how to position the forearm in internal or external rotation. The elbow is flexed to 90° then the amputee is instructed to rotate the forearm to the desired degree of internal or external rotation by passively moving the forearm medially (toward the body) or laterally (away from the body).

Use training for AE and BE amputees

Once controls of the prosthesis are mastered, use training is commenced. The first stage in use training is prepositioning the TD. This involves rotating the TD to the best position to grasp an object or perform a given activity. The BE amputee is instructed to rotate the TD into the desired degree of pronation or supination to accomplish the activity. For the AE amputee this involves flexing and locking the elbow and rotating the turntable to the desired degree of rotation before prepositioning the TD. The goal of prepositioning the TD should be to allow the amputee to approach the object or activity with as near normal a movement as one would with a normal hand and to avoid awkward body movements used to compensate for poor prepositioning.[5]

Along with prepositioning, prehension training should begin, first using large, hard objects, such as blocks, cans, and jars, and progressing to soft, then to crushable objects, such as rubber balls, sponges, paper boxes, cones, and paper cups. These objects should be placed at various heights and positions that demand prepositioning and opening and closing the TD, as well as elbow flexion, locking and unlocking, at various heights.[7]

A training board with common household hardware attached or actual hardware found in the training facility may be used as the next step in use training. Items, such as a pencil sharpener, door lock, padlock and key, jar and lid, and bottle opener, should be used to challenge the amputee. The amputee should be encouraged to use a problem-solving approach to these and other tasks to determine the best position for the TD, as well as appropriate use of the sound arm and the prosthesis in bilateral activities (Table 4). The prosthesis should be regarded as an assistive device and not as a primary member.

Use training should progress to performance of necessary ADL. The amputee is encouraged to analyze and perform the activities of personal hygiene and grooming, dressing, feeding, home management, communication and environmental hardware, avocation, and vocation as independently as possible. The therapist may help the amputee analyze and accomplish a task when needed or aid in task achievement through the use of a special method or gadget or repetitious practice to achieve the desired level of speed and skill.[6]

Prevocational evaluation may be included in the use training phase of the rehabilitation of the amputee. The

Table 4. Use training suggestions for the unilateral UE amputee[3,4,6]

Activity	Suggestion	
	Sound arm	Prosthesis
Dressing		
Tie shoes	Use one-handed methods or elastic shoelaces	
	Tie double knot, complete bow	Hold one loop of bow
Necktie	Manipulate knot	Hold and stabilize short end of necktie
Shirt, blouse	Insert in sleeve second, adjust shirt	Insert in sleeve first
Button and unbutton shirt or blouse	Manipulate buttons	Hold fabric taut
Button shirt cuff on sound arm	Hold cuff fabric taut	Button, using amputee buttonhook, if necessary
Don trousers	Tuck in shirt; fasten waist; zip zipper	Hold trousers up; hold bottom of zipper
Hang clothes on hanger	Place hanger in garment and hang in closet	Hold garment
Feeding		
Cut meat	Cut with knife (procedure may be reversed)	Hold fork with handle resting on TD thumb
Butter bread	Hold bread (procedure may be reversed)	Spread butter (TD at neutral, knife stabilized between TD fingers and over thumb)
Fill glass	Hold glass	Turn faucet handle
Open bottle	Open, remove, or unscrew cap	Stabilize carton or bottle
Carry tray	Hold one side of tray	Hold other side of tray, TD in neutral position
Sharpen pencil	Hold pencil	Operate crank
Read book	Turn pages	Hold book
Open envelope	Tear or cut open	Hold envelope
Home management		
Open jar	Unscrew lid	Hold jar
Wash dishes	Hold dish	Hold dish mop or sponge
Dry dishes	Hold dish	Hold towel
Iron	Maneuver iron	Stabilize and adjust garment
Use egg beater	Turn handle	Stabilize beater

Continued.

Table 4. Use training suggestions for the unilateral UE amputee—cont'd

Activity	Suggestion	
	Sound arm	Prosthesis
Home management — cont'd		
Use mop or broom	Guide or push implement	Hold implement
Hammer nail	Use hammer	Hold nail
Hygiene and grooming		
Shave (safety razor)	Insert blade; shave	Hold razor
Apply toothpaste	Hold tube and turn (procedure may be reversed)	Hold cap
Communication and environmental hardware		
Use phone	Dial phone; write message	Hold receiver
Write	Hold pen (if dominant arm); hold paper (if nondominant arm)	Hold pen with TD in 90° pronation (if dominant arm); hold paper (if nondominant arm)
Type	Use one-handed method	Hold typing stick with TD in 90° pronation to operate keys, space bar, and shift key

therapist will need to assess the client's potential for returning to his former occupation or consider a change of occupation. Work sample testing, simulated job tasks, or actual short-term job trials may be used to make these decisions. Work tolerance may need to be improved through the use of increasingly long periods at job samples. Alternate but related occupations may be considered or training or education for new jobs may be necessary. Home management skills and child care should be included as part of the amputee's assessment when appropriate to life roles.[4]

Duration of training

The average adult unilateral BE amputee who is otherwise healthy and well-adjusted will require approximately 6 to 10 hours of training to master control and use of the prosthesis for daily living. The unilateral AE amputee, under the same conditions, will require approximately 15 to 25 hours of training.

The initial training session should be about 1 hour long, and subsequent sessions should steadily increase in time duration in accordance with the client's increasing tolerance for the prosthesis, capabilities in use of the prosthesis, and physical endurance for activity until a full day of wear can be tolerated.

The prosthesis should remain in the training facility until use training is mastered and wearing tolerance is 3 to 4 hours. When the amputee is first allowed to take the prosthesis home, it should be for an overnight trial, so that the therapist can check for problems and correct faulty use habits before they become well established. Use of the prosthesis over the weekend should follow before the amputee makes the prosthesis a part of his regular daily life.[6]

THE LE AMPUTEE

The preprosthetic exercise program, prosthetic fitting, and ambulation training for the LE amputee are usually carried out by the physical therapist. However, occupational therapy can play an important role in the amputee's rehabilitation.

Stump conditioning in the preprosthetic training period, through purposeful activity, can be carried out in occupational therapy if the amputee has a temporary prosthesis applied at the time of surgery or through the use of a temporary pylon or working prostheses described by Mary Jones[1] in *An Approach to Occupational Therapy*. These devices, which can be constructed according to the specifications described by Jones, can be adapted for use on the floor loom, bicycle jigsaw, and treadle-operated machines. Use of the stump with the pylon or working prosthesis can promote circulation and healing, strengthen stump and proximal musculature, maintain joint ROM, and afford the amputee the senses of pressure, position, motion, and weight that may be similar to the actual prosthesis. In addition, the pylon or working prosthesis can be used to build standing tolerance when used with the stand-up table or can be worn while performing activities that require standing.

When the prosthesis is actually received and adequate ambulation skill has been achieved, the LE amputee can be engaged in ADL, such as dressing, hygiene and grooming, and home management tasks. Transfer and transportation skills may be an integral part of the occupational therapy program. Assessment of the client's vocational role and the need for change or modification should be part of the occupational therapy evaluation.

The temporary pylon or working prosthesis cannot be used until there is sound healing of the surgical site. Clients whose amputations resulted from circulatory disorders may need special adaptations, such as additional padding around the stump or the use of an above-knee device on a below-knee amputee, to prevent undue pressure on vulnerable blood vessels and circulatory compromise. These devices should be used only when medical clearance is obtained. Their benefits and the effects of use should be evaluated after every treatment session. Signs of circulatory disturbance and spasms are contraindications for their use.[1]

SAMPLE TREATMENT PLAN

Case study

Mr. K. is 41 years old. He is a member of a minority group who has lived in poverty all of his life. He is intellectually limited, although some of this may be due to poor educational advantage. Mr. K. recently sustained a left AE amputation due to a traumatic injury. The stump is well healed, and there is good stump shrinkage. There are no medical complications.

Mr. K. is receiving state aid and a prosthesis and vocational training have been authorized for him. He has done janitorial work and tobacco picking in the past. He reads the basic vocabulary necessary for everyday life at home and in the street (for example, signs and simple newspaper headlines). When employed Mr. K. is a steady and hard worker. He is married and has four children, all living at home. His interests are watching television, playing cards, and light gardening.

The client is accepting the prosthesis and is no longer depressed about the loss of his arm. Strength in the stump musculature is good to normal. He was referred to occupational therapy as an outpatient for prosthetic training and vocational evaluation. He will be scheduled for daily treatment sessions.

Treatment plan

A. Statistical data.
1. Name: Mr. K.
   Age: 41
   Diagnosis: Traumatic injury to left arm
   Disability: Left AE amputation
2. Treatment aims as stated in referral:
   Prosthetic training
   Vocational evaluation
B. **Other services.**
   Medical
   Social service
   Vocational counseling
   Sheltered employment and community social groups (possibly)
C. **OT evaluation.**
   Strength: Manual muscle test to muscles of stump
   ROM: Left shoulder, test
   Sensation (touch, pain, temperature) of end of stump: Test
   Physical endurance: Observe
   Manual dexterity, unilateral: Observe
   Speed of movement and motor planning skill: Observe
   Judgment: Observe

Problem-solving skills: Observe
Language skills: Observe
Potential work skills: Observe, test
Work habits and attitudes: Observe
Self-care independence: Test, observe
Independent travel: Observe or test
D. **Results of evaluation.**
1. Evaluation data.
   a. Physical resources.
      (1) Shoulder strength: G to N
          Rotators: G
          Flexors: N
          Extensors: N
          Adductors: G
          Abductors: N
      (2) ROM: All ranges normal
   b. Sensory-perceptual functions. Stump sensation (touch, pain, temperature): intact
   c. Cognitive functions. Limited reading skills prohibit following written directions. Client needs assistance with problem solving but succeeds with some verbal guidance.
   d. Psychosocial functions. Client tends to be quiet, cooperative, and compliant. He socializes when drawn into group interaction, but is somewhat hesitant and shy in interactions with therapist. He appears to be well motivated for prosthesis use and wear and return to employment.
   e. Prevocational potential. Client appears to have potential for unskilled work similar to that which was performed in the past. Janitorial tasks, assembly work, and simple use of tools will be part of the last phases of the prosthesis use training program.
   f. Functional skills. Mr. K. is performing most self-care activities independently, using the sound right arm, except for bilateral activities, such as cutting meat, buttoning shirt, applying deodorant, carrying large objects, and tying shoes. He needs some assistance in analyzing methods for one-handed performance.
2. Problem identification.
   a. Weakness in left shoulder rotators and adductors
   b. Limited problem-solving skills
   c. Partial self-care dependence
   d. Loss of vocational role, family provider
   e. Inability to use AE prosthesis

Continued.

SAMPLE TREATMENT PLAN—cont'd

E Specific OT objectives	F Methods used to meet objectives	G Gradation of treatment
With daily exercise the strength of shoulder rotators and adductors will increase from good to normal	PRE to shoulder adductors, using wall pulleys; PRE to shoulder rotators, using weighted cuffs on stump; client holds stump in 90° shoulder flexion, then 90° shoulder abduction and rotates shoulder internally and externally	Increase resistance by adding weight; increase number of repetitions from 10 to 30 per day
The client will achieve proficiency in stump care within the first week of the treatment program, so that stump care is carried out independently on a daily basis at home	Washing and drying stump; application and removal of stump socks; washing out stump socks; daily change of stump socks	Decrease amount of direction and assistance as proficiency is achieved
The client will know the names and functions of all the parts of the prosthesis by the end of the first week of training	Teach names and functions of parts of prosthesis; review repetitively during remainder of first week of training	
The client will be able to put on and remove the prosthesis smoothly and efficiently within 5 minutes at the end of the first week of training	Repetitive application and removal of prosthesis for practice	Decrease amount of supervision and assistance
The client will achieve proficiency in controls of elbow flexion, elbow locking, and TD opening and closing, so that each control motion is performed when needed with little or no hesitation by the end of the second week of training	Practice in elbow flexion control, elbow locking, and TD opening and closing; practice in performing these tasks in sequence	From need for assistance and direction to *independent* functioning, increase time spent in training sessions and wearing prosthesis
The client will be able to preposition the TD when using practice objects, so that he can preposition the TD and pick up 75% of the objects with little or no hesitation by the end of the second week of training	Grasp and release of objects of various weights, textures, sizes, and shapes in a variety of positions, for example, cans, jars, wood cylinders, blocks, pencils, door knob, and cabinet handles	Grasp and release large, hard objects to soft, light objects. Progress from table surface to grasp and release at side, overhead, and on floor
The client will achieve moderate skill in performance of bilateral ADL, so that he is performing 75% of these activities independently at home within the fourth week of training	Fasten trousers; handle wallet; tie shoes; clean fingernails; apply deodorant; tie necktie; button shirt; use phone; cut food	Increase number of simple to complex activities client is expected to perform; decrease amount of supervision and assistance
The client's potential for employment will be evaluated during the fifth and sixth weeks of the training program so that specific information about potential work skills, work habits and attitudes, and work tolerance can be conveyed to the vocational counselor	Janitorial work—floor cleaning, emptying trash Assembly jobs—electronic parts assembly Use of hand tools in light woodwork, such as sawing, hammering, drilling, using a screwdriver, planing, and sanding	Increase complexity and speed of work, time spent at work samples, and amount of manipulation required of prosthesis; decrease amount of instruction and supervision

---

SAMPLE TREATMENT PLAN—cont'd

H. **Special equipment.**
  1. Ambulation aids.
     None required
  2. Splints.
     None required
  3. Assistive devices.
     Amputee buttonhook to button right shirt cuff

REVIEW QUESTIONS

1. What do the following abbreviations mean?
   a. AE
   b. TD
   c. BE
2. Which arm function is lost and which functions are maintained in a long BE amputation?
3. Name two common problems of amputees that can interfere with prosthetic training. How is each solved?
4. What are the purposes of preprosthetic training?
5. Describe activities and exercises suitable for the preprosthetic period.
6. List the five major steps in prosthetic training.
7. What is the sequence of training in learning controls of the AE prosthesis?
8. What is the sequence of training in learning use of the prosthesis?
9. What motion of the arm accomplishes elbow locking on the AE prosthesis?
10. Before an AE amputee can operate the TD, what must he do?
11. What motions accomplish TD opening?
12. How is the TD prepositioned by the amputee?
13. Name two types of TDs. Which is more frequently prescribed and used?
14. How is use training graded?
15. When is the proper time for the amputee in a prosthetic training program to take his prosthesis home?
16. The best position for the TD when holding a coffee cup is at _____° _____.
17. When using an eggbeater the _____ holds the top of the beater while the _____ cranks the handle.
18. Describe the role of occupational therapy in the rehabilitation of LE amputees.

REFERENCES

1. Jones, M.S.: An approach to occupational therapy, ed. 2, London, 1964, Butterworth & Co. Ltd.
2. Larson, C.B., and Gould, M.: Orthopedic nursing, ed. 8, St. Louis, 1974, The C.V. Mosby Co.
3. Santschi, W.R., editor: Manual of upper extremity prosthetics, ed. 2, Los Angeles, 1958, University of California Press.
4. Spencer, E.A.: Amputations. In Hopkins, H.L., and Smith, H.D., editors: Willard and Spackman's occupational therapy, ed. 5, New York, 1978, J.B. Lippincott Co.
5. Trombly, C.A., and Scott, A.D.: Occupational therapy for physical dysfunction, Baltimore, 1977, The Williams & Wilkins Co.
6. Wellerson, T.L.: A manual for occupational therapists on the rehabilitation of upper extremity amputees, Dubuque, 1958, Wm. C. Brown Co., Publishers.
7. Wright, G.: Controls training for the upper extremity amputee, film, San Jose, Calif., Instructional Resource Center, San Jose State University.

SUPPLEMENTARY READING

Adams, I.L.: Bilateral lower extremity dressing frame, Am. J. Occup. Ther. 29:547, 1975.
Bailey, R.B.: An upper extremity prosthetic training arm, Am. J. Occup. Ther. 24:357, 1970.
Butts, D.E., and Goldberg, M.J.: Congenital absence of the radius, Am. J. Occup. Ther. 31:95, 1977.
Friedman, L.: Bilateral upper extremity amputee sandwich holder, Am. J. Occup. Ther. 28:358, 1974.
Kerstein, M.D., et al.: Successful rehabilitation following amputation of dominant versus nondominant extremities, Am. J. Occup. Ther. 31:313, 1977.
Marker, M.A.: Adapted living aids for the bilateral shoulder disarticulation, Am. J. Occup. Ther. 31:584, 1977.
Van Laere, M., et al.: A prosthetic appliance for a patient with a brachial plexus injury and forearm amputation: a case report, Am. J. Occup. Ther. 31:309, 1977.
Wendt, J., and Shaperman, J.: A study of development of prehension patterns: the infant with a cable-controlled hook, Am. J. Occup. Ther. 24:393, 1970.
Willard, H.S., and Spackman, C.S., editors: Occupational therapy, ed. 4, Philadelphia, 1971, J.B. Lippincott Co.
Wright, G.: Meet Jerry Leavey, film, San Jose, Calif., 1968, Instructional Resources Center, San Jose State University.

Chapter 8

Burns

The burn injury is the result of thermal damage to the skin and possibly to underlying structures. It is one of the most severe forms of trauma to the body. It may be due to contact with flame, hot fluids, steam,[13] chemicals, or electricity. The extent and seriousness of the injury depend on the amount of skin surface area involved and the depth of the burn.

Possible disabilities that can result from a burn injury include (1) loss of joint motion due to contractures of overlying skin; (2) loss of muscle strength due to disuse or nerve involvement; (3) loss of sensation due to destruction of the sense receptors in the skin or concomitant nerve damage; (4) loss of body parts, especially common to fingers; (5) disfigurement; and (6) associated injuries, such as loss of vision, neurovascular damage, and fractures.

The injury can result in serious psychosocial problems that rehabilitation workers should be aware of and deal with in their treatment of the client. These include depression and withdrawal; adverse reactions to disfigurement; anxiety and uncertainty about the ability to resume work, family, community, and leisure roles; financial difficulties; and concern about being accepted by family and friends.

MEDICAL MANAGEMENT

Following the burn injury the extent and depth of the burn must be medically evaluated to determine its severity. The patient's age, general health, past medical history, and part of the body that was burned will also be important factors in determining the severity of the burn injury.[7]

The surface area of the burn is usually measured by the rule of nines in adults over 16 years of age. The measurements are modified for children to accommodate the difference in proportion of limbs to trunk to head. The rule of nines is used to estimate the percentage of body area that has been injured. It divided the body surface into areas of 9% or multiples of 9%[7] (Fig. 8-1).

The depth of the burn is measured by degrees or thickness of the skin injured. The first-degree burn is relatively superficial and is a partial thickness burn of the epidermis only. It is characterized by pain and red-

ness and usually heals in 2 to 4 days without scarring. Treatment consists of measures to relieve discomfort.[1]

Second-degree burns, also referred to as partial thickness and deep partial thickness burns,[1,7] involve destruction of the full thickness of the epidermis and some portion of the dermis. The burn injury extends below the basal layer of the epidermis.[8] The burn is painful, and there is blister formation and subcutaneous edema.[1,7] Healing usually takes place in 2 to 4 weeks, and the amount of scarring is related to the depth of the burn. Healing occurs as a result of regeneration from epithelium-lined skin appendages, which are the hair follicles and sebaceous and sweat glands. Infection can convert the second-degree burn to a third-degree burn.[1]

The third-degree burn, or full thickness burn, destroys all layers of the skin and skin appendages down to the subcutaneous tissue.[1] There may be muscle, tendon, or bone damage as well.[7] The burn is not painful, since all skin receptors have been destroyed. Spontaneous healing is not possible, and there is regeneration of the epidermis only at the margins of the wound. Skin grafting is required to effect wound healing and minimize scarring and contracture.[1]

Recovery from burn injury may be divided into three phases. The first is the shock phase, which is the first 48 hours after the injury. During this period there is increased permeability of blood vessels, causing rapid leakage of protein-rich fluid to extravascular tissue thus resulting in edema.[1,7] The lymphatic system, which would normally carry away the excess fluid in the tissues, becomes overloaded.[7] Treatment includes intravenous fluid replacement with electrolyte and colloid solutions.[1,13] The fluid volume required is determined by a formula based on the extent of the burn and the weight of the patient.[13] The rate of fluid infusion is monitored by pulse rate, urinary output, central venous pressure, hematocrit, and state of consciousness.

During the shock phase a tracheostomy may be required to establish an adequate airway. Removal of burn eschar may be necessary to prevent constriction of the chest or of a limb, which can result from excessive edema. Escharotomy can improve ventilation and blood flow to a part.[13] Debridement is carried out to remove debris and loose epidermis. Additional medical measures include wound dressings and topical and systemic antibiotic therapy during this phase.[13]

The infection phase is the second recovery phase and begins about 5 days after the burn wound occurs and continues until the burn is less than 20% of the body area. During this period normal bacterial flora may be replaced by gram-negative organisms, usually *Pseudomonas aeruginosa,* that live on dead tissue.[1,8,13] The burn wound invasion syndrome is characterized by listlessness, bradycardia, hypothermia, and hypotension.[1,8] Infection is treated with topical antibiotics, such as silver sulfadiazine cream, silver nitrate, gentamycin, and Sulfamylon cream. Debridement is also carried out surgically or through the use of Travase ointment, which acts enzymatically to digest dead tissue. Hydrotherapy and skin grafting are also used in this phase of recovery.[1,8]

During the shock and infection phases, positioning, splinting, and exercise are used to prevent contracture and deformity.

The third phase of treatment is the rehabilitation phase. This is the after grafting period when the patient is medically stable. The goals of treatment are increased self-care independence, prevention of deformity and scarring, recovery of strength and ROM, prevocational exploration, and psychosocial adjustment.

The rehabilitation team is composed of the physician, psychiatrist or psychologist, physical and occupational therapists, nurse, nursing aides, social workers, recreation therapist, vocational counselor, client, and family.

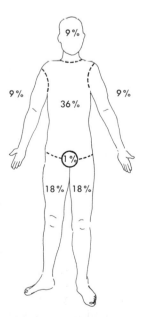

Fig. 8-1. Rules of nines.

THE ROLE OF OCCUPATIONAL THERAPY
Before grafting stage

During the before grafting stage of treatment the occupational therapy evaluation should include a review of the medical history to determine the degree and depth of the burn and the general medical status of the client. If possible the therapist should interview the client to begin to establish rapport and understand his life roles, goals, and needs. Active and passive ROM should be measured or estimated if possible. The need for special splints and positioning to prevent contracture and deformity should be ascertained.[9]

In cooperation with the aims of the other members of the rehabilitation team, the treatment aims of occupational therapy are to prevent deformity from skin contractures, prevent loss of ROM and strength in affected and unaffected parts, achieve maximum self-care independence possible at this stage, and provide psychological support.

Treatment is conducted in a sterile environment, using aseptic techniques. Early treatment includes maintaining antideformity positions of affected parts through splinting and positioning. Positioning techniques are listed in Table 5. Depending on the area involved some splints that may be used to maintain antideformity positions are the neck conformer (Fig. 8-2), axillary or airplane splint (Fig. 8-3), elbow or knee conformer (Fig. 8-4), antideformity splint (Fig. 8-5), three-point extension splint for the elbow or knee, and finger flexion or extension splints. Splints are made of low-temperature thermoplastics that can be gas autoclaved. They should be carefully washed and dried before each application, which is after wound cleansing, debridement, and dressing, at least twice a day. Night splinting is used until spontaneous healing occurs or, if there has been grafting, until the grafted areas have set, which is usually in 7 to 10 days. Splints must be revised frequently.[7]

In addition to splinting and positioning the occupational therapy program should include active ROM exercises for frequent short periods until pain and fatigue tolerance levels are reached. These may be carried out during dressing changes or hydrotherapy.[7] If there are dorsal burns of the hands, fist making should be avoided. Resistive exercises may be used for unaffected areas to maintain strength and ROM. They may also be used for burned areas if the hands are not burned, and the exercise equipment can be used without macerating the burned areas.

Simple craft activities and self-care activities that are within the client's ability may be used to encourage purposeful use of affected parts, promote independence, enhance self-esteem, and divert attention from the dysfunction to functional capacities.[9]

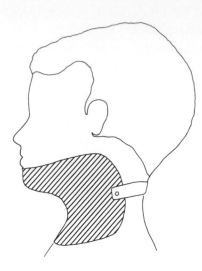

Fig. 8-2. Neck conformer splint to prevent flexion contracture of neck skin.

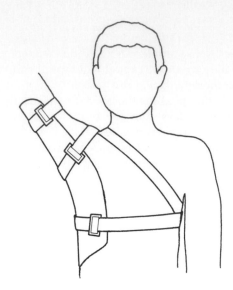

Fig. 8-3. Axillary or airplane splint to prevent adduction contracture of shoulder.

Table 5. Antideformity positioning and splinting[3,7,13]

Body part and splint	Position		
	Supine	Prone	Side lying
Neck			
Neck conformer, soft cervical collar	Slight extension; no pillow, except small roll behind neck may be used	Extension; small roll under forehead or head turned to side	Extension; pillows can be used to maintain position as needed
Shoulders			
Axillary or airplane splints	Abducted at least 90° with slight internal rotation	Same as for supine position	Position free shoulder at or near 90° flexion
Elbows			
Elbow conformer, three-point extension splint	Position in full extension and forearm in supination when anterior surface is involved	Alternate between 40° flexion and full extension	Extension; splints may be used to maintain extended position
Wrist and hand			
Antideformity splint	Splint to maintain antideformity position or maintain wrist extension by placing roll between thumb and fingers	Same as for supine position	Splint to maintain antideformity position
Hips			
No splints used	Extension with approximately 15° of abduction to separate thighs	Same as for supine position	Alternate extension of hips
Knees			
Three-point extension splint or knee conformer	Extension; splinting if knee, posterior thigh, or leg are burned	Extension; same as for supine position	Alternate extension of knees
Ankles and feet			
Footboard, foot drop splints	Ankles at neutral position with no pressure at heel and the plantar surface supported; posterior leg splint to maintain position	Hang feet over edge of mattress to maintain the position	Maintain neutral position; splint if necessary

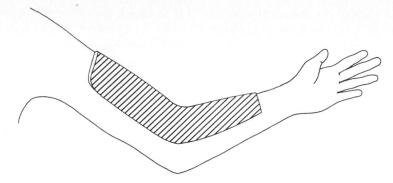

Fig. 8-4. Elbow conformer splint to prevent elbow flexion contracture.

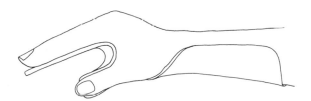

Fig. 8-5. Antideformity splint for dorsal burn of hand to prevent clawhand deformity.

The occupational therapist needs to offer the client reassurance and psychological support. Physical proximity to other people and facilitation of the relationship between the client and important others in his life can help to overcome feelings of revulsion and aversion to self.[10]

Grafting stage

During the grafting stage prevention of loss of ROM and deformity continue as important treatment aims. Additional aims are to preserve muscle strength in affected areas, prevent loss of ROM and strength in unaffected areas, prevent dependence, and alleviate depression.

These aims are achieved through several modalities. Appropriate splints are applied immediately after grafting to maintain desired position and prevent motion of the grafted area. No motion to grafted areas, adjacent areas, and donor sites is allowed for 5 to 7 days.[5,6] Isometric exercises to muscles in the grafted area may be used to maintain strength. Gentle, active exercise is commenced after 5 to 7 days. After 7 to 10 days active-assisted or resistive exercises may be started.[4] Pressure dressings are applied as soon as the skin can tolerate pressure. Their purposes are to hasten scar maturation and prevent hypertrophic scarring. They are worn 23 hours per day.[5] Active and resistive exercises, which do not produce stretching or motion of grafted and adjacent areas, may be used to maintain strength and ROM of involved parts while grafts are setting.

Environmental stimulation, self-care, and avocational activities should be continued and increased if possible, commensurately with the client's physical abilities and tolerance level.

Activities that can be used include leather lacing, ceramic tile work, floor loom weaving, peg games, and puzzles.[6] Activities that require irritating substances or potentially hazardous tools or equipment such as clay modeling or chip carving should be avoided.[10]

After grafting stage, extended rehabilitation

When grafts are healed and more activity is possible, a more thorough occupational therapy evaluation can be carried out with greater emphasis on assessment of performance skills.

Active and passive ROM measurements should be taken. Muscle strength can be measured by the manual muscle test, although this should be done only if the graft has taken well and with extreme caution when applying resistance on skin surfaces.[5] Performance of self-care and home management activities should be evaluated, including the need for assistive devices.[5] Psychological adjustment should be assessed by observation, interview, and consultation with other members of the rehabilitation team, especially the psychologist or psychiatrist and the social worker. Some clients may require driving evaluation. Evaluation of vocational potential should be undertaken in the later stages of rehabilitation if residual dysfunction necessitates a change in former vocational role.[5]

During the extended rehabilitation period the treatment aims are to (1) increase ROM of affected joints, (2) improve strength and physical endurance for return to community and employment, (3) increase skin tolerance level of grafted areas, (4) prevent hypertrophic scarring, (5) achieve independence in ADL, (6) explore vocational potential, and (7) aid psychological adjustment, including the restoration of self-confidence, social adjustment, and community reentry.[5]

To achieve these goals active and resistive exercises are continued for involved and uninvolved areas. Therapeutic activities are used for increasing strength, ROM, and endurance, as well as for psychological release, development of self-esteem, and evaluation of work-related skills.

Simulated work activities or work sample testing may be used to evaluate vocational potential. Training in self-care and home management activities and use of assistive devices as needed are carried out. Training in mobility, transfers, and ambulation is appropriate if wheelchair or other ambulation aids are required.

Hypersensitivity of grafted areas may be decreased through the self-application of handling, touch, and pressure stimuli,[12] and activities using tools and materials may be graded from soft to hard.[10]

Pressure splints and bandages and Jobst pressure garments are used to prevent hypertrophic scarring.[5] The occupational therapist is often responsible for the measurement and fitting of the pressure garments.[6] These are designed to conform to the burned part with the desired amount of pressure at different points in the garment.[10] They are used from approximately 2 weeks after grafting and have proved to be effective in reducing hypertrophic scars and contractures. The Jobst Institute, Inc. in Toledo, Ohio, provides diagrams and instructions for measurement. Willis[14] describes and illustrates a variety of Jobst garments and the directions for their use.

The occupational therapist should maintain a supportive and reassuring approach, yet not give excessive or false praise or demonstrate pity. Activities that require gradually increasing amounts of decision making,[12] responsibility, and initiative can increase self-determination and self-confidence.

The burned hand

A burn injury of the hand requires special consideration, since it is a common injury, can result in serious dysfunction if not treated appropriately, and is a primary concern of the occupational therapist.[7]

Dorsal burns are more common than those on the palmar surface. A dorsal burn can result in a clawhand deformity. A contracture of the skin on the dorsal surface of the hand will tend to flatten the metacarpal transverse arch and pull the MP joints into extension with associated flexion of the IP joints, and the thumb will assume the adducted and extended position. The wrist will be pulled into flexion and radial deviation.[7,8] The extensor tendons, which lie superficially on the dorsum

of the hand, are especially vulnerable to injury as they cross the PIP joint. The central slip of the extensor tendon, inserting at the PIP joint, may rupture. If this occurs, a boutonnière deformity will result.[2,7]

Serious palmar burns are uncommon because of the thickness of the palmar skin and because the hands are used instinctively to protect the face or body.[2,13] Palmar burns usually result from direct contact with a hot object, electricity, or chemical substance. The deformity that could result from the palmar burn is severe flexion and adduction contractures of the fingers and thumb.[13]

Treatment of the dorsal burn. The elements of treatment of a dorsal burn of the hand consist of active exercise, or active-assisted exercise if the client is incapable of active motion, from the first day after the injury occurs; elevation of the hand above heart level; and splinting. The hand is splinted in the antideformity position, which is 30° of wrist extension, 70° to 90° of MP flexion, complete PIP and DIP extension, and extension and palmar abduction of the thumb.[2,7] This position prevents contracture of the collateral ligaments and intrinsic muscles, protects the central slip of the extensor tendon over the PIP joint from rupture, and maintains the dorsal skin and thumb web space fully stretched.[2,8]

In first-degree or mild second-degree burns splinting may not be necessary unless there is edema and resulting tendency to revert to the claw position. Active exercise is initiated on the first day with no restrictions of motion. Fist making is allowed. In moderate to deep second- to third-degree burns continuous splinting is necessary when there is edema in the before grafting stage, except during exercise periods. When edema has subsided, the splint may be worn at night and during periods of inactivity. Functional activities and exercise are used during the day to encourage motion. Passive PIP and DIP flexion are contraindicated, as is fist making. Active PIP and DIP flexion are allowed if the MP joints are stabilized in extension. Full finger extension and abduction and wrist and thumb motions are allowed. A Jobst pressure glove to control hypertrophic scarring is used after healing has taken place.[2]

Treatment of the palmar burn. The treatment of the full thickness palmar burn is similar to that for the dorsal burn. The antideformity position is 15° to 20° of wrist extension, full extension and abduction of the fingers, and extension and radial abduction of the thumb.[2,7] This position can be maintained by a "banjo splint" applied to the dorsal surface of the hand.[2] Dressmaker's hooks, glued to each fingernail with a polymer adhesive, allow the fingers to be held in gentle traction by fastening rubber bands from each of them to the distal end of the splint.[11]

SAMPLE TREATMENT PLAN

Case study

Mr. B. is a 45-year-old automobile assembly worker who was burned in an automobile accident. He sustained deep second- and third-degree burns in the region of the left shoulder, left axilla, anterior surface of the left arm, and dorsum of the hand.

Mr. B. is considered a well-adjusted family man. He lives with his wife and two teenaged children in their own home. He is the sole support of his family. His leisure activities include spectator sports, card playing, gardening, golf, and home repairs.

He has been admitted to the burn unit of a rehabilitation center. Occupational therapy has been called on to treat Mr. B. through all phases of rehabilitation. The objectives are to prevent contractures and deformity, restore maximum functional independence, and aid with adjustment to disability.

Treatment plan

A. Statistical data.
  1. Name: Mr. B.
     Age: 45
     Diagnosis: Burn injury to left upper extremity
     Disability: Potential axillary contracture, elbow flexion contracture, and clawhand deformity
  2. Treatment aims as stated in referral:
     Prevent contractures and deformity
     Restore to maximum functional independence
     Aid with adjustment to disability
B. Other services.
  Physician: Prescribe medication; perform debridement or escharotomy as needed; supervise rehabilitation therapies; grafting
  Nursing: Nursing care; positioning; administer medications; change dressings; carry out ADL
  Physical therapy: Prevent contractures through ROM and strengthening exercises; hydrotherapy procedures
  Psychologist: Evaluate psychological status; counsel; consultant to staff
  Social worker: Explore financial problems; counsel client and family
  Family: Provide support, acceptance, encouragement, and assistance
  Vocational counseling: Explore feasibility of return to same or similar job; explore job alternatives, if needed
  Recreation therapy: Mental stimulation; activities for enjoyment and diversion; function of affected and nonaffected parts

C. OT evaluation.
  Before grafting.
    Active and passive ROM: Observe
    Muscle strength: Observe for function
    ADL: Observe
    Need for splints and positioning: Observe
    Psychological status: Observe, interview, and consult with psychologist
  After grafting.
    Active and passive ROM: Measure
    Muscle strength: Test with precautions
    ADL: Evaluate performance
    Pressure garments: Assess need, measure
    Psychological adjustment: Observe
    Sensory modalities: Test for touch and thermal sensitivity; hypersensitivity
    Vocational exploration: Evaluate simulated work skills
    Assistive devices: Observe need
D. Results of evaluation.
  1. Evaluation data.
    a. Physical resources.
       Before grafting: Active ROM limited to approximately 90° of shoulder flexion and abduction; full active extension of elbow, wrist, and fingers possible; muscle strength observed to be at least at good level
       After grafting: Shoulder ROM increased to 130°; full motion possible at elbow, wrist, and fingers; strength in left arm rated good in all muscle groups
    b. Sensory-perceptual functions.
       Before grafting: Not tested
       After grafting: Hypersensitivity to light touch and thermal stimuli; normal perceptual functions
    c. Cognitive functions. Within normal limits for a 45-year-old adult
    d. Psychosocial functions. Initial depression and withdrawal are gradually being replaced by increasing motivation to recover and resume former life roles; active involvement and participation in the rehabilitation program is increasing; client realistic about injury, medical status, and future potential
    e. Prevocational potential. Since a good recovery is expected, client will probably be able to return to former place of employment at a less demanding job on the line; physical endurance, work speed, and use of power tools will be evaluated during the stage of extended rehabilitation

Continued.

SAMPLE TREATMENT PLAN—cont'd

f. Functional skills.

Before grafting: Client able to do most hygiene and grooming, feeding, and dressing activities with uninvolved hand, using one-handed techniques, except for washing and combing hair

After grafting: Client independent in all self-care activities and light home management activities and able to handle garden tools and do light gardening (raking and planting); he cannot play golf because of sudden stretching movements required; he can handle minor woodworking tools without difficulty and can hold cards with left hand, although it tires easily and he prefers to use a card holder

2. Problem identification.

Before grafting:

a. Potential contracture and deformity of left shoulder, elbow, wrist, and hand

b. Depression and withdrawal, initially

c. Anxiety about hospitalization and potential disability

After grafting:

d. Decreased physical endurance

e. Slight limitation of strength in left arm

f. Limited range of shoulder flexion and abduction

g. Changed vocational and leisure roles

h. Potential hypertrophic scarring

i. Hypersensitivity of grafted areas

3. Assets/functions.

Normal right arm and lower extremities

Good coping skills

Supportive family

Good potential for reemployment

Severe deformity prevented in before grafting and grafting stages of treatment

Intelligent, realistic outlook

Good motivation and cooperation with medical and rehabilitation efforts

E Problem	F Specific OT objectives	G Methods used to meet objectives	H Gradation of treatment
Before grafting stage a	Through splinting, positioning, and exercise, contracture and deformity will be prevented at shoulder, elbow, wrist, and fingers	Positioning and splinting the shoulder in 90° of abduction, elbow in full extension, and hand with wrist extended, MPs flexed to 90°, PIP and DIP in complete extension, thumb abducted and extended Elevate arm above heart to reduce edema Active ROM exercise, if possible for all joints, frequently for very short periods of time	Revise splints as edema decreases to maintain maximum anti-deformity positions Passive to active exercise if active ROM is not possible initially
b, c	Through a supportive and accepting approach and environment and appropriate activities, the client's depression will subside, and he will participate more actively in the rehabilitation program	Therapist uses supportive, reassuring approach to client Procedures are carefully explained and guided Therapist explains potential disability and preventive measures to client and family Card and board games with other clients are used to enhance discussion of feelings, reactions to injury, anxieties about disfigurement, and acceptance; therapist acts as guide and facilitator	Increase interaction with staff and other clients Increase independent decision making regarding activities and topics of discussion

SAMPLE TREATMENT PLAN—cont'd

E Problem	F Specific OT objectives	G Methods used to meet objectives	H Gradation of treatment
Grafting stage a	Through appropriate splinting and positioning, grafted areas will be prevented from moving to promote healing	Axillary splint with shoulder abducted to 135° Elbow conformer splint to maintain full extension Antideformity splint for hand Splints worn 24 hours per day for 5 to 7 days	
a	Through isometric exercise during immobilization, muscle strength will be maintained at good grade	Isometric exercise without resistance to shoulder flexors, extensors, and abductors; elbow flexors and extensors; and wrist and finger flexors and extensors	
After grafting stage a, d, e, f	Through exercise and functional activities, ROM and strength in left arm will be maintained or increased	Gentle, active exercise to all joints of left arm against gravity Independent performance of self-care activities Board games or leather lacing positioned for maximum possible reach overhead, in front, and out to side of body	Increase to light resistive exercise as strength and tolerance improves Add gardening activities when well healed Add woodwork when fully healed
h	Through pressure garments, hypertrophic scarring will be minimized or prevented over grafted areas	Jobst pressure garment for left arm and hand to be worn 22 hours per day for 6 to 9 months	
i	Through graded tactile stimulation, grafted areas will be desensitized so that touch, light rubbing, and pressure can be tolerated in everyday living	Self-application of touch and pressure stimuli and rubbing with own fingers, then with fabrics and brushes graded in texture	Grade from satin to velvet to felt to cotton to muslin to denim Soft, fine brush to coarse paint brush

I. **Special equipment.**
   A. Ambulation aids.
     None required
   B. Splints.
     Axillary splint: Maintain abduction at shoulder
     Elbow conformer: Maintain extension
     Antideformity splint: Prevent claw deformity for dorsal burn of the hand
   C. Assistive devices.
     None required

REVIEW QUESTIONS

1. What is the role of the occupational therapist in the before grafting stage of treatment of the burn patient?
2. What is the purpose of splinting after burn injury?
3. What kind of exercise is appropriate to maintain muscle strength during immobilization in the grafting stage? What is the rationale for this?
4. Describe or demonstrate the antideformity position for bedrest in the supine position.
5. What types of exercise are commenced 7 days after grafting?
6. What is the precaution for exercising a hand with a dorsal burn? Why is this so?
7. What measures can be taken to desensitize hypersensitivity of healed graft areas?
8. What is the purpose of pressure garments?
9. In which position is the hand with palmar burn splinted?
10. Which important tendon can be ruptured when there is a dorsal burn? How can this be prevented?
11. How can the occupational therapist help the patient accept himself and prepare him for return to the community?
12. What are some of the social and psychological problems that the burn injured patient may experience? Discuss how occupational therapy can help to prevent or minimize these problems during early phases of treatment and later during the extended rehabilitation program.

REFERENCES

1. Anonymous: Aims of the American Burn Association: prevention, care, teaching, and research. Mimeographed.
2. Anonymous: Hand protocol, San Jose, Calif., 1972, Department of Plastic and Reconstructive Surgery, Burn Unit, Santa Clara Valley Medical Center. Mimeographed.
3. Anonymous: Positioning, San Jose, Calif., 1972, Department of Plastic and Reconstructive Surgery, Burn Unit, Santa Clara Valley Medical Center. Mimeographed.
4. Cervelli, L.: O.T. for the burn patient, lecture, San Jose, Calif., 1974, Department of Occupational Therapy, San Jose State University.
5. Gorham, J.: O.T. for the burn patient, lecture, San Jose, Calif., 1975, Department of Occupational Therapy, San Jose State University.
6. Krocker, C., Denor, B., and Nicoud, B.: Occupational therapy in the rehabilitation of burn patients, Milwaukee, 1977, St. Mary's Hospital.
7. Malick, M.H.: Burns. In Hopkins, H.L., and Smith, H.D., editors: Willard and Spackman's occupational therapy, ed. 5, Philadelphia, 1978, J.B. Lippincott Co.
8. Pardoe, R.: Wound healing and burns, lectures, San Jose, Calif., 1978, Department of Occupational Therapy, San Jose State University.
9. Schiff, W.: O.T. for the burn patient, lecture, San Jose, Calif., 1977, Department of Occupational Therapy, San Jose State University.
10. Trombly, C.A., and Scott, A.D.: Occupational therapy for physical dysfunction, Baltimore, 1977, The Williams & Wilkins Co.
11. Von Prince, K., Curreri, W., and Pruitt, B.A.: Application of fingernail hooks in splinting burned hands, Am. J. Occup. Ther. 24:556, 1970.
12. Von Prince, K.: O.T. for the burn patient, lecture, San Jose, Calif., 1971, Department of Occupational Therapy, San Jose State College.
13. Von Prince, K., and Yaekel, M.: The splinting of burn patients, Springfield, Ill., 1974, Charles C Thomas, Publisher.
14. Willis, B.A.: Burn scar hypertrophy: a treatment method, Galveston, Tex., 1973, Shriners Burn Institute.

SUPPLEMENTARY READING

Curreri, P.W., and Pruitt, B.A., Jr.: Evaluation and treatment of the burned patient, Am. J. Occup. Ther. 24:475, 1970.
Fishwick, G.M., and Tobin, D.G.: Splinting the burned hand with primary excision and early grafting, Am. J. Occup. Ther. 32:182, 1978.
Gorham, J.A.: A mouth splint for burn microstomia, Am. J. Occup. Ther. 31:105, 1977.
Petersen, P.: A conformer for the reduction of facial burn contracture: a preliminary report, Am. J. Occup. Ther. 31:101, 1977.
Rivers, E.A., Strate, R.G., and Solem, L.D.: The transparent face mask, Am. J. Occup. Ther. 33:108, 1979.
Willis, B.: The use of orthoplast isoprene splints in the treatment of the acutely burned child, Am. J. Occup. Ther. 24:187, 1970.

Chapter 9

Rheumatoid arthritis

Rheumatoid arthritis is a chronic systemic disease that can affect the lungs, cardiovascular system, and eyes in some clients. However, joint involvement resulting from inflammatory disease of the synovium is the primary clinical feature.[4,11,12] The disease may range from mild to severe and can result in joint deformity and destruction of varying degrees.[11]

Although rheumatoid arthritis occurs most frequently between the ages of 20 and 40[4] and about three times more frequently in women than in men, it can occur from infancy to old age.[4,11,12]

The cause of the disease is unknown, however, there appears to be a continued immune reaction in the synovium that results in its inflammation and pannus formation.[4] This can progress to erode the joint capsule, tendons, ligaments, and eventually cartilage and bone.[4,12]

Diagnosis

The diagnosis is usually made by an analysis of the initial symptoms, the presence of rheumatoid nodules usually over bony prominences, radiologic evidence of cartilage destruction or bony erosions, and presence of the rheumatoid factor in the blood serum.[12] Certain macroglobulins or antiglobulins constitute the rheumatoid factor.[4]

The number of clinical features present determines the classification of the disease. It can be designated as *possible*, *probable*, *definite*, or *classic* rheumatoid arthritis.[2,12]

Course

The onset of rheumatoid arthritis is usually gradual or insidious, although it may be abrupt. It is characterized by bilateral, symmetrical involvement of the small joints of the hands and feet.[2,12] The joints are typically painful, stiff, tender, hot, and occasionally, red.

Muscles that act on the involved joints may decrease in strength and size fairly early in the course of the disease due to disuse. ROM is limited because of edema and pain in the early stages and later may be due to destructive changes in the joint.[2]

The systemic manifestations should not be overlooked. Signs, which may be present in varying degrees, include fever, weight loss, weakness, fatigue, and generalized stiffness.[2] There may be an apparent depression and lack of motivation that may be related to the fatigue and organic symptoms and should be differentiated from the same symptoms that can be psychogenic.[12]

The course of the disease is unpredictable. Some individuals experience a single, brief episode and others experience multiple episodes of varying severity. A small percentage of patients experience a gradual and continuous progression to severe joint deformity and dysfunction.[2]

The course is usually characterized by exacerbations and remissions. The client's level of function and independence can fluctuate from independent to completely dependent, varying with the stage and severity of the disease process.[11,12]

Drug therapy

Drugs used include aspirin and aspirin-like analgesics, intra-articular steroids, systemic steroids, gold salts, antimalarials, and cytotoxic agents.[9,12] Aspirin is the drug of choice because of its analgesic and anti-inflammatory properties.[2,9,12] Nonsteroidal, anti-inflammatory agents that can be used are indomethacin, phenylbutazone, ibuprofen, naproxen, and tolectin. Some of these have potentially serious side effects that are, fortunately, rare. They act to relieve inflammation, but do not alter the course of the disease.[9,12]

Steroids are used as anti-inflammatory agents, which usually are very effective. However, because of the multiplicity and potential seriousness of their side effects, they are reserved for patients who would become severely disabled without them.[12]

Gold salts also act as effective anti-inflammatory agents. The mechanisms of their action is unknown. Because of the close monitoring of the patient, which is required to identify potential toxicity, and the seriousness of the possible side effects, the use of gold salts is reserved for patients who are dependable and have failed to respond to more conservative forms of treatment.[2,12]

Antimalarial drugs such as chloroquine and plaquenil sulfate and cytotoxic agents, such as Cytoxan, Imuran, and penicillamine, are used infrequently and can benefit selected patients. Their undesirable side effects are serious considerations and may preclude their use.[9,12]

Surgical procedures that may be of benefit to patients with rheumatoid arthritis include synovectomy, tendon repair and transplant, tightening of ligaments, joint replacement, bone resection, and joint fusion.[2,9,12]

Psychological factors

It has been suggested that rheumatoid arthritis is "psychosomatic," stress induced, or somehow related to specific personality variables. However, the research has not been adequate to produce definite associations between personality variables and the disease.[12,14]

Personality factors seen in patients with rheumatoid arthritis are found in persons with other chronic diseases and in the healthy population. The psychological factors are probably a response to chronic disease rather than a predisposing cause.[12] The patient may have suffered a serious change in physical function and life roles, and even appearance may be altered by deformity and drug side effects. These changes evoke an adjustment process akin to the grief process after a death. The patient may respond to the disability with depression, denial, a need to control the environment, and dependency.[12]

Some aspects of the illness that may contribute to the psychological state include constant pain and fear of pain; changed body image and perception of self as a sick person; continuous uncertainty about the course and prognosis of the disease; sexual dysfunction because of pain or deformity; and altered social, family, vocational, and leisure roles.

Rehabilitation workers need to be aware of the client's response to his disability and the adjustment that is in progress. All of the factors and behaviors just cited will have an influence on rehabilitation. The interaction of personnel with the client can facilitate the development of healthy coping mechanisms and acceptance of disability. The reader is referred to Melvin[12] for a more detailed discussion of this subject.

SPECIFIC JOINT PROBLEMS AND DEFORMITIES*[6,10]
Pathogenesis of joint destruction

The initial event and prime cause of joint destruction is proliferation of the synovial membrane. The cause of the onset of proliferation is unknown, but infection is suspected. The synovial membrane becomes so proliferated that it grows over and into cartilage, bone, and tendons and secretes enzymes that destroy them. The major microscopic fibers that hold the tissues of bone, cartilage, and tendons together are called collagen. The destruction of collagen is a major event, causing joint damage. This destruction is caused by the abnormal secretion of the enzymes collagenase and elastase by the abnormal synovium. The abnormal synovium also produces a thin, watery synovial fluid that is a poor lubricant and nutrient.

Polymorphonuclear white blood cells produced by the inflamed synovium bathe the joint by the millions, and when they break down, they release lysosomal enzymes and other enzymes that further alter the synovial fluid viscosity, cartilage, bone, and tendons to create a vicious cycle.

Specific joint problems

DIP and PIP joints of second to fifth fingers

Swan-neck deformity. Swan-neck deformity results when synovitis weakens or destroys the lateral slips of the extensor tendon that insert into the base of the distal phalanx or weakens the intrinsic interossei and lumbrical muscles that insert into this tendon. The result is incomplete and weak to absent extension at the DIP joint with overbalanced contraction of the central slip of the extensor tendon that inserts at the base of the middle phalanx with hyperextension of the PIP joint (Fig. 9-1).

The process can result in swan-neck deformity of the intrinsic plus type. If there is chronic, incomplete extension of the DIP, a contracture will ensue. Complete extension will be impossible, even passively. The overbalanced pull of the extensor central slip will result in more degrees of hyperextension of the PIP joint. The tendency toward resting hyperextension will result in gradual reduction of the range of flexion of the PIP joint.

Direct surgery involving the lateral slips of the extensor tendons is rarely done because of poor technical results. Sometimes synovectomy is indicated early to remove the invading synovium at the MP joints. Daily passive ROM and gentle stretching are indicated for the DIPs. Active ROM should be done daily to the MPs, PIPs, and DIPs to prevent contractures. A small, short *dynamic* splint may be applied to the PIPs during daily activity to prevent progressive hyperextension.* Flex-

---

*Adapted primarily from Lages, W.: Pathogenesis of joint destruction, San Jose, Calif., 1976 and 1980, Santa Clara Valley Medical Center. Mimeographed.

*EDITOR'S NOTE: Melvin[12] described a three-point finger splint that is sometimes used to maintain range of PIP flexion and relieve stress to the volar aspect of the PIP joint resulting from severe hyperextension.

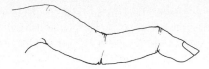

Fig. 9-1. Swan-neck deformity results in PIP hyperextension and DIP flexion.

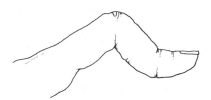

Fig. 9-2. Boutonnière deformity results in DIP hyperextension and PIP flexion.

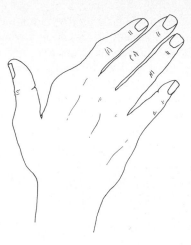

Fig. 9-3. MP joint ulnar drift.

ion contractures of the MPs, PIPs, and DIPs should be treated by active muscle contraction with stretch and not with passive or device stretch.

Isotonic and isometric resistive exercise to the finger extensors will not strengthen damaged tendons and may damage them further.

Boutonnière deformity. Boutonnière deformity can occur when synovitis at the wrist, MP, or PIP joints weakens or destroys the central slip of the extensor tendon that inserts into the base of the middle phalanx. There is often associated PIP joint arthritis. The result is incomplete and weak to absent extension at the PIP joint with overbalanced contraction of the lateral slips of the extensor tendon that insert into the base of the distal phalanx with hyperextension at the DIP joint (Fig 9-2). The central slip of the extensor tendon is the major extensor of the finger, and if this problem is recent (days) and if *the physician does not know of it,* he or she should be informed immediately. Invariably a flexion contracture of the PIP joint and hyperextension of the DIP joint with loss of flexion range will ensue. Function of the finger will be seriously compromised.

Direct surgery of the central slips is often done if caught early enough, but there may be severe damage to the extensor tendon by the synovium, which may require a tendon graft from another site or may be irreparable. Because of this the fourth and fifth fingers are rarely operated on, whereas the second and third fingers often are operated on because of hand function priorities. Synovectomy will not restore tendon integrity but may be indicated to prevent the invasion of others in proximity. Daily passive ROM is indicated for the MPs, PIPs, and DIPs to correct or prevent deformity. Active ROM exercises should be done daily to the MPs, PIPs, and DIPs to preserve joint ROM and muscle

tone. *Dynamic* extension splints of the second and third fingers may be indicated to improve function and opposition.

Isotonic and isometric exercise or resistive exercise to the extensors will not help this deformity and may further damage tendons.

MP joints of second to fifth fingers

MP ulnar drift. Synovitis of the MP joints leads to weakness or destruction of the MP ligaments. The MP ligaments, particularly when the MPs are flexed at 45°, give medial and lateral stability. Both the extensor and flexor tendons to the fingers are bowed to produce an ulnar drift tendency of the tendons at the MP joints during normal contractions. Forced contraction and especially forceful hand grip accentuate this force. With MP ligaments weakened the normal forces result in ulnar drift. The fifth MP joint buttresses the remainder of fingers from static, postural ulnar drift, but when the fifth MP ligament loses stability, ulnar drift can occur with gravity and posture even at rest (Fig. 9-3).

The result is that if the MP ligament damage is mild or if the stability of the fifth joint is preserved, the ulnar drift may occur only dynamically with finger extension-flexion. This gives weak pinch, which may result in thumb adduction and lateral pinch being substituted for true opposition. If the MP ligament damage is severe or if the stability of the fifth MP joint is lost, there will be ulnar drift even at rest, posturally, and the problem of opposition will be severe.

The dynamic and static ulnar drift plus lifting of the extensor hood by MP synovitis will result in dislocation of the extensor tendons from the extensor hood over the metacarpal heads into the space between the heads, leading to possible tendon injury and loss of ability to completely extend the MP joints. The lateral pinching of the thumb will result in radial subluxation and deformity of the IP joint of the thumb.

Treatment consists of early synovectomy, which may prevent progressive MP ligament damage. Extensor tendons dislocated ulnarly may be able to be replaced surgically with excision of MP synovial tissue. Severe problems may require replacement of the MP joints, since the MP ligaments cannot be successfully repaired surgically. Daily passive ROM exercises of the MP joints are indicated only if daily active ROM does not produce full flexion and extension. A joint protection program is strongly indicated to prevent forceful flexion and extension in ADL. *Dynamic* ulnar deviation splints during the day coupled with *static* splints with the MPs in neutral deviation and 45° of flexion at night may halt progression of deformity and improve opposition.

Isotonic and isometric exercise or resistive exercise of the fingers will not help this deformity and may produce further MP ligament damage.

MP palmar subluxation-dislocation. Synovitis of the MPs results in MP ligament damage. Since finger flexors are much stronger and much more used than extensors, palmar dislocation will result. Palmar dislocation is often associated with ulnar drift but may occur by itself. Loss of effective MP extension is the usual isolated problem, as well as the shortening and weakening of the intrinsic muscles. Complete dislocation can occur (Fig. 9-4).

Early, complete surgical replacement or repair of the MP joints is the only effective treatment. Passive ROM exercises of the MPs to prevent loss of ROM are indicated, as well as active ROM. No exercises or splints are effective in correcting or treating this problem. A joint protection program is strongly indicated to prevent further progressive damage during ADL.

Thumb[10,12]

Flexion of MP joint with hyperextension of the IP joint (type I deformity). Chronic MP synovitis causes attenuation of the joint capsule, MP collateral ligaments, and the overlying extensor mechanism. Pain and distention of the joint capsule cause damage of the intrinsic muscles of the thumb. This may progress to MP palmar subluxation and ulnar-volar displacement of the extensor

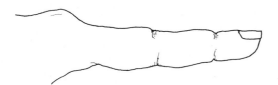

Fig. 9-4. MP palmar subluxation.

pollicis longus tendon. Once displaced this tendon acts as an MP flexor and with intrinsic muscle damage, causes hyperextension of the IP joint. The result is MP flexion and IP hyperextension.

Flexion of the MP joint with IP hyperextension and CMC involvement (type II deformity). Type II deformity appears similar to type I deformity, but CMC joint damage and subluxation, due to chronic synovitis of this joint, are the major factors. Once there is subluxation of the CMC joint, the adductor pollicis muscle pulls on the first metacarpal, which can result in a fixed adduction contracture with hyperextension of the *distal* phalanx.

MP hyperextension, IP flexion, and CMC joint involvement (type III deformity). The dynamics of type III deformity are initially the same as those described for type II deformity. However, type III deformity will result if there is a natural or pathological laxity of the MP joint with hyperextension of the proximal phalanx.

These problems may be treated surgically by extensor tendon repair, synovectomy, arthrodesis, or joint replacement. A joint protection program is indicated, and a CMC stabilization splint may be helpful to relieve pain and increase hand function.

Wrist joint

Wrist synovitis. Wrist synovitis can result in a variety of problems, which are discussed here.

Carpal tunnel syndrome. The carpal tunnel under the transverse flexor carpal ligament is a tightly closed space, and inflammation can lead to high pressure on the median nerve, which runs in the carpal tunnel. This produces pain and sensory disturbances over the median nerve distribution in the hand and median nerve motor weakness and atrophy of the opponens pollicis, abductor pollicis brevis, and thenar atrophy. *If not already known by the physician, this should be promptly brought to his attention for treatment.* Sensory and motor deficits over the median nerve distribution and severe pain in the hand can result that can progress to permanent loss of feeling in the hand and weak to lost thumb opposition, which are serious impairments to hand use.

Until treatment any exercises of the wrist other than active ROM are contraindicated, as is heat. The hand should be kept elevated to reduce swelling, even at night. A cock-up splint to immobilize the wrist may also help and should be worn as much as possible during the day and all night. If splints, elevation, and corticosteroid injection fail to promptly resolve the problem, surgical release of the transverse carpal ligament is indicated.

Synovial invasion of the extensor tendons. Dorsal swelling can be seen and felt in cases of invasion of the extensor tendon sheaths. This can lead to their weakness or rupture, resulting in weak to lost extension of the fingers at the MP, PIP, and DIP joints, flexion contractures, and loss of hand function, which is serious.

As soon as discovered, surgical synovectomy can correct and prevent further problems. Tendon repair may be done if caught promptly. Active ROM exercises at the wrist and night splints for the wrist can preserve function prior to surgery but are not substitutes for surgery. Passive and active ROM of the MP, PIP, and DIP are indicated to prevent flexion contracture.

Isotonic and isometric exercise or resistive exercise of the wrist extensors are of no value and may produce further damage.

Synovial invasion of the carpal bones. Synovial invasion of the carpal bone results in erosion and destruction of the intercarpal ligaments and joints. It can result in progressive loss of wrist motion, contracture of the wrist in a nonfunctional position, or in flexion subluxation-dislocation of the wrist (Fig. 9-5).

Loss of ROM can be minimized by active ROM exercise. Passive ROM should be gentle to avoid damaging ligaments. Night splints of the wrist in the position of function (neutral radioulnar position and slight wrist extension) can prevent contracture in nonfunctional positions. Surgery is not feasible except to fuse in more functional positions. Since all surgery has to offer is wrist fusion in the position of function, *static* wrist splints in the position of function produce the same end result. Splints causing loss of pronation-supination are contraindicated. Active pronation-supination ROM exercise and gentle passive ROM are indicated several times a day with the wrist out of the splint to prevent this. Joint protection of forceful flexion is strongly indicated. Isometric strengthening of wrist extensors is indicated.

Isotonic and isotonic resistive exercise may lead to subluxation-dislocation.

Synovitis of the radioulnar joint. Synovitis of the radioulnar joint, causing erosion of joint cartilage, usually results in progressive loss of pronation and supination at the wrist, particularly if there is associated elbow

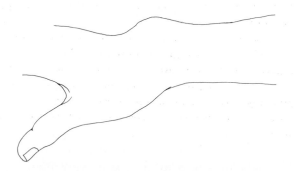

Fig. 9-5. Flexion subluxation of wrist.

disease. It can result in partial to complete loss of pronation and supination of the wrist with severe functional impairment.

Surgical resection of the distal ulna can be done to restore lost pronation-supination. Active pronation-supination ROM exercises and passive ROM are indicated daily to prevent loss. Pronation-supination in ADL is encouraged.

Isotonic or resistive exercises are contraindicated.

Elbow joint

Elbow synovitis. The humeroulnar joint is a hinge joint, and synovitis results in loss of ROM. Disease of the radiohumeral joint can result in loss of pronation-supination at the elbow.

Loss of flexion can result in contracture that prevents feeding and many other ADL. Loss of extension can result in contracture that makes ADL and crutch use difficult and some tasks impossible. Loss of pronation-supination severely compromises the use of the hands and wrists in ADL. A dominant arm with severe loss of extension and pronation makes writing and other activities extremely difficult.

Flexion and extension contractures of the elbows are extremely difficult to improve surgically. Both elbows with severely limited flexion seriously impair ADL and functional activities; both elbows with severely limited extension make transfers and crutch use extremely difficult. The radial head can be resected to improve pronation-supination. With disease in the elbows splints and slings limiting movement are contraindicated unless daily ROM is preserved by a therapist or nurse. Active and passive ROM exercises are strongly indicated daily for the elbow. Isometric exercise is indicated for strengthening only if isotonic exercise is too painful. Isotonic exercise is best given through proper ADL instruction. Pain that may limit exercise can be reduced by corticosteroid injection. Loss of ROM is a greater concern than is joint damage, since the only surgical corrections for contractures are destructive of joints. Sometimes surgery is aimed toward improving extension at the expense of flexion in the dominant arm to permit crutch use and writing and improving flexion at the expense of extension in the nondominant extremity for feeding and personal grooming.

Shoulder joint. The shoulder is a ball-and-socket joint that has some susceptibility to subluxation and instability but very great susceptibility to loss of motion.

Shoulder synovitis. The main result of synovitis is loss of some planes of ROM. A complication of shoulder synovitis is "frozen shoulder," which means very restricted ROM, and, unfortunately, is common. This results in major problems in ADL and in crutch ambulation. With shoulder contracture there is extremely severe restriction of ADL and other functions. Surgery is of little value in treating this problem. Corticosteroid injection early is very effective in reducing pain and restricted motion. Aggressive active and passive ROM and isotonic exercise are imperative, expecially preceded by hot packs. A joint protection program is strongly indicated. Slings are a hazard and should be avoided.

PRINCIPLES OF REHABILITATION

Conservative management of rheumatoid arthritis is the preferred approach to its treatment. The long-term prognosis, using conservative methods, is usually as good as with more radical approaches. There is less risk of side effects using salicylates, appropriate rest, and rehabilitation measures than from drugs such as gold salts, steroids, and cytotoxic agents.[4]

The goals of the basic treatment regime are to decrease inflammation and pain, preserve function, and prevent deformity. The treatment methods used include systemic, emotional, and joint rest; drug therapy; and appropriate exercise[4] and activity. In some instances surgery is required.[9]

Joint rest in non-weight-bearing positions and prone lying to prevent hip and knee flexion contractures are part of the program of rest. Splints to provide temporary rest of individual joints are used.[9]

The amount of rest required varies with the individual patient. In some instances complete bed rest will be necessary, whereas in others the patient may continue with normal daily living, incorporating 2 hours of rest into the daily schedule.[4]

It is of primary importance in the treatment program to preserve function of the hips, knees, elbows, and MP joints. Therefore exercise to other joints must not interfere with functions of these joints or be done at their expense. Complete joint rest is applicable to acutely involved joints only.

Self-care activities are permitted to pain tolerance, even in acute arthritis. Splinting should be maintained for as short a period as possible to prevent loss of ROM.[8]

Indications for splinting

Splinting is indicated for the wrist, MP and IP joints, and the ankle if it is acutely painful. Splinting is contraindicated at the shoulder and hip joints; at the elbow, except when weight bearing; and at the knee, unless there is joint instability.[8]

Splints and other orthoses must be removed regularly for ROM exercises to the involved joints.

The reader is referred to *Rheumatic Disease: Occupational Therapy and Rehabilitation* by Jeanne L. Melvin[12] for a full discussion and description of a wide variety of hand splints and their uses in the treatment of rheumatoid arthritis.

Indications for exercise

The concomitant use of the appropriate therapeutic exercise along with rest, in proper balance, is basic to the management of rheumatoid arthritis. The objectives of the exercise program are to preserve joint motion, muscle strength, and endurance. Active-assistive exercises are most useful and can be performed, within limits of pain tolerance, from the outset in the treatment program. As disease activity subsides and tolerance for exercise increases, gradation of the program may be increased to include active and resistive exercises.[4]

Acute stage. During the acute stage, involved joints are inflamed and swollen. There may be systemic signs and symptoms, and bed rest may be required. Splints, braces, and positioning are used to provide joint rest and prevent deformity.

Active ROM exercise is started after 1 week and is gradually increased to active exercise to tolerance. Passive ROM exercise may be used only if the client is unable to complete the ROM with active motion. The purpose of these exercises is to improve or maintain joint mobility.

Isometric exercise without resistance (muscle setting) may be used to maintain muscle tone. Active exercise in water (hubbard tank or whirlpool) can be used to provide active exercise with a minimum of joint stress for maintenance of joint ROM and muscle tone.[1,8]

Active ROM exercises should be repeated 3 to 10 times once or twice daily. Isometric exercise should be repeated 3 to 10 times several times daily.[4] Active exercises should be performed in a manner to prevent active stretching and joint stress. Pain or discomfort that results from exercise and lasts more than 1 hour indicates that the exercise was too stressful and should be decreased.[12]

Active resistive exercise, isometric exercise against resistance, and stretching exercise are contraindicated during the acute stage of the disease.[8]

Subacute stage. During the subacute stage of the disease a few joints are actively involved, and there may be mild systemic symptoms. Short periods of rest and splints for corrective or preventive purposes are used.

Gentle passive stretch and active isotonic exercise with minimal joint stress may be added to the passive or active ROM exercise program. Their purpose is to regain lost ROM in those joints that have become limited. Graded isometric exercise twice daily for 5 to 10 minutes may be used to maintain or increase muscle strength and endurance.[1,8]

Chronic-active and chronic-inactive stages. During the chronic-active and chronic-inactive stages, stretch at the end of the ROM during exercise is recommended to increase ROM.[12] Active ROM, isometric, and isometric resistive exercises may also be continued.[8]

Isotonic resistive exercise should seldom be used.[4] It is thought to produce excessive and undesirable joint stress.[8] Melvin[12] outlines circumstances under which resistive exercises are used by some practitioners and describes specific exercise procedures.

A home exercise program that is designed for the particular client should be carried out. It is best for the therapist to write out the directions for exercises for the client to follow. The exercises should be done when the client is feeling his best, often after a warm shower or bath and analgesic medication. Application of heat or cold for muscle relaxation and analgesic effect may be of benefit to some clients.[4,12]

Indications for activity

Treatment principles that apply to the therapeutic exercise just cited also apply to therapeutic activities. The activities that are selected should be nonresistive and provide opportunities for the maintenance or increase of ROM and strength. They should be meaningful and interesting to the client. Joint protection principles, to be discussed subsequently, should be employed during leisure and work activities, as well as during ADL.

Crafts and games as therapeutic modalities are not as frequently or effectively used as therapeutic exercise regimes. However, they can be of value and interest to some clients and should not be overlooked as a purposeful application of therapeutic exercise procedures. Activities that can be useful in the treatment of rheumatoid arthritis include weaving, Turkish knotting, macrame, and peg games.[12]

The use of crocheting, knitting, and similar traditional needlecrafts is controversial. In principle they are to be avoided because they involve the use of prolonged static contraction of hand muscles in the intrinsic plus position for holding tools and material. They also facilitate MP ulnar drift and MP volar subluxation through the forces in the hand during the performance of the activity. Melvin[12] points out that in general the only conditions in which knitting and crocheting can be harmful are when there are active MP synovitis, beginning swan-neck deformity caused in part by intrinsic tightness, and degenerative joint disease of the CMC joint of the thumb.

Adverse effects can be prevented by using an MP extension splint, performing intrinsic stretching exercises, and using a thumb CMC stabilization splint, depending on the specific potential problem. Frequent rest breaks during the activity or performing the activity for short, intermittent periods may also be helpful in preventing adverse effects. These are important considerations for those clients who would derive much pleasure and psychological benefit from these traditional and readily available avocational activities.[12]

ADL, including self-care and home management skills, is an important part of the rehabilitation program for the client with rheumatoid arthritis. Self-care activities to pain and fatigue tolerance should be performed even during early acute stages of the disease episode. The number and types of activities are gradually increased as the client's endurance and strength improve and pain and discomfort subside.[12]

These activities can be used to maintain or improve joint ROM, muscle strength, and physical endurance. Joint protection, work simplification, and energy conservation principles should be applied during the performance of these activities. The client, with the aid and direction of the therapist, needs to work out a daily schedule of intermittent rest and activity that is suitable for the stage of the disease, activity tolerance, and any special systemic or joint problems that affect performance.

These principles apply to work activities. Since there are more women than men affected by arthritis, there has been an emphasis in the literature on home management activities, and joint protection principles related to these focused on the traditional role of woman as homemaker. The therapist must not lose sight of the facts that men also perform homemaking tasks and that a substantial percentage of women are employed outside of their homes. Therefore job analysis and application of joint protection and energy conservation principles may be an important part of the rehabilitation program for both men and women. Prevocational evaluation may be necessary if a job change is necessitated by the disability.

For juvenile rheumatoid arthritis, school and leisure activities need to be considered and appropriate pacing of activities employed.

Assistive equipment

Assistive devices and equipment are used to reduce pain, decrease joint stress, and increase independence.[12]

In general the purposes of various devices are to (1) facilitate grasp (built-up soft handles on tools); (2) compensate for lost ROM (dressing sticks or reachers); (3) facilitate ease of performance (lightweight equipment or electric appliances); (4) stabilize materials or equipment (nonskid mats or suction brushes); (5) prevent deforming stresses (extended faucet handles or adapted key holder); (6) prevent prolonged static contraction (book stand or bowl holder); (7) compensate for weak or absent motor

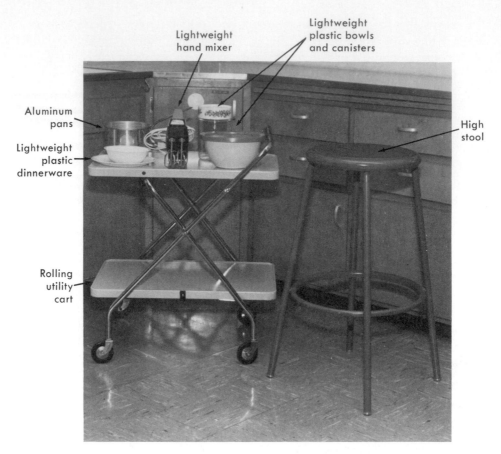

Fig. 9-6. Equipment designed to ease housework for client with arthritis.

function (universal cuffs or stocking devices); and (8) prevent accidents (bathtub grab bars and nonskid mats for shower or bathtub).

Some of these devices are discussed in Chapter 4 of this text. Melvin[12] outlines a long list of assistive devices for specific joint involvement. Some suggestions to ease home management are shown in Fig. 9-6.

Principles of joint protection[3,12,15]

The purpose of joint protection training is to instruct the client in methods of reducing joint stress, decreasing pain, preserving joint structures, and conserving energy.[12]

The arthritic joint is predisposed to deterioration from abuse that can lead to reduced performance abilities.[3] Clients with rheumatoid arthritis need to employ joint protection principles in all of their daily activities to maintain maximum function and prevent joint damage and deformity.

Maintain muscle strength and joint ROM.[3] During daily activities each joint should be used at its maximum ROM and strength consistent with the disease process. For example, long, sweeping, flowing strokes to main-tain and increase ROM can be employed when ironing. The arms should be straightened as far as possible, especially on flat work (Fig. 9-7). When vacuuming or mopping the floor a long, forward stroke of the implement, then pulling it in close to the body so the arm is first fully straightened, then fully bent, will achieve full or nearly full range of elbow flexion and extension and some shoulder motion. The use of dust mitts on both hands keeps fingers straight and prevents the static contraction and potentially deforming forces of holding a dust cloth. Light objects, such as cereal, oats, or sugar, can be kept on high shelves so that full ROM in the shoulder can be used with reaching.[15]

Avoid positions of deformity and deforming stresses. Internal, that is, tight grasp around an object, and external, that is, propping up chin on side or back of fingers, forces in the direction of deformity should be avoided during daily activities. Some applications of this principle include always turning the fingers toward the thumb side, such as turning a doorknob toward the thumb or opening a door with the right hand and closing it with the left. Jars should be opened with the right hand and closed with the left. When wringing out hand

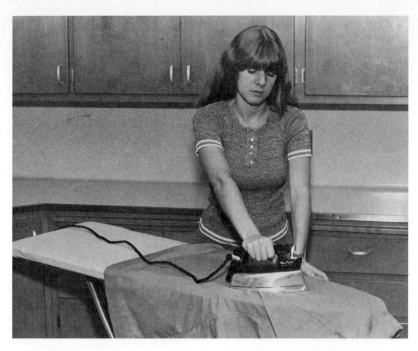

Fig. 9-7. During ironing full extension at elbow can be practiced.

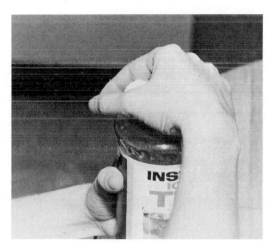

Fig. 9-8. Jar cap is twisted off, using palm of hand, and opened with right hand to prevent ulnar drift.

laundry the object should be held steady with the left hand and twisted with the right in the direction of the thumb.[15]

Pressures along the thumb side of fingers should be avoided. These pressures contribute to ulnar deviation. This position of ulnar deviation decreases the use of the hands. Pressure can be prevented by (1) avoiding leaning chin on fingers or palm of hand; (2) picking up coffee cup with two hands instead of with index, middle finger, and thumb; (3) twisting a jar cap off and on with the palm of the hand and not with the fingers (Fig. 9-8); (4) installing lever extensions on faucet handles to avoid use of fingers to turn on and off; and (5) using electric can opener instead of hand-operated type, since this device requires sustained grasp of one hand and forced motion of the thumb and fingers of the other hand for operation.

Tight grasp should be avoided. This position increases the strength of the muscles that allow grasp and therefore, contributes to ulnar deviation and dislocation of joints. This happens in activities such as carrying pails and baskets; using pliers, scissors, and screwdrivers; and holding spoons to stir or mix foods.

When standing up the client should be instructed to take the body weight through the wrist with fingers straight rather than on the fingers. "This will help reduce the pressure against the backs of the fingers. Excessive pressure in this area will contribute to dislocation of the knuckles"[15] (Fig. 9-9). The palm of the hand, rather than the fingers, should be used when taking down or hanging clothes in the closet. The palm can be used to lift the hanger at the exposed area in its apex. This method is most useful with heavy coats and jackets.

Excessive and constant pressure against the pad of the thumb should be avoided. For example, pressure against the pad of the thumb to open a car door, sew through thick fabric, and rise to a standing position all contribute to dislocation of the thumb joints.[15]

Use each joint in its most stable, anatomical, and

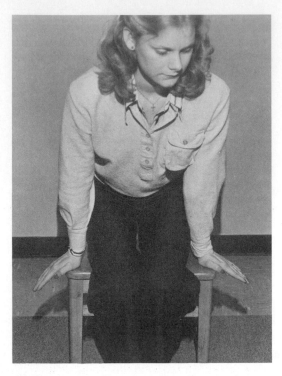

Fig. 9-9. Pushing off chair, using palms, helps prevent dislocation of finger joints.

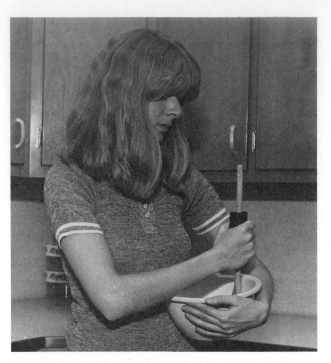

Fig. 9-10. Mixing bowl is stabilized with forearm. Spoon with soft, built-up handle is held so that pressure is toward radial side of hand.

functional plane.[3] The client should be instructed to stand up straight from any sitting position. He should stand or position himself directly in front of a drawer to open it and not pull while standing to one side. In reaching for objects on a shelf he should stand or position himself directly in front of or under the shelf, not at the side. The wrist and fingers should always be used in good alignment.[15]

Use the strongest joints available for the activity.[3] Applications of using the strongest joints include using the hips and knees, not the back, when lifting and using the entire body to move heavy things. Carts and chairs should be pushed from behind; use straps for opening and closing heavy doors and drawers; and roll objects on counters and floors rather than lifting them. If any objects must be lifted, they should be scooped up in both hands, palms upward. This technique can be used when handling baking pans and casseroles if long oven mitts are used and in handling dishes, packages, books, and laundry.[15]

Avoid using muscles or holding joints in one position for any undue length of time. Sustained muscle contraction is fatiguing and can contribute to joint subluxation and dislocation. Applications of this principle include (1) using a book stand instead of holding the book while reading; (2) when mixing, stabilizing the bowl with the palm of the hand and fingers against the body

or a wall or in an open drawer to avoid holding the bowl with the fingers and thumb; (3) holding the mixing spoon with the thumb side pointing upward, not with the thumb pointing downward, and using a built-up handle to decrease the force of grasp (Fig. 9-10); (4) using the palm to scour pans, not with the fingertips; (5) using the palm of the hand or the bend in the elbow instead of fingers in carrying handbags and coats; (6) using the side of the hand to push, as in shutting drawers, or using the little finger side of the hand in smoothing sheets on a bed; (7) squeezing the toothpaste tube with the palm of the hand, not between the thumb and fingers; and (8) holding objects such as a vegetable peeler or knife parallel to MP joints and not across the palms.[15]

Never begin an activity that cannot be stopped immediately if it proves to be too taxing. In climbing up and down stairs, standing balance should be adequate to allow stopping and resting. In transferring from bed to wheelchair a sliding board should be used for less stress and to allow for stopping, if necessary. In getting in and out of a bathtub graded platforms to ascend and descend gradually at individual speed and tolerance can be used.

Respect pain. Some discomfort during treatment and activity may be tolerable and acceptable. If rest produces rapid relief, the level of activity need not necessarily be excessive.[3] However, pain lasting 1 or more hours after activity is a sign that the activity needs to be stopped or modified.[12,15] Pain can evoke protective muscle spasm and inhibit muscle contraction.[3]

Energy conservation and work simplification

Since prevention of fatigue is an important consideration in the management of rheumatoid arthritis, methods of simplifying work to save energy should be employed. One of the most important means to the end is to determine and carry out an appropriate balance between rest and play. The recommended amount of rest is 10 to 12 hours of rest per day, including a 1- to 2-hour nap in the afternoon.[12]

Short rest breaks of 5 to 10 minutes during daily activities can be very helpful in increasing overall endurance.[12] In general, 5 to 10 minutes of rest to 30 or 40 minutes[5] of activity is adequate. It may be difficult for the client to accept the notion of these short rest breaks, since it is often the desire to get work or housekeeping over with as quickly as possible. However, intermittent rest can actually save energy for more enjoyable tasks.[12] Work can be planned for an entire week and month. Light and heavy tasks can be alternated and work paced throughout the week, instead of doing a lot of work in 1 day. Work should be planned so that it is efficient, that is, not requiring getting up and down and moving to and fro repeatedly.

Time management needs to be explored if rushing is a tendency of the client. Rushing increases tension and fatigue. Most importantly the client should learn an energy-saving program and work schedule that prevent pushing to exhaustion.[15]

Other suggestions for conserving energy include (1) avoid bending and stooping by using long handle reachers and flexible handle dust mops; (2) avoid long periods of standing during activities such as ironing and food preparation; rather, use a high stool; (3) avoid extra trips by using a utility cart to convey as many items as needed at once; and (4) relax homemaking standards by using prepackaged foods and by air drying dishes, for example.

Work may be simplified by adjusting the work height for maximum comfort. The elbows should be flexed to 90°, and shoulders should be in a relaxed position. This can be accomplished without expensive home modification by using an adjustable ironing board as a work surface, placing a board over an open drawer, or using a high stool with a backrest to work at counters. A rack may be placed in the sink bottom to elevate the dishpan and thus prevent stooping during dish washing.

Work areas can be rearranged so that frequently used tools, equipment, and supplies are stored nearby and at easily reached levels. Counter tops may be used for convenient storage of small appliances. Commercial organizers such as step shelves and revolving turntables can make work easier.[15]

OCCUPATIONAL THERAPY FOR RHEUMATOID ARTHRITIS

The client with rheumatoid arthritis is usually seen for occupational therapy services when many joints are involved, after surgery, or when the disease is severe enough to cause hospitalization or moderate to severe performance limitations.[13]

Evaluation

The occupational therapy evaluation includes active and passive ROM measurements. These may take 45 to 60 minutes per upper extremity if there is discomfort or pain in the joints. It may be necessary to perform the measurements gradually over two or three treatment sessions. The therapist should be aware of how the joints feel, that is, stiff, unstable, or crepitant. A major discrepancy between active and passive ROM may indicate significant muscle weakness.[13]

Muscle strength should be assessed by a functional muscle test, and strength should be estimated by muscle groups. Muscle grades are likely to be in the fair to good range because of weakness from disuse or pain. The use of the manual muscle test is controversial, since some physicians prohibit any resistance that can cause harm to diseased tissue and joints and place deforming forces on the joint.[10]

Hand function testing is important. Pinch and grip strength testing with instruments is controversial for the reasons just stated. Grip and pinch can be tested with an adapted blood pressure cuff and measured in millimeters of mercury.[5,12] A test of hand function that evaluates grasp and prehension patterns should be administered.

The occupational therapist should observe the appearance of the hand for heat, redness, edema, deformity, deforming tendencies on motion, skin quality, and joint enlargement. In the early stages of the disease joints may appear puffy and soft. If the disease is active, joints may be red and hot. Later in the disease process enlarged joints may appear bony and hard.[5,13]

Tests for specific deformities or potential deformities of the hand should be administered as appropriate. Some of these are described in Chapter 2. The therapist might evaluate for possible carpal tunnel syndrome, swan-neck deformities, boutonnière deformities, flexor tendon nodules, ulnar drift, MP and wrist subluxation, intrinsic and extrinsic muscle tightness, ruptured tendons, extensor tendon displacement, and laxity of the MP collateral ligaments.[5]

Sensory evaluation is indicated if there is potential nerve compression due to swelling. Modalities that should be tested are senses of touch, pain, temperature, and position. Paresthesias should be noted.

The client's physical endurance should be evaluated by observation and an assessment of the daily or weekly schedule. Specific LE evaluation is usually carried out by the physical therapist; however, the occupational therapist should observe the gait pattern and mode of rising and sitting. She should observe the client's posture during ambulation and when sitting. She should observe for any obvious joint limitations and weakness in the lower extremities and have data from the physical therapy evaluation regarding ROM, strength, and deforming tendencies in the legs. These factors are important considerations in planning treatment and presenting joint protection and energy conservation techniques, as well as positioning to prevent loss of ROM in the lower extremities.

Assessment of performance is a very important part of the occupational therapy program. Evaluation of ADL, including self-care, child care, home management, and work activities, should be carried out by interview and observation. A home evaluation should be carried out to assist the client in learning new methods and in making modifications to simplify work, save energy, and protect joints from undue stress. Job performance may be evaluated by observation in a real or simulated situation. The job tasks can be analyzed, and joint protection principles can be applied, if possible. Pacing of work responsibilities may be a consideration to incorporate the required rest periods into the working day.

Treatment objectives

The general objectives of treatment for clients with rheumatoid arthritis are to (1) maintain or increase joint mobility; (2) maintain or increase muscle strength; (3) increase physical endurance; (4) prevent or correct deformities, if feasible; (5) minimize the effect of deformities; (6) maintain or increase ability to perform daily life tasks; (7) increase knowledge about the disease and the best methods of dealing with physical performance and psychosocial effects; and (8) aid with stress management and adjustment to physical disability.

Treatment methods

Methods used by occupational therapists to minimize the dysfunction that can result from rheumatoid arthritis include a variety of exercises, just described, tailored to the client's needs and stage of the disease. For clients not in the acute stage of the disease, exercise should be incorporated into daily activity as much as possible to reduce the need for a formal and rigid program of daily exercise.[13]

Training in ADL is an important aspect of the occupational therapy program for many clients. This includes training in joint protection, energy conservation techniques, and use of assistive devices and special equipment. Self-care, child care, home management, and work activities may be included in the ADL training program. Joint protection principles and energy-saving techniques should be introduced gradually, and the number and complexity of procedures should be increased as the client incorporates previously learned skills into his daily life. For some clients arts and crafts or games, as described earlier, can be a meaningful part of the treatment program. This will depend on the client's needs, interests, and life-style and should be explored with him and not overlooked.

Splints to protect joints and prevent or retard the development of deformity are usually made by the occupational therapist. She may recognize the need for splints and recommend them to the physician in some instances. Some splints that may be of benefit in the treatment of rheumatoid arthritis include the resting, cock-up, ulnar drift, MP extensor assist, flexor assist, CMC stabilization, and three-point finger extension splints.[12]

Psychosocial factors may be treated by exploring with the client his attitude toward the disability, his goals, how he deals with pain and fear, and his performance priorities and objectives. Activity groups, such as movement or exercise classes, home management classes, or arthritis education classes, can serve as mutual support and problem-solving groups. Occupational therapists may lead or participate with other rehabilitation specialists in such activity groups. Sexual counseling may be necessary to teach joint protection techniques during sexual activity and explore attitudes about body image, self-acceptance, and acceptance by the partner as a sexual being.

Education of the client and his family about the disease, potential disability, treatment, and home program to achieve maximum function is essential. Such education can be provided through classes and literature available from the Arthritis Foundation. Family roles may need to be changed or modified as a result of one member's physical dysfunction. Therefore it is important for families to understand and support the disabled member and lend aid for tasks the client cannot or should not do.[13]

The occupational therapist should assist in designing a home program for the client. This should include a suitable work and rest schedule, activities, and exercises that will maximize function and minimize deformity and dysfunction. The home program should be outlined for the client in writing.

Treatment precautions

Fatigue should be avoided, and pain should be respected. It may be difficult for the client to do things in the morning due to stiffness of "gelling" of joints. A warm shower may be helpful to begin moving. Static, stressful, or resistive activities should be avoided. The use of a ball, putty, or clay for squeezing should be avoided, since these involve forceful flexion of the fingers, which can produce ulnar deviation, MP subluxation, and extensor tendon displacement.[5] If sensation is impaired, techniques to prevent injury to the desensitized part must be taught and observed by client and therapist.[13] If warmth is used to relax muscles and increase mobility, it should be limited to 20 minutes. Longer periods of warmth can increase inflammation and, later, produce increased swelling and pain. Resistive exercises for strengthening muscles do *not* improve joint stability and should not be used with this as an objective. Joint instability is usually due to ligamentous laxity, and resistive exercises can make this worse.

SAMPLE TREATMENT PLAN

Case study

Mrs. J. is a 36-year-old woman with a diagnosis of rheumatoid arthritis. The onset was 3 years ago. She is a wife and the mother of an 8-year-old girl. She lives with her husband and daughter in a three-bedroom single-level tract home. Mrs. J.'s primary role is that of homemaker. However, she has held a part-time job at a florist shop doing wreath design and construction and flower arranging. She both enjoys this work and sees her salary as a necessary adjunct to the family income.

Mrs. J. experiences intermittent acute disease episodes that have primarily involved the elbows, wrists, MP, and PIP joints bilaterally. There are slight losses of ROM and strength at all involved joints.

To date there is no permanent deformity, but ulnar deviation, MP subluxation, boutonnière deformity, wrist subluxation, and further limitation of ROM at all involved joints are possible deformities.

Medical management has been through rest and salicylates. Medical precautions are no strenuous activity, no resistive exercise or activity, and avoidance of fatigue.

She was referred to occupational therapy during the acute phase of her most recent episode for prevention of deformity and loss of ROM and maintenance of maximum function. She continued with occupational therapy services during the subacute period with the same goals.

Treatment plan

A. **Statistical data.**
   1. Name: Mrs. J.
      Age: 36
      Diagnosis: Rheumatoid arthritis
      Disability: Limited ROM, strength, and potential deformity of elbows, wrists, MP, and IP joints bilaterally
   2. Treatment aims as stated in referral:
      Prevent deformity
      Prevent loss of ROM
      Maintain maximum function
B. **Other services.**
   Medical services: Supervise medical management and rehabilitation therapies
   Physical therapy: May be used for specific exercise program
   Social services: Client and family counseling, if needed; financial arrangements, if appropriate
   Vocational counseling: Explore feasibility of return to same or modified occupation in floral work.
C. **OT evaluation.**
   Active and passive ROM: Test
   Muscle strength: Observe, functional testing
   Sensation: Test
   Carpal tunnel syndrome: Test
   Boutonnière deformity: Test
   MP stability: Test
   Ulnar drift: Measure
   Wrist subluxation: Observe
   MP subluxation: Observe
   Hand function: Test
   ADL: Interview, observe
   Endurance: Interview, observe
   Prevocational skills: Observe
   Adjustment to disability: Observe
   Interpersonal and coping skills: Observe
D. **Results of evaluation.**
   1. Evaluation data.
      a. Physical resources. ROM measurements are equal for active and passive motion and bilaterally.
         Joint measurements are
         Elbows 10° to 130°
         Wrists
            Extension: 0° to 40°
            Flexion: 0° to 70°
         MP joints: 10° to 80°
         PIP joints: 10° to 110°

Continued.

SAMPLE TREATMENT PLAN—cont'd

Strength is estimated as
  Elbow flexors: G
  Elbow extensors: F+
  Wrist extensors: F+
  Wrist flexors: G
  Grasp: G
  Finger extensors: F+
  Thumb muscles: N

All other joint motions and muscle groups within normal limits. MP joints are slightly unstable with 10° of ulnar drift on active motion. There is no evidence of wrist or MP subluxation, boutonnière deformity, or carpal tunnel syndrome at this time. Hand function testing reveals difficulty with fingertip prehension, and pinch and grip are good but not normal in strength. Forceful use of the thumb in opposition enhances ulnar drift and produces MP discomfort.

b. Sensory-perceptual functions. Sensory modalities of touch, pain, temperature, and position are intact. Perceptual functions are normal for a 36-year-old adult.

c. Cognitive functions. Cognition is normal. Client appears alert, intelligent, and interested in her progress.

d. Psychosocial functions. Client interacts comfortably with staff and other clients. She is cooperative and helpful. Her husband reported that she withdrew from social situations somewhat after her last disease episode. She interacts comfortably with him and with her daughter, although her patience is very limited when she is fatigued or in pain. Her daughter has some understanding of her mother's problems and is usually willing to help with light chores.

e. Prevocational potential. Observation of the job performance of another worker by the occupational therapist and observation of Mrs. J. in simulated job tasks revealed that some aspects of the job would contribute to development of deformity. Cutting and twisting floral wire, forcing stems and stem support into Styrofoam, and binding wreaths were thought to be likely to enhance ulnar drift and MP subluxation because of the resistance and direction of joint forces. However, wreath design and layout and fresh flower arrangement are possible alternatives. Mrs. J.'s employer is willing to retain her on a part-time basis to perform these duties.

f. Functional skills. During acute episodes Mrs. J. is severely limited in ADL. She leaves all home management to her husband and daughter during these periods and is not able to work. She only manages to do light self-care activities independently. During inactive periods, Mrs. J. is independent in light housekeeping, self-care, and work activities. She fatigues after 2 hours of light to moderate activity and requires a 20-minute rest period.

2. Problem identification.
  a. Muscle weakness
  b. Limited ROM
  c. Potential deformity
  d. Fluctuating vocational role
  e. Limited ADL independence
  f. Fluctuating role as wife and mother
  g. Tendency to social withdrawal
  h. Limited endurance

3. Assets-functions.
  a. No lower extremity involvement
  b. Good preservation of function
  c. Supportive and intact family unit
  d. Potential job skills, flexible employer
  e. Intelligence, motivation

E Problem	F Specific OT objectives	G Methods used to meet objectives	H Gradation of treatment
Acute stage a	Through appropriate exercise to elbows and wrists, muscle strength will be maintained	Isometric exercise without resistance to biceps, triceps, and flexors and extensors, carpi radialis and ulnaris, 3 to 10 repetitions 3 times daily	Increase number of exercise sessions

SAMPLE TREATMENT PLAN—cont'd

E Problem	F Specific OT objectives	G Methods used to meet objectives	H Gradation of treatment
b	Through appropriate exercise, ROM of affected joints will be preserved at present level	Active or active-assisted ROM exercises to elbow, MP and PIP flexion and extension, wrist flexion and extension, radial and ulnar deviation; active ROM exercise may be carried out in warm whirlpool bath	Grade to active exercise and add gentle active and passive stretching during subacute stage
b, c	Through splinting, joints will be rested to prevent damage and potential deformity	Hand resting splints in the position of function for night wear and use during periods of inactivity; short cock-up splint to protect the wrist may be useful when hands are active or being exercised	Decrease use of splint; remove splint for exercise and during self-care activities
e	Given instruction in joint protection, client will perform self-care to tolerance during acute episode	Self-feeding, using built-up, soft handle utensils; oral hygiene with electric toothbrush or built-up toothbrush; sponge and tub bathing, using wash mitt; self-dressing, using loose, slipover garments	Increase number of activities as disease activity subsides
Subacute or inactive stage a	Through exercise and daily activities, muscle strength of affected joints will increase to one-half grade higher than initial evaluation	Isometric exercise with resistance to elbow and wrist flexors and extensors, MP and PIP extensors, 3 to 10 repetitions 5 times daily; manual resistance is applied Light ironing, dust mopping, and dish washing	Maintain at light resistance; increase number of exercise periods, if tolerated Increase amount of activity, within physical tolerance
b	Through appropriate exercise and activity, ROM of affected joints will be increased or maintained	Active ROM exercise to elbow, wrist, MP and PIP motions; gentle passive stretching to elbow flexion and extension, MP flexion and extension, and PIP extension	
c	Given instruction in joint protection techniques, deformity will be prevented or retarded in development	Individual and group instruction in techniques of joint protection applied to home management and work activities	Increase number of techniques as each is mastered and applied in daily life
d	Explore potential for return to same or modified job in floral wreath design and construction	Client describes all steps of the involved tasks Therapist observes normal worker performing tasks; analyzes activity for potential deforming forces; determines need for job modification and application of joint protection and energy conservation principles in the workplace; modifies job to floral design and fresh flower arrangement; provides built-up pencil and protective ulnar deviation splint to be used during drawing, writing, and handling of flowers and clippers	Begin with one or two simple job tasks to be performed at home; job trial for 2 to 4 hours a day with 10 minutes of rest for every 40 minutes worked

Continued.

SAMPLE TREATMENT PLAN—cont'd

I. **Special equipment.**
   1. Ambulation aids.
      None required
   2. Splints.
      Hand resting splints: For joint rest and maintenance of optimal position during acute episodes
      Short cock-up splint: For rest and protection of wrist when hand is in use during acute and possibly subacute stages
      Protective ulnar deviation splint: To prevent ulnar drift during housekeeping and work activities

   3. Assistive devices.
      a. Electric mixer, can opener, toaster oven
      b. Lightweight dust mop with flexible handle
      c. Lever handles on faucets
      d. Fabric loops on oven doors so they may be opened with arm movement and not fingertips
      e. Utility cart
      f. High stools with backrest for kitchen and for work place
      g. Adapted key holders
      h. Wash mitts
      i. Dust mitts
      j. Foam rubber tubing to build handles on utensils and pencils

---

REVIEW QUESTIONS

1. What is the outstanding clinical feature that produces joint limitation and deformity in arthritis?
2. What sex and age groups are most frequently affected by arthritis?
3. What is meant by "rheumatoid factor"?
4. List four systemic signs of rheumatoid arthritis.
5. What is the characteristic course of the disease?
6. Describe the appearance and mechanics of two common finger deformities that may affect the DIP and PIP joints in rheumatoid arthritis.
7. What are the deformities that can result at the MP joints? How are they treated or prevented?
8. What are the major problems at the elbow and shoulder in arthritis? How can they be prevented?
9. What kinds of exercises are appropriate for arthritis clients in the acute stage of disease?
10. When is stretching exercise indicated?
11. When is joint rest indicated in treatment of arthritis?
12. Which joints should not be splinted in treatment of arthritis?
13. Which joints are frequently splinted in treatment of arthritis?
14. What is the role of the occupational therapist in splinting for arthritis?
15. List appropriate occupational therapy evaluation procedures for rheumatoid arthritis.
16. What are the general objectives of occupational therapy in treatment of arthritis?
17. What kinds of activities are contraindicated for the arthritis client during the acute stage of disease?
18. What kinds of activities are appropriate during the acute stage?
19. When the acute stage of the disease has abated, how can the client's activity be graded?
20. Discuss some of the ways work can be simplified for the arthritic client.
21. List some of the principles of joint protection directed toward maintaining ROM of the elbow and shoulder joints. Give some practical examples of methods of application of the principles to household tasks.
22. List five assistive devices for self-care or home management that could be useful to an arthritic client, and give the rationale for each.

REFERENCES

1. Arthritis Foundation: Guidelines for treatment of adult rheumatoid arthritis: exercise guide for physicians. Adapted by Dr. William Lages, San Jose, Calif., 1972, Santa Clara Valley Medical Center. Mimeographed.
2. Arthritis Foundation: Arthritis manual for allied health professionals, The Professional Manual Subcommittee of the Education Committee, Allied Health Professions Section, New York, 1973, The Arthritis Foundation.
3. Cordery, J.C.: Joint protection: a responsibility of the occupational therapist, Am. J. Occup. Ther. 19:285-294, 1965.
4. Engleman, E., and Shearn, M.: Arthritis and allied rheumatic disorders. In Krupp, M., and Chatton, M., editors: Current medical diagnosis and treatment, Los Altos, Calif., 1980, Lange Medical Publications.
5. Kasch, M.: O.T. for rheumatoid arthritis, lecture, San Jose, Calif., 1975, Department of Occupational Therapy, San Jose State University.
6. Lages, W.: Pathogenesis of joint destruction, San Jose, Calif., 1976 and 1980, Santa Clara Valley Medical Center. Mimeographed.
7. Lages, W.: Principles of treatment program for rheumatoid arthritis, San Jose, Calif., 1976, Santa Clara Valley Medical Center. Mimeographed.
8. Lages, W.: Rheumatoid arthritis: indications for exercise, San Jose, Calif., 1976, Santa Clara Valley Medical Center. Mimeographed.
9. Lages, W.: Arthritis and connective tissue diseases, lectures, San Jose, Calif., 1977, Department of Occupational Therapy, San Jose State University.
10. Lages, W.: Specific joint problems in rheumatoid arthritis, San Jose, Calif., 1976 and 1980, Santa Clara Valley Medical Center. Mimeographed.
11. Larson, C.B., and Gould, M.: Orthopedic nursing, ed. 8, St. Louis, 1974, The C.V. Mosby Co.
12. Melvin, J.L.: Rheumatic disease: occupational therapy and rehabilitation, Philadelphia, 1977, F.A. Davis Co.
13. Paterson, M.: O.T. for rheumatoid arthritis, lectures, San Jose, Calif., 1977, Department of Occupational Therapy, San Jose State University.

14. Pelletier, K.R.: Mind as healer: mind as slayer, New York, 1977, Dell Publishing Co., Inc.

15. Quan, P.E., and English, C.: Principles of joint protection and energy conservation, San Jose, Calif., Department of Occupational Therapy, Santa Clara Valley Medical Center. Mimeographed. (Adapted from Cordery, J.C.: The conservation of physical resources as applied to the activities of patients with arthritis and connective tissue diseases. In Rothenberg, E., editor, and Kandel, D., editorial chairman: Dynamic living for the long-term patient, World Federation of Occupational Therapists, study course III, 1962, Dubuque, Iowa, 1964, Wm. C. Brown Co., Publishers.)

16. Trombly, C.A., and Scott, A.D.: Occupational therapy for physical dysfunction, Baltimore, 1977, The Williams & Wilkins Co.

SUPPLEMENTARY READINGS

Bland, J.H.: Arthritis, medical treatment and home care, London, 1969, Collier Macmillan Ltd.

Brown, D.M., DeBacher, G.A., and Basmajian, J.V.: Feedback goniometers for hand rehabilitation, Am. J. Occup. Ther. 33:458-463, 1979.

Coley, I.L.: The child with juvenile rheumatoid arthritis, Am. J. Occup. Ther. 26:325-329, 1972.

English, C.B., and Nalebuff, E.A.: Understanding the arthritic hand, Am. J. Occup. Ther. 25:352-359, 1971.

Gruen, H.: A postoperative dynamic splint for the rheumatoid hand, Am. J. Occup. Ther. 24:284, 1970.

Kales-Rogoff, L.: Community skills experience for rheumatic disease patients, Am. J. Occup. Ther. 33:394-395, 1979.

MacBain, K.P., and Hill, R.H.: A functional assessment for juvenile rheumatoid arthritis, Am. J. Occup. Ther. 27:326-330, 1973.

Millender, L., and Philips, C.: Uses of the proximal interphalangeal joint gutter splint, Am. J. Occup. Ther. 27:8-13, 1973.

Moore, J.W.: Adapted knife for rheumatoid arthritics, Am. J. Occup. Ther. 32:112-113, 1978.

Spelbring, L., et al.: The use of activities in rheumatic disease, Am. J. Occup. Ther. 19:259-263, 1965.

Spencer, E.A.: Functional restoration. In Hopkins, H.L., and Smith, H.D., editors: Willard and Spackman's occupational therapy, ed. 5, Philadelphia, 1978, J.B. Lippincott Co.

Quest, I.M., and Cordery, J.: A functional ulnar deviation cuff for the rheumatoid deformity, Am. J. Occup. Ther. 25:32-37, 1971.

Wynn-Parry, C.B.: Rehabilitation of the hand, London, 1966, Butterworth & Co. Ltd.

Chapter 10

Occupational therapy for acute hand injuries

MARY C. KASCH, O.T.R.

The hand is vital to human function and appearance. It flexes, extends, opposes, and grasps thousands of times daily, allowing the performance of necessary daily tasks. The hand's sensibility allows feeling without looking, protects, and perceives of minute contrasts in texture and temperature. The hand is adorned with jewels and paint. The hand touches, gives comfort, and expresses emotion. Consequently, loss of hand function through injury touches every aspect of a person's life. It may jeopardize a family's livelihood and upset the balance of many lives.

Treatment of the injured hand is a matter of timing and judgment. Early treatment before physical deformity or development of poor motor patterns is the ideal. Standard treatment of a variety of hand injuries and a timetable for that treatment have been outlined in this chapter, but the therapist should always coordinate the application of any treatment with the hand surgeon. Surgical techniques may vary, and inappropriate treatment of the hand patient can result in the failure of a surgical procedure. Communication between the surgeon, therapist, and patient is especially vital in this setting. The creation of a comfortable atmosphere is essential to success in treating hand patients. The presence of the therapist as an instructor and evaluator is essential, but without the patient's cooperation limited gains will be achieved. Dealing with the psychological loss suffered by the patient who has a hand injury is an integral part of rehabilitative therapy as well.

EXAMINATION AND EVALUATION

When approaching a patient who has a hand injury for the first time the therapist must take many factors into account. The injured structures must be identified and evaluated. Identification of injury or disease is often done by consulting with the hand surgeon, whereas more detailed evaluation is performed by the therapist. X-ray films should be consulted to determine the location and extent of the injury and repair to the bone. Tendons and muscle function should be evaluated, using the standard manual muscle test. The presence and absence of sensation and sensory or nerve function must be ascertained. The skin should be examined for edema, wrinkles, moisture, scars, and skin lesions.[5]

The patient's age, occupation, and hand dominance should be taken into account in the initial evaluation. The type and extent of medical and surgical treatment that have been received as well as the length of time since such treatment are all important in determining a treatment plan. Any further surgery or conservative treatment that is planned should also be noted.

FRACTURES

In treating a hand or wrist fracture the surgeon will attempt to achieve good anatomical position through either a closed (nonoperative) or open (operative) reduction. Internal fixation with Kirschner wires, metallic plates, and/or screws may be used to maintain the desired position. The hand is usually immobilized in wrist extension and MP joint flexion with extension of the distal joints, whenever the injury allows this position. Trauma to bone may also involve trauma to tendons and nerves in the adjacent area. Treatment must be geared toward the recovery of all injured structures, and this fact may influence treatment of the fracture.

Occupational therapy may be initiated during the period of immobilization, which is usually 3 to 5 weeks. Uninvolved fingers of the hand must be kept mobile through the use of active motion. Edema should be carefully monitored, and elevation is required at all times.

As soon as there is sufficient bone stability, the surgeon will allow mobilization of the injured part. The surgeon should provide guidelines for the amount of resistance or force that may be applied to the fracture

---

□ Director of Hand Therapy, Hand Surgery Associates, Sacramento, Calif.

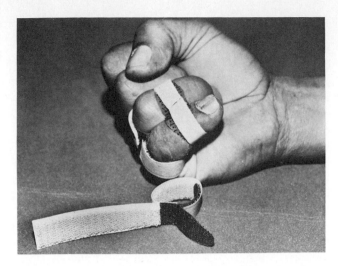

Fig. 10-1. Velcro "buddy" splint may be used to protect finger following fracture or encourage movement of stiff finger. (Available from Smalley and Bates, Inc., 85 Park Avenue, Nutley, N.J.)

site. Activities that correct poor motor patterns and encourage use of the injured hand should be started as soon as the hand is pain free. Early motion will prevent the adherence of tendons and reduce edema through massage of the lymphatic and blood vessels. As soon as the splint is removed, the presence of edema should be evaluated through the use of a volumeter. A baseline ROM should be established, and the application of appropriate splints may begin. A splint may be used to correct a deformity that has resulted from immobilization or it may be used to protect the finger from additional trauma to the fracture site. An example of this type of splinting would be the application of a Velcro "buddy" splint (Fig. 10-1) or the use of a splint to block full extension. A dynamic splint may be used to achieve full ROM and prevent the development of further deformity under certain circumstances. Evaluation of hand function and ADL should be performed to determine if a patient is neglecting the formerly injured hand.

Stiffness and pain are common complications of fractures, but the control of edema coupled with early motion and good patient instruction and support will minimize these complications.

NERVE INJURIES

Injuries to peripheral nerves are quite common and are often treated by the occupational therapist because of the effect nerve injury has on the function of the hand. Nerve injury may be classified into the following three categories:

1. Neurapraxia is contusion of the nerve without wallerian degeneration. The nerve recovers function without treatment within a few days or weeks.

2. Axonotmesis is an injury in which nerve fibers distal to the site of injury degenerate, but the internal organization of the nerve remains intact. No surgical treatment is necessary, and recovery usually occurs within 6 months. The length of time may vary, depending on the level of injury.

3. Neurotmesis is a complete laceration of both nerve and fibrous tissues. Surgical treatment is required. Microsurgical repair of the fascicles is common. Nerve grafting may be necessary in situations where there is a gap between nerve endings.[2]

Peripheral nerve injuries may occur as a result of disruption of the nerve by a fractured bone, laceration, or crush injury. Symptoms of nerve injuries will include weakness or paralysis of muscles that are innervated by motor branches of the injured nerve and sensory loss to areas that are innervated by sensory branches of the injured nerve. Before evaluating the patient for nerve loss the therapist must be familiar with the muscles and areas that are innervated by the three major forearm nerves.

Radial nerve

The radial nerve innervates the extensor-supinator group of muscles of the forearm, including the brachioradialis, extensor carpi radialis longus, extensor carpi radialis brevis, extensor digitorum communis, extensor digiti quinti, extensor indicis, extensor carpi ulnaris, supinator, abductor pollicis longus, extensor pollicis brevis, and extensor pollicis longus. The sensory distribution of the radial nerve is a strip of the posterior upper arm and the forearm, dorsum of the thumb, and index and middle fingers and radial half of the ring finger to the PIP joints. Sensory loss of the radial nerve does not usually result in dysfunction.

Clinical signs of a high-level radial nerve injury (above the supinator) are pronation of the forearm, with loss of wrist extension, and thumb adduction.[3] Clinical signs of a low-level radial nerve injury (below the elbow) include incomplete extension of the MP joints of the fingers and thumb. The intrinsic muscles will substitute for some finger extension, and the patient must be carefully evaluated.

Ulnar nerve

The ulnar nerve in the forearm innervates only the flexor carpi ulnaris and the median half of the flexor digitorum profundus. It travels down the volar forearm through the canal of Guyon, innervating the intrinsic muscles of the hand, including the palmaris brevis, abductor digiti quinti, opponens digiti quinti, flexor digiti quinti, interossei dorsales, interossei volares, lumbricales manus, adductor pollicis, and half of the flexor pollicis brevis.

The sensory distribution of the ulnar nerve is the dorsal and volar surfaces of the little finger ray and the ulnar half of the dorsal and volar surface of the ring finger ray.

Clinical signs of a high-level ulnar nerve injury may include clawhand with a loss of the hypothenar and the interosseous muscles. In a low-level ulnar nerve injury the flexor digitorum profundus and flexor carpi ulnaris will be present and unopposed by the intrinsic muscles. When attempting lateral or key pinch the IP joint of the thumb will flex instead of extend because of paralysis of the intrinsic muscles. This is also known as Froment's sign. Long-standing compression of the ulnar nerve in the canal of Guyon will result in a flattening of the hypothenar area and conspicuous atrophy of the first dorsal interosseous muscle.[3]

Sensory loss of the ulnar nerve results in frequent injuries to the ulnar side of the hand, especially burns.

Median nerve

The median nerve innervates the flexors of the forearm and hand and is often called the "eyes" of the hands because of its importance in sensory innervation of the volar surface of the hands. Median nerve loss is often secondary to lacerations as well as compression syndromes of the wrist such as the carpal tunnel syndrome.

Motor distribution of the median nerve is to the pronator teres, palmaris longus, flexor carpi radialis, radial portion of the flexor digitorum profundus, flexor digitorum superficialis, flexor pollicis longus, pronator quadratus, abductor pollicis brevis, opponens pollicis, half of the flexor pollicis brevis, and lumbricales manus.

Sensory distribution of the median nerve is to the volar surface of the thumb, index and middle fingers, and radial half of the ring finger and dorsal surface of the index and middle fingers and radial half of the ring finger distal to the PIP joints. Clinical signs of a high-level median nerve injury are loss of flexion of the wrist and fingers, supination of the forearm, and poor opposition of the thumb. A low- or wrist-level median nerve injury will result in decreased thumb flexion, abduction, and opposition. Sensory loss associated with a wrist-level median nerve injury is the inability to use the hand for pinch without watching the objects being manipulated. The patient, when blindfolded, will substitute pinch to the ring or little fingers to compensate for this loss. An injury in the forearm that involves the anterior interosseous branch of the median nerve will not result in sensory loss.[3]

Following nerve repair the hand is placed in a position that will minimize tension on the nerve. For example, following repair of the median nerve, the wrist will be immobilized in a flexed position. Immobilization usually lasts for 2 to 3 weeks, after which gradual stretching of the joints may begin. The therapist must exercise great care not to put excessive traction on the newly repaired nerve.

Correction of a contracture may take 4 to 6 weeks. Active exercise is the preferred method of gaining full extension, although a light dynamic splint may be applied with the surgeon's supervision. Splinting to assist or substitute for weakened musculature may be necessary for an extended period during nerve regeneration. Splints should be removed as soon as possible to allow for active exercise of the weakened muscles. However, it is important to instruct the patient in correct patterns of motion so that substitution does not occur.

Initially treatment is directed toward the prevention of deformity and correction of poor positioning during the acute and regenerative stages. Patients must be instructed in visual protection of the anesthetic area. ADL should be evaluated, and new methods or devices may be needed for independence. Use of the hand in the patient's work should be evaluated, and the patient should be returned to employment with any necessary modifications of his job or adaptations of equipment as soon as possible.

Careful muscle, sensory, and functional testing should be done frequently. As the nerve regenerates, splints may be changed or eliminated. Exercises and activities should be revised to reflect the patient's new gains, and adapted equipment should be discarded as soon as possible.

Detailed sensory testing will indicate when sensory reeducation should begin. Sensory testing may include pain testing (pinprick), light touch and deep pressure, two-point discrimination, warm-cool temperature discrimination, object identification, and proprioception. A more thorough sensory evaluation may be performed with the Semmes-Weinstein pressure-sensitive monofilaments.[1] The skin should be examined for trophic changes, which may result in a shiny, smooth appearance and loss of sweating ability. Dellon, Curtis, and Edgerton[6] have shown that perception of pinprick is the first sensation to return distally, followed by perception of vibration at 30 cps, the perception of constant touch, and, finally, the perception of vibration at 256 cps. They have used this information to develop a program of sensory reeducation of the hand. The sensory exercises do not change the status of the nerves themselves but help the patient to sharpen his perception of stimuli. The exercises are designed to use the level of sensibility available at the time of the evaluation. Maynard[8] describes the details of a sensory reeducation program.

Nerve recovery is a long process that requires a great deal of patience and cooperation between the injured person and the medical team. The patient usually finds the process frustrating, painful, and endless. As with other types of disabilities, activity groups will often help by providing exposure to others who have been through similar injuries. If nerve recovery is incomplete and is not improved by sensory reeducation, the patient may not be able to return to his former employment. Vocational rehabilitation counselors may assist in retraining, and they will consult with the therapist as to the patient's functional abilities.

TENDON INJURIES

Injuries to tendons may be isolated or may occur in conjunction with other injuries, especially fractures or crushes. Flexor tendons injured in the area between the distal palmar crease and the insertion of the flexor digitorum superficialis are considered to be the most difficult to treat, because the tendons lie in their sheaths in this area beneath the fibrous pulley system, and any scarring will cause adhesions. This area is often referred to as "no-man's-land" or "zone 2". Tendons injured in this area may be repaired shortly after injury and placed in a traction splint by the surgeon. While the wrist is in 20° to 30° of flexion a rubber band is attached to a fingernail suture and held at the wrist by a safety pin, allowing full passive flexion with active extension within the limits of the dressing. The MP joints should be kept in 70° to 90° of flexion to allow full PIP joint extension (Fig. 10-2). The splint is removed 21 days after the repair, and the patient begins active flexion and extension. A protective dorsal splint is continued for 1 or 2 weeks. PRE may be started in the fifth postoperative week.

If the damage to the finger is too extensive for primary tendon repair, a two-stage tendon reconstruction operation may be done. At the first stage a Silastic rod is inserted to make a new scar sheath for the tendon. The pulley system is also reconstructed at that time. Rubber band traction as just described is again used. At the second stage a free tendon graft is inserted and the rod removed 3 or 4 months later. The controlled passive flexion and active extension that are achieved in the elastic traction during the first 3 postoperative weeks allow for gliding of the tendon within the sheath, a minimum degree of scar formation, and no tension on the repaired tendon itself. However, excessive exercise may be an impediment to tendon healing as well.

In the fourth to sixth postoperative weeks passive flexion is continued and active flexion is initiated. When active flexion begins, the patient is instructed to block flexion at the MP joint and the PIP joint, allowing motion at the DIP joint. The PIP joint should be flexed approximately 15° during this blocking[10] to avoid excessive traction on the long flexor tendon. After a few days of isolated DIP flexion the patient is allowed to begin protected flexion at the PIP joint. Thus motion begins distally and moves proximally as more joint excursion is achieved. The MP joint continues to be blocked so that the intrinsic muscles that act on it cannot overcome the power of the repaired flexor tendons. Blocking can be performed with a small, wooden block (Fig. 10-3), the other hand (Fig. 10-4), or a variety of devices that are available on the market or from patterns. A Velcro "buddy" splint may be provided to attach the involved finger to the adjacent finger.

After 6 weeks dynamic splinting may be necessary to correct a flexion contracture at the PIP joint. Gentle dynamic extension is preferred at this point. If a per-

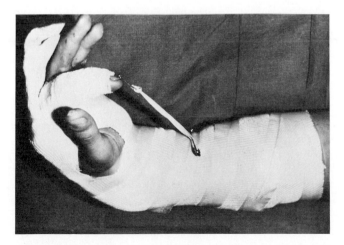

Fig. 10-2. Following flexor tendon repair wrist is placed in 30° of flexion with rubber band from fingernail to wrist, allowing full passive IP joint flexion and active extension. Note that MP joints maintain full flexion in dressing.

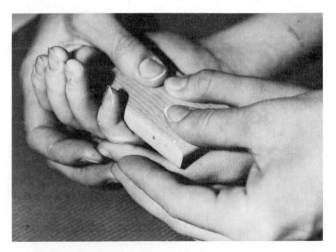

Fig. 10-3. Bunnell block is used to exercise each joint individually, allowing full tendon excursion, following surgical repair.

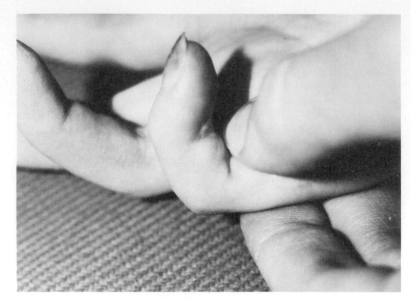

Fig. 10-4. Manual blocking of MP joint during flexion of PIP joint.

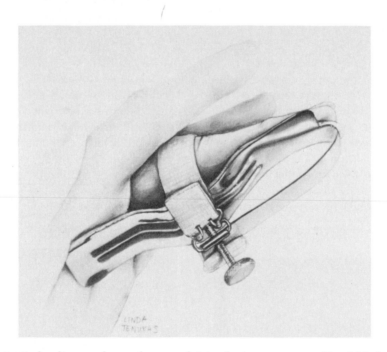

Fig. 10-5. Joint-Jack splint may be used to stretch joint flexion contracture (Available from Joint-Jack Co., 198 Millstone Road, Glastonbury, Conn.)

sistent flexion contracture is present after 8 weeks, a splint with greater tension such as a Joint-Jack may be applied (Fig. 10-5). Night splinting in extension is often necessary to maintain extension gains made during the day. Dynamic flexion splinting may be necessary if the patient has difficulty regaining passive flexion.

At about 8 weeks the patient begins light resistive exercises and activities. The hand should now be used for light ADL, but the patient should continue to avoid heavy lifting with or excessive resistance to the affected hand. Sports activities should be discouraged. However, activities such as clay work, woodworking, and macrame are excellent.

When evaluating a hand that has sustained a tendon injury, passive versus active limitations of joint motion must be evaluated. Limitations in active motion may indicate joint stiffness or muscle weakness. If passive motion is greater than active motion, the therapist

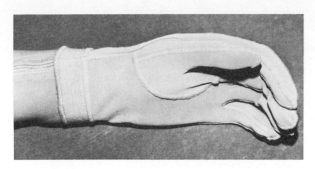

Fig. 10-6. Jobst pressure garment is used to reduce edema and prevent hypertrophic scarring.

should consider that tendons may be caught in the scar tissue. The therapist should be able to determine if a tendon is adhering and causing a flexion contracture or if the tendon is free, but the joint itself is stiff. Treatment should be based on this type of evaluation.

ROM, strength, function, and sensation testing (if digital nerves were also injured) should be performed frequently with splints and activities geared to progress. Although performance of ADL is generally not a problem, the therapist should ask the patient about any problems he may have or anticipate. Disuse and neglect of a finger, especially the index finger, are common and should be prevented.

Gains in flexion and extension may continue to be recorded for 3 to 4 months postoperatively. A finger with limber joints and minimum scarring preoperatively will function better after repair than one that is stiff and scarred and has trophic skin changes.[1] It is important therefore that all joints, skin, and scars be supple and movable before reconstructive surgery is attempted. A "functional" to "excellent" result is obtained if the combined loss of extension is less than 40° in the PIP and DIP joints of the index and middle fingers and is less than 60° in the ring and little fingers[10] and if the finger can flex to the palm.[4]

INJURIES TO SKIN

Hypertrophic scarring may occur after injury involving skin loss, skin grafts, thermal and electrical burns, and lacerations or after surgery.

If large areas are affected, Jobst pressure garments may be necessary (Fig. 10-6). Smaller scars respond to dynamic splinting, lanolin or friction massage, application of gauze and plastic splints (as in the thumb web space), and full active motion. Stretching a scar should be done extremely gently so that small ruptures do not occur, causing increased scar formation.

PAIN SYNDROMES

Pain syndromes, frequently referred to as sympathetic reflex dystrophy, often occur following nerve injury

and may occur after any injury, especially fractures and crushes. An abnormal cycle of pain, edema, vasospasm, lack of use, atrophy, deposition of fibrous tissue, and stiffness develops. The patient may exhibit symptoms of hysteria or describe an intensity of pain that is unbearable, although the pain does not follow peripheral nerve roots.[9]

Treatment should be initiated early and aggressively by a sympathetic but persistent therapist. An analysis of activities that increase or decrease pain and the times of day when pain occurs should be done. Painkillers or tranquilizers may be prescribed by the surgeon, who may also prescribe stellate ganglion blocks. If the patient responds to the stellate ganglion blocks, active and complete ROM must be obtained during the painfree period. The use of crafts that require shoulder, elbow, and finger motions, such as macrame hung from a hook in the ceiling, will be most beneficial, since they will not only exercise the affected joints and muscles but will also take the patient's mind off the pain. A warm atmosphere, less pain, and more activity will often help these patients through this difficult pain cycle.

Following fingertip amputation a scar or neuroma may become hypersensitive. In these cases massaging the scar or neuroma with lanolin, rubbing gently with cotton balls or terry cloth, or immersing in sand will decrease the sensitivity. A facilitation brush and electric vibrator have also been found to be useful. As the finger becomes less sensitive, activities may be initiated within the patient's tolerance level. Progression to manipulation of objects used in the patient's vocation is also indicated. The therapist should observe the patient's use of his hand and note any tendency to ignore the involved fingers. Finger guards should never be used after the wound has achieved initial healing.

THE STIFF HAND

Joint stiffness can occur after any type of hand injury. Stiffness is one of the most common and difficult challenges the therapist faces in the treatment of the patient who has a hand injury. Treatment must be performed frequently at home and in the clinic. Patients will often require care for several weeks or more.

Stiffness begins with edema, which leads to fibrosis, limitation of full ligamentous and tendinous excursion, pain, abnormal positioning of the hand, and disuse. Preventative measures should always be taken by instructing the patient in hand care after the injury, because the cycle is difficult to break once it is established. Treatment of the stiff hand will be discussed in the sample treatment plan that follows.

SAMPLE TREATMENT PLAN

Case study

E.M. is a 36-year-old right-handed punch press operator. He sustained a severe crush injury to the right hand with fractures of the fourth and fifth metacarpal bones, proximal phalanx of the little finger with MP joint disruption and multiple lacerations, disruption of the extensor mechanism of the little finger, and compression of the intrinsic muscle compartments. The patient was referred to occupational therapy to (1) increase passive and active motion of the right hand, (2) increase strength of the right hand, and (3) assess functional capabilities.

Treatment plan

A. Statistical data.
　1. Name: Mr. E.M.
　　Age: 36
　　Diagnosis: Crush injury to right hand
　　Disability: Metacarpal and phalangeal fractures; lacerations; disruption of extensor mechanism of little finger; and compression of intrinsic compartments, resulting in decreased ROM and use of the right hand

　2. Treatment aims as stated in referral:
　　　Increase passive and active motion and strength of right hand
　　　Assess functional capabilities

B. Other services.
At the time of injury patient underwent surgery with open reduction, internal fixation of all fractures, repair of the extensor mechanism, and release of the intrinsic compartments.

C. OT evaluation.
Patient was referred to therapy 6 weeks postoperatively after the removal of pins. Until that time he elevated the hand and had begun active flexion and extension at 2 weeks.
　Hand volume measurement: Test
　Complete evaluation of passive and active ROM of all joints of the fingers, thumb, and wrist: Test
　Sensation: Test
　　Touch
　　Pinprick
　　Two-point discrimination
　　Object discrimination
　ADL: Observe
　Jebsen-Taylor Test of Hand Function: Test

ROM of E.M.*

Affected hand	Active ROM Extension-flexion		Tips from palm (cm)	Passive ROM Extension-flexion		Tips to palm (cm)
Index finger						
MP	−35/65	30	2.0	−35/65	30	2.0
PIP	0/75	75		0/75	75	
DIP	−20/45	25		−20/45	25	
TAM†		130		TPM‡	130	
Middle finger						
MP	−15/35	20	2.8	−15/35	20	2.8
PIP	0/80	80		0/80	80	
DIP	−20/40	20		−20/40	20	
TAM		120		TPM	120	
Ring finger						
MP	−20/30	10	5.5	−20/45	25	2.5
PIP	−45/55	10		−45/65	20	
DIP	−10/30	20		−10/45	35	
TAM		40		TPM	80	
Small finger						
MP	−10/15	5	6.0	−10/15	5	6.0
PIP	−30/35	5		−30/35	5	
DIP	−25/35	10		−25/35	10	
TAM		20		TPM	20	

*As described by American Society for Surgery of the Hand, recommendations of the Clinical Assessment Committee, 1976.
†TAM, total active motion
‡TPM, total passive motion.

SAMPLE TREATMENT PLAN—cont'd

D. Results of evaluation.
1. Evaluation data.
    a. Physical resources.
        (1) Right hand volume was noted to be great-er than that of the left hand. A baseline measurement was made of hand volume for later comparison.
        (2) Active and passive ROM are reported in the accompanying table. Notice the loss of flexion and extension in all fingers, with the ring and little fingers being the most involved. The ring finger could passively be brought to within 2.5 cm of the mid-palmar crease, and it was felt that the flexor tendons were adhering in the pal-mar scar. Observation of the hand indi-cated scarring in the thumb web space between the index and middle fingers and across the palm in the area of the fourth and fifth metacarpal bones. All tendons were noted to be intact with trace motion in the little finger. The thumb was able to abduct 35°, and limitation was felt to be due to severe scarring in the thumb web space.
        (3) Sensation was intact in all areas tested.
        (4) The ADL evaluation revealed that the pa-tient had not been using his hand for any self care activities and was surprised to learn that he was indeed able to perform some activities.
        (5) The Jebsen-Taylor Hand Function test was not administered at this time.
    b. Psychosocial functions. During the course of administering the objective evaluations the therapist was able to elicit information about family and vocational interests. It was, at first, thought that the patient, whose major language was not English, was not able to understand the language or converse in it adequately. However, it was later determined that he had a good knowledge of English but was very uncomfortable and withdrawn in this setting. He arrived cradling his hand and was very nervous in the initial interview. Over the course of his treatment the patient re-vealed himself to be a warm and receptive individual who was extremely anxious to re-turn to his former employment and very co-operative in using all the equipment and ac-tivities given to him in therapy. Through his initial treatment, pain was decreased and motion was increased sufficiently that many of his anxieties about not being able to support his family were quickly put to rest. Any gains in motion, strength, and dexterity were thoroughly discussed with the patient, and he was constantly congratulated on his accom-plishments.
    c. Prevocational potential. The patient wished to return to his former employment as a punch press operator. It was felt that after a period of therapy, if physical gains were sufficient, the patient would be returned to that employ-ment. If he was not able to return to his for-mer job, a more thorough prevocational eval-uation and conference with the vocational re-habilitation counselor would be necessary to find appropriate employment or retraining. After initial treatment had begun, the Jebsen-Taylor Test of Hand Function was admin-istered to the patient. His times for com-pleting the activities, which required small dexterity, were only slightly below the stand-ard norms. The activities that caused him the most difficulty were moving large objects and moving weighted large objects. There-fore because of the physical demands of his job the patient was returned to light duty work 3 months after the injury occurred. His employer was most cooperative in giving him jobs that were within his physical capabilities, and, as his improvements continued, the pa-tient gradually returned to his normal job tasks.
2. Problem identification.
    a. Presence of edema
    b. Loss of passive motion of all finger joints
    c. Decreased active motion, especially in the ring and little fingers
    d. Contraction of the thumb web space due to scar tissue
    e. Scar adhesions of the palm onto the flexor tendons
    f. Tight extensor mechanism of the little finger
    g. Loss of abduction of all fingers
    h. Decreased grip strength of the right hand

Continued.

A

B

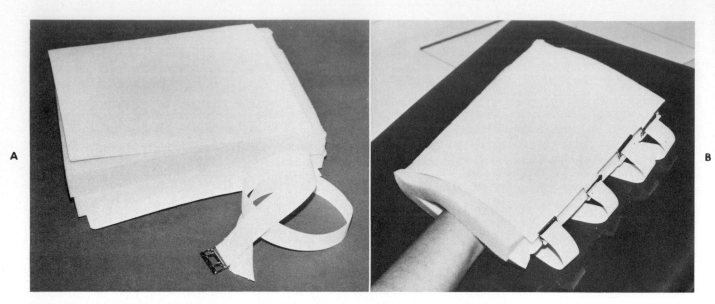

Fig. 10-7. A, Temper-foam sandwich splint is fabricated by splitting to one edge a 2-inch rectangle of temper-foam, placing sheets of plastic splinting material on each side, and securing tightly. Hand should be elevated and left in splint about 15 minutes. (Available from Alimed, 138 Prince Street, Boston, Mass.) **B,** Temper-foam sandwich splint in place on hand.

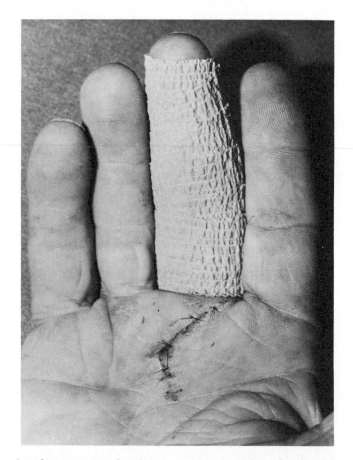

Fig. 10-8. One-inch Coban is wrapped with minimum pressure from distal end to proximal crease of digit. Patient is instructed to be aware of vascular compression or "tingling." Coban may be worn several hours a day to reduce edema. (Available from Medical Products Division/3M, St. Paul, Minn.)

SAMPLE TREATMENT PLAN—cont'd

E Problem	F Specific OT objectives	G Methods used to meet objectives	H Gradation of treatment
a	Decrease edema	Elevation except during use (may use Gardner Arm Elevator [Zimmer Orthopedic Products]) Contrast baths (alternate 96° warm/66° cool soaks each for 30 seconds; start and end with cool) Flex and extend to maximum in each bath (use sponge) Active motion through full range Isotoner glove worn constantly If edema persists, treat with "temper-foam sandwich" splint (Fig. 10-7) three to four times a day or use other pressure gradient garment For edema localized to one finger, a nonrestrictive wrapping with coban or lampwick for several hours will reduce edema (Fig. 10-8)	Methods are graded, for example, if elevation and active motion do not reduce edema, attempt contrast baths, then pressure wrapping; all may not be needed
b	Increase joint mobility	Refer to physical therapy for paraffin or hot packs prior to occupational therapy Passive ROM to fingers Immediately follow with active ROM Dynamic flexion splints to alternate with extension splint for ring finger 3 to 4 hours a day at home; a variety of splints may be used, including lampwick or web straps, commercially made splints, and polyform splints with outriggers An electric hand exercise splint is now available[7]	Increase time of activity Increase dynamic forces and length of time worn
c	Increase excursion and strength of affected tendons and muscles	Full controlled active range of each finger; observe hand to note any neglect or substitution of any muscles; allow active muscle pull to stretch soft tissue and remodel scar Allow isolated pull through of any tendons that appear to be stuck in scar tissue, that is, block MP and PIP flexion in ring finger and use full DIP (FDP) motion to pull free of scar Light resistance in grasping with Play doh, temper-foam blocks, or foam sponges; working against resistance helps the patient to feel active motion through pressure and proprioceptive feedback, as well as increases muscle strength Place ruler perpendicularly to palm; have patient attempt to get closer to palm each exercise session; patient measures and records best measurement; for extension, patient can attempt to touch a ruler projecting distally from dorsal surface of hand Work with Bunnell block to isolate PIP and DIP joints	Increase repetition Passively assist motion; then ask patient to "hold" position at end point of passive range Increase resistance Always attempt to decrease measurement Increase repetition

Continued.

SAMPLE TREATMENT PLAN—cont'd

E Problem	F Specific OT objectives	G Methods used to meet objectives	H Gradation of treatment
c	Increase excursion and strength of affected tendons and muscles—cont'd	Exercise with graduated dowel rods or rolling pin for grasp and release and pronation-supination, twisting with other hand Use activities that promote needed motions, always positioning properly	Decrease dowel size Increase difficulty of activity or strength required; gross to fine prehension (grasp and pinch)
d	Stretch web space; soften scar	Splint that applies constant, uniform pressure to scar and places thumb in maximum abduction (wear 23 hours a day) Massage scar with lanolin or tacky ointment if patient is allergic to wool (lanolin is made from sheep fat and will cause a rash in patients with wool allergy); gentle massage with low-intensity vibrator combined with stretching Active motion four times a day for 15 minutes each Friction massage with no ointment, using Dycem pad between thumb and skin, for friction may also be used to break up scar adhesions (combine with active motion)	As web stretches, new splints are made always to maximum abduction (serial splinting)
e	Pull tendons free of adhesions	Dynamic extension splinting Isolated DIP (FDP) and PIP (FDS) active motion Pressure bandage or glove if scar is extensive and hypertrophic	Increase force of traction; work against resistance
f	Increase mobility of soft tissue	Dynamic flexion splint (a variety might be necessary as gains are made) Active motion to maintain gains made by splinting	Increase traction; increase time spent in splint
g	Increase MP mobility (MP tightness limits abduction); increase strength of interossei and long extensors (assists in abduction)	Passive stretching of joints into abduction with fingers extended Lay hand flat and draw around fingers (have patient try to go beyond pattern) Isolate abduction and work on each finger individually (also do isolated MP joint extension) Resist abduction-adduction with theraplast splint or other device; resist MP extension (may use other hand)	Increase force (limit by pain and swelling); make new patterns Increase repetitions Increase resistance
h	Increase grip strength	Exercises and activities that provide resistance, allow full active ROM, and utilize hand use as needed in vocation (may also utilize avocation interests if appropriate); as strength increases, evaluate need for forearm and shoulder strength; evaluate and treat the entire extremity (see also methods for problem c)	Increase resistance; increase time of activity; increase variety of activities

REVIEW QUESTIONS

1. Name four structures that should be evaluated in a patient who has a hand injury.
2. List two complications that commonly occur with fractures.
3. How is the presence of edema evaluated? List three methods used to reduce edema.
4. Explain the three classifications of nerve injuries.
5. What are two symptoms of nerve injury?
6. Discuss the pattern of motions that would be lost in a high-level radial nerve injury.
7. Name three clinical signs of injury to the ulnar nerve in the hand.
8. Discuss the significance of the median nerve to hand function.
9. Discuss the role of splinting following nerve injury.
10. List five sensory tests.
11. What is the goal of sensory reeducation following nerve repair?
12. Define the area referred to as "no-man's-land". What is the significance of injury in this area?
13. What is the purpose of rubber band traction of the finger following tendon repair?
14. How soon after tendon repair would dynamic splinting for a flexion contracture begin?
15. Is motion begun proximally or distally following tendon repair?
16. What is the meaning of trophic skin changes?
17. What are the symptoms of a sympathetic reflex dystrophy?
18. List three modalities that would be used in treatment of a pain syndrome.
19. How would sensitivity of a painful neuroma be decreased?
20. Discuss the pathology of joint stiffness.
21. List three different objectives of splinting.

REFERENCES

1. Bell, J.A.: Sensibility evaluation. In Hunter, J.M., et al., editors: Rehabilitation of the hand, St. Louis, 1978, The C.V. Mosby Co.
2. Bora, F.W.: Nerve response to injury and repair. In Hunter, J.M., et al., editors: Rehabilitation of the hand, St. Louis, 1978, The C.V. Mosby Co.
3. Boyes, J.H.: Bunnell's surgery of the hand, ed. 5, Philadelphia, 1970, J.B. Lippincott Co.
4. Boyes, J.H., and Stark, H.H.: Flexor tendon grafts in the fingers and thumb, J. Bone Joint Surg. 53:1332-1342, 1971.
5. Burton, R.I., et al.: The hand: examination and diagnosis, Aurora, Colo., 1978, The American Society for Surgery of the Hand.
6. Dellon, A.L., Curtis, R.M., and Edgerton, M.T.: Reeducation of sensation in the hand after nerve injury and repair, Plast. Reconstr. Surg. 53:297-305, 1974.
7. Ketchum, L.D., Hibbard, A., and Hassanein, K.M.: Follow-up report on the electrically driven hand splint, J. Hand Surg. 4:474-481, 1979.
8. Maynard, J.C.: Sensory reeducation following peripheral nerve injury. In Hunter, J.M., et al., editors: Rehabilitation of the hand, St. Louis, 1978, The C.V. Mosby Co.
9. Omer, G.E.: Management of pain syndromes in the upper extremity. In Hunter, J.M., et al., editors: Rehabilitation of the hand, St. Louis, 1978, The C.V. Mosby Co.
10. Peacock, E.E., Madden, J.W., and Trier, W.C.: Post-operative recovery of flexor tendon function, Am. J. Surg. 122:686-692, 1971.

SUPPLEMENTARY READING

A.A.O.S.: Symposium on tendon surgery in the hand, St. Louis, 1975, The C.V. Mosby Co.

Bevan, G., and Perry, J.: Evaluation procedure for patients with hand injuries, Phys. Ther. 54:593-598, 1974.

Cailliet, R.: Hand pain and impairment, ed. 2, Philadelphia, 1975, F.A. Davis Co.

Flatt, A.E.: The care of minor hand injuries, ed. 3, St. Louis, 1972, The C.V. Mosby Co.

Hunter, J.M., et al., editors: Rehabilitation of the hand, St. Louis, 1978, The C.V. Mosby Co.

Lister, G.: The hand: diagnosis and indications, London, 1977, Churchill Livingstone.

Malick, M.H.: Manual on static splinting, Pittsburgh, 1973, Harmarville Rehabilitation Center.

Malick, M.H.: Manual on dynamic hand splinting with thermoplastic materials, low temperature materials and techniques, Pittsburgh, 1974, Harmarville Rehabilitation Center.

Moberg, E.: Evaluation of sensibility in the hand, Surg. Clin. North Am. 40:357, 1960.

Onne, L.: Recovery of sensibility and sudomotor activity in the hand after nerve suture, Acta Chir. Scand. Suppl., 300:1-69, 1962.

Spinner, M.: Injuries to the major branches of peripheral nerves of the forearm, Philadelphia, 1972, W.B. Saunders Co.

Thurber, P.: Evaluation of industrial disability, New York, 1960, Oxford University Press, Inc.

Wynn-Parry, C.B., et al.: Rehabilitation of the hand, ed. 3, London, 1973, Butterworth & Co. (Publishers) Ltd.

Chapter 11

Lower motor neuron dysfunction[1]

GUY L. McCORMACK, M.S., O.T.R.

The lower motor neuron system[1] includes the anterior horn cells of the spinal cord, spinal nerves and their associated ganglia, and 10 pairs of cranial nerves and their nuclei, which are housed in the brain stem (cranial nerves 1 and 2 are fiber tracts in the brain).[4] The motor fibers of the lower motor neurons are divided into the somatic and autonomic components. The somatic motor components include the alpha motor neurons, which innervate skeletal (extrafusal fibers) muscles, and gamma motor neurons, which innervate muscle spindles (intrafusal fibers). The autonomic component innervates the glands, smooth muscles, and heart musculature.[5,7,19] A lesion to any of these neurologic structures constitutes a lower motor neuron dysfunction.[5]

Lower motor neuron dysfunction can result from several different causes, including traumatic injury, such as bone fractures and dislocations, contusions, compression of nerve roots, lacerations, traction (stretching), penetrating wounds, and friction. Vascular deficiencies may also cause lower motor neuron dysfunction. Examples of these deficiencies include arteriosclerosis, diabetes mellitus (sensory loss), peripheral vascular anomalies, and polyarteritis nodosa.[3] Furthermore toxic agents such as lead, phosphorus, alcohol, benzene, and sulfonamides can cause lower motor neuron dysfunction. Other contributing factors may include neoplasms such as neuromas and multiple neurofibromatosis and inflammatory processes such as polyneuritis or mononeuritis. Degenerative diseases of the CNS and congenital anomalies can also produce lower motor neuron dysfunction.[6,23]

Since the occupational therapist traditionally treats a variety of lower motor neuron dysfunctions that affect the upper extremities, this chapter will deal with the conditions most likely to be seen in clinical practice.

DISEASES OF THE LOWER MOTOR NEURON
Poliomyelitis

Poliomyelitis is a contagious viral disease that affects the anterior horn cells of the gray matter of the spinal cord and the motor nuclei of the brain stem. The cervical and lumbar enlargements of the cord are affected the most. Because of the active immunization program (Salk and Sabin vaccines) in the United States, new cases of poliomyelitis are rare. However, the recent complacency about immunization has created some new cases, and "old cases" are frequently referred to occupational therapy for rehabilitation or improvement of the quality of life.[9]

Clinically patients who have poliomyelitis initially have flaccid paralysis that may be local or widespread. The lower extremities, accessory muscles of respiration, and muscles that promote swallowing are primarily affected. Marked atrophy may be seen in the involved extremities, and deep tendon reflexes may be absent. Sensation is often intact. Contractures can occur very early in the course of the disease. In cases of local paralysis the asymmetry of muscles pulling on various joints may promote deformity complications, such as subluxation, scoliosis, and contractures. In severe cases osteoporosis (bone atrophy) may weaken the long weight-bearing bones, and pathologic fractures can occur.[13]

The medical treatment for poliomyelitis during the acute phase includes bed rest, positioning, and applications of warm packs to reduce pain and promote relaxation. Since there is no known cure for poliomyelitis, the disease must run its course. There is an incubation period of 1 to 3 weeks, and the recovery is dependent on the number of nerve cells destroyed. Paralysis may begin in 1 to 7 days after the initial symptoms. The medical aspects of rehabilitation may include reconstructive surgery, such as tendon transfer; arthrodesis; and surgical release of fascia, muscles, and tendons. Other medical procedures may include therapeutic stretching, casts, muscle reeducation, and bracing for standing or stability.[11]

□ Assistant Professor, Department of Occupational Therapy, San Jose State University, San Jose, Calif.

Occupational therapy intervention. During the acute phase the patient receives symptomatic treatment and is confined to bed. The therapist should assist the nurse in providing good bed positioning to prevent contractures and protect weakened joints. Since the poliomyelitis virus is infectious during this stage, isolation procedures should be carefully followed. The therapist should provide gentle passive ROM at the patient's physical tolerance level to prevent contractures, joint stiffness, and deformities. Care should be taken not to grasp the involved muscle bellies, because they will be extremely tender and painful. The muscles may also be prone to spasms when painfully stimulated.[9]

The primary emphasis should be placed on the avoidance of muscle fatigue. Fatigue at this point can result in further residual weaknesses. If the patient has bulbar poliomyelitis, which affects the muscles of respiration, a respirator may be used to facilitate ventilation of the lungs or a tracheostomy may be performed. If the muscles necessary for swallowing are impaired, tube feeding may also be prescribed. The therapist should collaborate treatment procedures with the nursing staff to ensure proper functioning of the equipment necessary for the life support systems.[4,9,11]

The treatment program should include psychological support. The patient's fears and anxieties about the crippling effects of the disease should not be underestimated. The patient may need encouragement and positive experiences to promote an optimistic outlook during the rehabilitation process. The family may also need assistance in adjusting to the patient's disability.

As the rehabilitation process progresses, the precautions against physical and body fatigue continue. Assistive devices, splints, and MASs may be used to gain independence in daily activities. The long-range rehabilitation program should follow a functional course of action. After the acute medical problems have subsided, the recovery stage may last as long as 2 years.[4] Since the damage to the anterior horn cells is permanent, the therapist should assist the patient in making the best possible use of whatever muscular function remains. Before treatment is started, an evaluation of the existing disability must be obtained. A thorough manual muscle test not only provides a baseline for muscle strength but detects joint deformities secondary to contracted muscles, ligaments, tendons, and joint capsules. Manual muscle tests should be repeated monthly for the first 4 months and bimonthly for the next 4 months. After 8 months of therapeutic exercises the average patient has probably responded to the maximum of his ability.[3,4,10] In short the therapeutic regime includes combinations of rest, movement, muscle reeducation, functional activities, and psychological support. Consequently the prognosis of poliomyelitis depends on the personality of the patient and the perseverance of the therapist.

Movement for the patient who is recovering from acute poliomyelitis proceeds from passive to active ROM, depending on the patient's level of voluntary control. Muscle reeducation should be preceded by gentle stretching exercises. For the upper extremity emphasis should be placed on stretching the pectoralis major and minor and latissimus dorsi to ensure free motion of the shoulder region. All active motions should be performed under careful supervision of the therapist. Compensatory movement should be avoided. A limited but correct movement is preferred to an ampler but incorrect movement. Active movements should be done in front of a mirror, which enables the patient to observe and correct motions accordingly.[9-11]

Muscle reeducation is accomplished in a graded fashion. At first the patient should learn "muscle-setting" exercises, that is, alternating contraction and relaxation of muscles without moving the joints. Isometric exercises and electromyographic (EMG) biofeedback may be beneficial at this juncture. As the patient progresses, light resistance can be applied manually by the therapist before the use of pulleys and weights. This allows the therapist to develop an empirical understanding of the patient's physical strengths and weaknesses. Weakened muscles must be protected at all times. Muscles that cannot resist the forces of gravity are supported during exercise as well as during rest periods. As a rule of thumb, resistive exercises are not attempted until the muscle is able to carry out a complete ROM against gravity. Weakened or flaccid muscles can be splinted at night to counteract the forces of gravity or the pull of the stronger antagonist muscles. During resistive exercises the therapist should stress correct body positioning, joint alignment, and energy conservation. Periods of rest should be included in the exercise program, as well as activities that incorporate the same movements and musculature.[10]

The rationales for resistive exercises in the rehabilitation of the patient who has poliomyelitis are to cause hypertrophy of the undamaged muscle fibers and give usefulness to the slightest contraction by integrating it into the global movement that permits the performance of a given activity. Emphasis is placed on strengthening individual weakened muscles. After the 8-month period if the muscle is unable to contract completely against gravity, it is doubtful that additional muscle strength will return. At this point the emphasis should be placed on maintenance of existing muscles and functional ADL. Again a self-care evaluation should be administered to achieve a baseline of function. Dressing activities may include putting on braces, prostheses, or orthoses. Assistive and adaptive devices should be tailored to the needs of the patient. The adaptation of assistive devices should begin where the patient's functional abilities are limited. Assistive and adaptive devices should provide the patient with the most ability within the limits of his disability.[18] It may also be advantageous to begin activities for prevocational and vocational exploration. The patient's quality of life can be improved if he is employed and productive.

Today therapists are seeing more "old polio" patients in rehabilitation centers. Some of the patients are experiencing additional weakness and paralysis. The phenomenon is not fully understood, but it is believed to be the normal loss of neurons in later life. Since the poliomyelitis victim has a diminished number of neurons in the anterior horn cells, further loss can be debilitating. This problem may pose some new challenges to the therapist in the future.

Guillain-Barré syndrome

Guillain-Barré syndrome, also known as either infectious polyneuritis or Landry's syndrome, is an acute inflammatory condition involving the spinal nerve roots, peripheral nerves, and, in some cases, selected cranial nerves. The Guillain-Barré syndrome often follows an afebrile illness. It is probably caused by a virus that produces a hypersensitive response that results in patchy demyelination of lower motor neuron pathways. The axons are generally spared, so recovery often follows a predictable course. In severe cases, however, wallerian degeneration of the axon results in a slow recovery process. This disease affects men and women equally from ages 30 to 50.*

Clinically Guillain-Barré syndrome is characterized by a rapid onset. Initially there is an absence of fever, pain and tenderness of muscles, and weakness and decrease in deep tendon reflexes. As the disease progresses, it produces motor weakness or paralysis of the limbs, sensory loss, and muscle atrophy. The prognosis is varied. In severe cases cranial nerves 7, 9, and 10 may be involved, and the patient may have difficulty speaking, swallowing, and breathing. If vital centers in the medulla are affected, the patient may experience respiratory failure.

In the majority of the cases the patient completely recovers within 3 to 8 months. Some slight exacerbation can occur, producing residual weaknesses and muscular atrophy.[11]

Occupational therapy intervention. Once the patient is medically stabilized, treatment goals should be coordinated with the nurse, physical therapist, and other members of the team to implement a comprehensive rehabilitation program. The occupational therapist should grade the activity to the patient's physical tolerance level. Physical fatigue should be avoided at all costs. Gentle, nonresistive activities can be introduced to alleviate joint stiffness and muscle atrophy and prevent contractures.[9,21]

Treatment should always begin with a thorough evaluation of the patient's level of functioning. During the early stages of recovery the evaluation process itself may be fatiguing. It is often best to spread the evaluation process over the course of a few days. For example, testing may begin by gently squeezing the muscle bellies of the large muscle groups to determine the extent of muscle tenderness and atrophy. Since the muscles of the limbs are usually affected symmetrically, this test can be grossly administered. Manual muscle testing should not be done in one session. It is best to test a few muscles at a time, and allow the patient periods of rest. Particular attention should be paid to the intrinsic muscles of the hands to determine residual weakness. If swallowing or speech is impaired, a tongue depressor may be used to apply light resistance against the tongue to estimate the motor involvement in the twelfth (hypoglossal) cranial nerve. Manual muscle testing is subjective, and the patient's prior physical condition and occupation should be taken into account when calibrating the muscle strength.[9] It is important to establish a baseline on all of the clinical findings and chart the progression of the affected muscles.

Sensory testing should also be conducted because the sensory pathways are often affected. Sensory tests should include light touch, stereognosis, pain and temperature, proprioception, and two-point discrimination. Test findings should be recorded and deficits should be noted.

Passive ROM should begin with gentle movement of the proximal joints and should proceed only to the point of pain. As the patient's tolerance level increases, active ROM and light exercises may be introduced. The program should stress joint protection, and the therapist should look for muscle imbalance and substitution patterns. PREs should be used conservatively. Throughout the course of recovery the therapist should guard against fatigue and irritation of the inflamed nerves. As the patient's strength and tolerance level increase, more resistance can be employed, but to a moderate degree. The therapist may also introduce sedentary or tabletop activities during the early stages of recovery. As the patient's strength increases, activities promoting more resistance, such as leather work, textiles, and ceramics, can be incorporated into the treatment regime. Grooming, self-care, and other ADL should be included as the need and

*References 3, 4, 9, 20, 23.

desire arise. Slings and MASs may be employed to alleviate muscle fatigue and gain independence.

Bell's palsy

Bell's palsy represents an acute inflammatory disorder that affects the seventh (facial) cranial nerve. The resulting symptoms depend on the location of the lesion. In most cases the patient experiences ipsilateral facial paralysis, which causes distortion of the face. The course of the disease is usually short in duration, lasting 2 to 8 weeks. Yet during the period of involvement the patient may have difficulty eating and speaking, and the eye on the affected side may produce tears.[4,5]

Occupational therapy intervention. The occupational therapist may play an important role in the treatment of the patient with Bell's palsy. The occupational therapist and the orthotist may be asked to fabricate a temporary facial splint to support impaired facial muscles. The affected facial muscles can also benefit from gentle, upward massage for 5 to 10 minutes 2 to 3 times a day to maintain muscle tone. Electrical stimulation and infrared treatments by the physical therapist may also be included in the patient's treatment regime. The therapist should assist the patient in carrying out his normal personal hygiene tasks. The lack of facial sensation on one side will require careful visual awareness while shaving. Brushing the teeth will require careful visual attention because food particles can collect on the affected side. Some patients may wear a patch over the affected eye, so visual awareness should be stressed to compensate for the temporary loss of sight and sensation.[4]

INJURIES TO PERIPHERAL NERVES
Clinical signs of peripheral nerve injuries

Regardless of the origin of the injury peripheral nerve lesions produce similar clinical manifestations. The most obvious manifestation is muscle weakness or flaccid paralysis, depending on the extent of the nerve damage. Because of the loss of muscle innervation atrophy will follow, and deep tendon reflexes will be absent or depressed. Sensation along the cutaneous distribution of the nerve will also be lost. Trophic changes, such as dry skin, hair loss, cyanosis, brittle fingernails, painless skin ulcerations, and slow wound healing in the area of involvement, may also be present as clinical signs. Occasionally minute muscle contractions called fasciculations may be seen on the surface of the skin overlying the denervated muscle belly. As a result of disturbances of sympathetic fibers of the autonomic nervous system, there will be a loss of the ability to sweat above the denervated skin surfaces. The patient may experience paresthesias, that is, sensations such as tingling, numbness, and burning or pain (causalgia), particularly at night. In

addition if the nerve damage was caused by trauma, edema will be a prominent clinical manifestation. EMG examinations may reveal extremely small muscle contractions called fibrillations.*

Extensive peripheral nerve damage may produce deformity if contractures, joint stiffness, and poor positioning are allowed to occur. Disfigurement of the hands is particularly noticeable and may produce some psychological complications. Other complications may include osteoporosis of the bony structures and epidermal fibrosis of the joints.

All of the clinical manifestations just discussed may not be present. The clinical findings may vary with the underlying cause of the lesion.

Clinical signs of peripheral nerve regeneration

Peripheral nerve regeneration begins about 1 month after the injury occurred. The rate of regeneration depends on the nature of the nerve lesion. If, for example, the nerve has been severed, the regeneration would occur at the rate of 1.35 cm (½ inch) per month.[16] Early medical treatment may require suturing the nerve and immobilizing the involved extremity to ensure good opposition of the severed nerves. In most cases rehabilitation begins about 7 weeks after the injury occurred. Full recovery of muscle function is not probable because regenerated fibers lose about 20% of their original diameter and conduct impulses at a slower rate.[5,15]

Since peripheral nerves have the capacity to regenerate, the course of recovery can be somewhat predictable. The clinical signs of regeneration do not always abide by a specific sequence. Yet one might expect to see the following clinical signs:

Clinical signs of regeneration
Skin appearance: As the edema subsides and collateral blood vessels develop, the circulatory system should become more normalized. The skin should improve in its color and texture.

Primitive protection sensations: The first signs of cutaneous sensation will usually be the gross recognition of crude pain, temperature, pressure, and touch.

Paresthesias (Tinel's sign): Tapping along the involved nerve route will produce crude sensations. The patient may also experience pain sensations, especially at night.

Scattered points of sweating: As the parasympathetic fibers of the autonomic nervous system regenerate, the sweat glands will recover their functions.

Discriminative sensations: The more refined sensations, such as the ability to identify and localize touch, joint movements (proprioception), recognition of objects in the three-dimensional form (stereognosis), speed of movement (kines-

*References 1, 2, 4, 5, 8, 12.

thesia), and two-point discrimination, should be returning at this juncture.

Muscle tone: As nerve fibers regenerate and tie into their respective musculature via their motor end-plates, flaccidity will decrease and tone will increase. An important principle is that paralyzed muscles must first sense pressure before tone and movement can be realized.

Voluntary muscle function: The patient will be able to move the extremity first with gravity eliminated, and, as strength increases, he may actively move the extremity through full ROM. At this point graded exercises can begin.

Full recovery of muscle power is not probable, because the possibility that thousands of regenerating fibers will find their previous connections is unlikely.*

Phelps and Walker[16] reported that for complete laceration of peripheral nerves, the two-point discrimination test and the wrinkle test are viable methods of monitoring sensory return. The two-point discrimination test provides a quantitative measure of sensation. An earlier study by Moberg reveals the normal distance to discriminate one point from two points on the distal fingertip is 2 to 4 mm. A two-point discrimination of greater than 15 mm denotes tactile agnosia (absent sensation). This test can be achieved with the use of a high quality caliper with blunted tips so that the pain sensation is not elicited. Light application of the calipers to the patient's skin in a random pattern can help the therapist map out the cutaneous, topographical areas that are innervated and denervated.

Another test that can be clinically significant is the wrinkle test. This test is performed by immersing the patient's hand in plain water at 42.2° C (108° F). The hand remains submerged for about 20 to 30 minutes until wrinkling occurs. At this point the patient's hand is dried, graded on a scale of 0 to 3, and photographed. The "0" on the scale represents an absence of wrinkling, whereas "3" represents normal wrinkling. The wrinkle test appears to provide an objective method of testing innervation of the hand with recent complete and partial peripheral nerve injuries. The actual physiological mechanism that causes the wrinkling is not fully understood, and the test is not appropriate for patients with traumatic peripheral nerve compression injuries.[16] Nevertheless the test can be significant in determining the rate of sensory regeneration and can provide a graphic record of denervated areas.

Medical management of peripheral nerve injuries

The medical-surgical management of peripheral nerve lesions depends on the type of injury that has occurred. Lacerations may be treated with microsurgery to suture the severed nerve. Exploratory surgery (neurolysis) may be conducted to remove unwanted scar tissue from the site of the lesion. Nerve grafts and transplants are performed for severe traumatic injuries. Alcohol injections, vitamin B_{12}, and phenol are used to alleviate the pain that might accompany peripheral neuropathy. For inflammatory processes high caloric diets with liberal use of vitamin B complex is the treatment of choice.[3,4]

Specific peripheral nerve injuries

Brachial plexus injury. The nerve roots that innervate the upper extremity originate in the anterior rami between C4 and T1. This network of lower anterior cervical and upper dorsal spine nerves is collectively called the *brachial plexus.* This very important nerve complex can be palpated just behind the posterior border of the sternocleidomastoid muscle as the head and neck are tilted to the opposite side.[3,4,11]

Lesions to the brachial plexus usually result from a variety of traumatic injuries. Most brachial plexus injuries in children are caused by birth defects. The more classic of these brachial plexus injuries are call Erb-Duchenne and Klumpke's paralyses. The Erb-Duchenne is indicative of lesions to the fifth and sixth plexus roots. Paralysis and atrophy occur in the deltoid, brachialis, biceps, and brachioradialis muscles. Clinically the arm hangs limp, the hand rotates inward, and functional movement is extremely limited.

Klumpke's paralysis affects the more distal aspect of the upper extremity. The disorder results from injury to the eighth cervical and first thoracic plexus roots. Consequently there will be paralysis to the distal musculature of the wrist flexors and the intrinsic muscles of the hand.[3,4]

Long thoracic nerve injury. The long thoracic nerve (C5-7) innervates the serratus anterior (magnus) muscle, which anchors the apex of the scapula to the posterior of the rib cage. Although injury to this nerve is not common, it has been injured by carrying heavy weights on the shoulder, neck blows, and axillary wounds. The resulting clinical picture is threefold: First, winging of the scapula occurs when the arm is extended and pressed against a stabilized object in front of the patient. Second, the patient will have difficulty flexing his outstretched arm above the level of his shoulder. Third, the patient will have difficulty protracting the shoulder or performing scapula abduction and adduction.

Injuries involving the long thoracic nerve are usually treated by stabilizing the shoulder girdle to limit scapula motion. The therapist must avoid using activities that promote shoulder movements. If nerve regeneration is not complete, surgery may be indicated to relieve the excessive mobility of the scapula. After medical treatment the occupational therapist encourages maximum

---

*References 1, 3-6, 12, 15.

functional independence and teaches the patient to use long-handle devices to compensate for shoulder limitations.

Axillary nerve injury. The axillary nerve is composed from the C5-6 spinal nerves and derived from the posterior region of the brachial plexus. The motor branches of the axillary nerve innervate the superior aspect of the deltoid muscle and the teres minor muscle. Although the axillary nerve is rarely damaged by itself, it is often damaged along with traumatic lesions to the brachial plexus. As a result, the patient will experience weakness or paralysis of the deltoid muscle, causing limitations in horizontal abduction and hyperesthesia on the lateral aspect of the shoulder. In addition to the loss of muscle power, atrophy of the deltoid muscle produces asymmetry of the shoulders. If the nerve damage is permanent, a muscle transplantation may be required to provide some abduction of the arm.[3,4,20]

The occupational therapist should maintain ROM to prevent deformity and improve circulation. Passive abduction of the shoulder should be done daily. The teres minor and deltoid muscles should be protected from stretch during the manual ROM activities. The patient may be taught to use long-handle assistive devices to compensate for the abduction deficit. If a surgical transplant is performed, the therapist should be familiar with the surgical procedure and assist in muscle reeducation. An EMG biofeedback machine can be beneficial in providing the patient with visual and auditory incentives during muscle reeducation sessions. The occupational therapist may also assist the patient in dressing activities. If the asymmetry of the shoulders presents a cosmetic problem when wearing shirts or jackets, a foam rubber or Orthoplast pad can be fabricated to fill in the space that was once filled by the deltoid muscle. The patient should be encouraged to learn self-ranging techniques and implement an exercise program to maintain the integrity of the unimpaired muscles of the involved extremity.

Radial nerve injury. The radial nerve represents the largest branch of the brachial plexus and descends along the humerus in the musculospiral groove. Below the elbow it bifurcates into the superficial radial nerve and the deep radial nerve. The superficial radial nerve terminates in the first, second, and third phalanges, whereas the deep radial nerve descends along the posterior region of the forearm, branching out to supply the extensor-supinator group of muscles.

The sensory branches innervate cutaneous receptors along the dorsal aspect of the arm and forearm and the posterior surface of the thumb, index and middle fingers, and half of the ring finger. The motor branches innervate the triceps, brachioradialis, anconeus, extensor digiti communis, extensor carpi ulnaris, supinator, ab-

ductor pollicis longus, extensor pollicis brevis, extensor pollicis longus, and extensor indicis proprius muscles.

The actions produced by the radial nerve are wrist extension, MP extension, thumb abduction and extension, ulnar and radial deviation, and release of grasping actions.

The most common types of injury to the radial nerve are fractures of the humerus or lacerations across the dorsum of the forearm.

The most blatant clinical feature of radial nerve injury is extensor paralysis. The patient will exhibit "wrist drop" and an inability to extend the thumb, proximal phalanges, and elbow joint. In addition the patient will have difficulty pronating the hand and grasping objects.*

Median nerve injury. The median nerve originates in the lateral and medial cords of the brachial plexus. The two cords unite, forming one nerve trunk that descends along the medial part of the arm to the anterior region of the forearm, branching out until it terminates in the hand.

The sensory branches of the median nerve innervate the cutaneous receptors of the palmar aspect of the thumb and the second, third, and half of the fourth fingers. The motor branches innervate the pronator teres, flexor carpi radialis, palmaris longus, flexor digitorum sublimis, flexor pollicis longus, half of the flexor digitorum profundus, and pronator quadratus muscles and lumbricales 1 and 2.

The actions produced by the median nerve are thumb opposition and abduction, IP flexion of the index finger, DIP flexion of the thumb, wrist flexion, forearm pronation, MP flexion of the second and third fingers, and IP flexion of the third, fourth, and fifth fingers.

The most common types of injury for the median nerve are forearm lacerations, wrist trauma, and deep lacerations to the flexor pollicis brevis muscle.[2,4,15,21]

Clinically one would expect to see loss of thumb opposition, thenar atrophy, and ape hand deformity. Furthermore the patient would have difficulty making a fist because the second and third fingers would remain extended while the fourth and fifth would flex.

Ulnar nerve injury. The ulnar nerve is the largest branch of the medial cord of the brachial plexus. It travels down the medial side of the arm and passes posteriorly to the medial epicondyle of the humerus. From the elbow it descends along the ulnar side of the forearm to innervate the small muscles of the hand.

The sensory branches of the ulnar nerve innervate cutaneous receptors in the little finger, half of the ring finger, and the medial portion of the hand. The motor branches innervate the flexor carpi ulnaris, half of the flexor digitorum profundus, adductor digiti quinti, op-

*References 2, 4, 14, 15, 21.

ponens digiti quinti, flexor digiti quinti, lumbricales 3 and 4, interossei, adductor pollicis, flexor pollicis brevis, and palmaris brevis muscles.

The actions produced by the ulnar nerve are finger adduction and abduction, wrist flexion, and MP extension. Grasp and pinch are achieved by PIP flexion of the fourth and fifth phalanges, and thumb adduction and opposition.

The usual sites of injury of the ulnar nerve are the posterior elbow region and the palmar region of the hand from the MP joint of the fifth phalanx to the carpal joint.[2,4,21]

Combined ulnar and median injury. Since the ulnar and median nerves are anatomically close to each other in the wrist region, they are often injured together. The clinical picture depends on the severity of the lesion and which nerve has undergone the most damage. If both nerves suffer a complete transection, ape hand deformity would be present, the wrist would be hyperextended, and flexor movements and abduction and adduction of the fingers would be greatly impaired.[2,4,15,21]

Volkmann's contracture. A fracture of the lower end of the humerus (supracondylar region) may result in a diminished supply of well-oxygenated blood to the muscles of the forearm. This phenomenon can occur when the fracture has been tightly cast and bandaged. Edema sets in near the site of the injury and shuts down the blood supply to the muscle bellies because the site of injury cannot swell outward. Ischemia will deprive tissues of oxygen and nourishment. The muscle can become necrotic, causing atrophy and contractures of the wrist, fingers, and forearm. The flexor digitorum profundus and flexor pollicis longus muscles are severely affected. The median nerve is often more impaired than the ulnar nerve.[3,11]

Shortly after a fracture of the humerus has been immobilized, the patient may have a cold, distal extremity with a smooth, glossy, or dusky appearance of the skin. If the therapist cannot detect a radial pulse, the physician should be informed immediately, and the cast should be removed. Early detection and prevention of this problem can eliminate a very severe deformity. If, for example, the ischemia lasts 6 hours, some contracture will follow. Ischemia lasting 48 hours or more will result in a permanent deformity of the forearm.

If mild ischemia has occurred, the physician may prescribe vigorous, active exercises to increase circulation, activate musculature, and prevent joint stiffness.

The occupational therapist may be involved in the treatment of acute peripheral nerve injury or may be involved later in the rehabilitation process. Treatment during the acute postoperative phase is aimed at the prevention of deformity. Initially static splints are used to immobilize the extremity and protect the site of injury.[9,21] During this phase the reduction of edema may be of primary importance. The first step in the reduction of edema is to elevate the extremity above the level of the heart. This will decrease the hydrostatic pressure in the blood vessels and promote venous and lymphatic drainage. Manual massage while the extremity is elevated may also reduce edema. The massage should entail centripetal strokes to gently force the excess fluids toward the proximal aspects of the body. Care must be taken not to disturb the healing process of the site of injury. External elastic support can also be used to alleviate the edema. Furthermore passive ROM will assist in the prevention of edema by promoting venous return.[22]

Occupational therapy intervention for peripheral nerve injuries

The treatment goals for peripheral nerve injuries are generally similar. The aim is to assist the patient in regaining the maximum level of function. The rate of return and the residual impairments depend largely on the severity of the lesion and the quality of care during the rehabilitation process.

For supracondylar fractures of the humerus the therapist should assist the health team in the prevention and detection of ischemic contractures. If ischemia occurs, acute treatment focuses on the restoration of blood circulation. Immediate surgical intervention may be required or the arm may be elevated in suspension. If surgery is performed, a loose postoperative dressing will be applied, and the arm will be elevated. The therapist may be asked to make a resting splint to maintain the functional position of the hand. The therapist should remove the splint periodically and gently apply passive ROM to the fingers to maintain the length of the intrinsic muscles and the integrity of the joints.

As the patient's muscle tone returns, a mild PRE program can be established. Resistive activities, such as woodworking, ceramics, leather work, and copper tooling, may be used in conjunction with isometric and isotonic exercises. The therapist should not overtax the returning musculature and should protect the weaker muscle groups from stretch and fatigue.

The peripheral nerve injury may create some challenging problems in ADL that the therapist and patient must overcome. If one upper extremity is impaired (flaccid paralysis), the therapist may design a temporary "static sling" to be worn during shower activities or anytime the extremity needs to be securely positioned so that the person can move about. Static slings have some disadvantages. They should not be worn for long periods because they hold the arm in a flexed position, interfere with the postural support of the arm during some activities, limit proprioceptive feedback, and change the body image. Some therapists are fabricating "dynamic slings." Elastic straps are used instead of webbing straps, and a cone is secured in the patient's hand to maintain a functional position. Tourniquet hosing has also been used in place of a rigid shoulder strap to allow some mobility of the joints, yet allow enough support to keep the arm flexed and close to the trunk. This elasticity allows better circulation to the extremity and better tactile, proprioceptive, and kinesthetic stimulation.

Assistive devices, such as long-handle reaching aids and one-handed kitchen tools used in the treatment of hemiplegia, have also been found to be beneficial.

SAMPLE TREATMENT PLAN

Case study

John is a 23-year-old man employed as a construction worker. He is a high school graduate, married, and has two children. Recently while working he sustained a deep laceration of the right anterior forearm. This injury resulted in a severed ulnar nerve and partial damage to the median nerve. The patient has undergone microsurgery and the severed nerves have been repaired with moderate success.

John is an energetic young man who has difficulty adjusting to the hospital environment and to a sedentary existence.

He was referred to occupational therapy for services during the acute and rehabilitation phases of his treatment program. The goals are to prevent deformity, restore joint and muscle function to maximum level possible, facilitate adjustment to hospital and disability, and evaluate potential for return to former employment.

Treatment plan

A. **Statistical data.**
1. Name: John
   Age: 23
   Diagnosis: Laceration to right forearm, peripheral nerve injury
   Disability: Ulnar and median nerve dysfunction; moderate to severe motor paralysis
2. Treatment aims as stated in referral:
   To prevent deformity
   To restore joint and muscle function to maximum level possible
   To facilitate adjustment to hospital and disability
   To evaluate potential for return to employment

B. **Other services.**
   Medical-surgical: Surgery, medication, supervision of rehabilitation program
   Nursing: Nursing care during acute phase of treatment, psychological support
   Physical therapy: ROM, muscle reeducation, edema control
   Social service: Financial arrangements, counseling to client and family
   Vocational rehabilitation counselor: Explore vocational potential, vocational counseling

C. **OT evaluation.**
   Sensation: Test (light touch, stereognosis, proprioception, 2 PD, pain)
   Nerve regeneration: Wrinkle test
   Muscle strength: Manual muscle test
   ROM: Measure
   Grip and pinch strength: Test with instruments
   Hand evaluation: Observation, Jebsen-Taylor Test of Hand Function; tests of speed and dexterity
   ADL: Observe performance
   Psychosocial adjustment: Observe
   Muscle function: EMG biofeedback evaluation to obtain quantitative information for baseline function.

D. **Results of evaluation.**
1. Evaluation.
   a. Physical resources.
      (1) Muscle strength
          Wrist flexors: P
          Finger adductors: P
          Finger abductors: P
          Opposition of thumb: P
          Marked muscle atrophy of web spaces (interossei)
          Moderate atrophy of thenar muscles
          Ape hand deformity
          Grasp strength: Right 10 lbs pressure, Left 130 lbs
          Palmar pinch strength: Right 4 lbs pressure, Left 24 lbs
          Hand function and fine dexterity: Below standard norms for age in gross grasp and fine prehension and movement speed
      (2) ROM: Within normal limits for wrist, thumb and finger joints; some tightness in long finger flexors when fingers are extended actively
   b. Sensory-perceptual functions.
      (1) Light touch, proprioception, and 2 PD: Absent in medial half of right hand; impaired in lateral aspect of right hand, especially thenar region
      (2) Stereognosis: Impaired

Continued.

SAMPLE TREATMENT PLAN—cont'd

D. **Results of evaluation**—cont'd.
  (3) Superficial pain sensitivity (pinprick):
    (a) Intact: Median cutaneous region
    (b) Absent: Ulnar nerve root distribution
  (4) Nerve regeneration: Absence of wrinkling along cutaneous sensory distribution of ulnar nerve; mild wrinkling along median nerve root distribution; photograph of results recorded for visual documentation
  c. Cognitive functions. Client's cognitive functions are considered normal for a 23-year-old man of average intelligence. During evaluation and early treatment he has demonstrated normal memory, good judgment, and problem-solving skills. He attends to the task at hand and shows ability to concentrate for long periods. Motivation for recovery and return to former life roles is very high.
  d. Psychosocial functions. John is married and has two children. The marriage is stable, and his wife is supportive. John has a high level of energy and is accustomed to being very active and moving about freely. The sedentary existence imposed by hospitalization has resulted in mild agitation, impatience, and mild depression. John's leisure interests were playing baseball and racquetball and racing sports cars. At home he enjoyed improving his home by painting, decorating, and light construction. John and his wife had many friends and engaged in social activities on weekends. Since John was injured on the job, his financial support and medical expenses are covered by workmen's compensation and disability insurance.

  e. Prevocational potential. If there is good to normal return of neuromuscular function, client is expected to resume his former occupation.
  If there is residual weakness that precludes employment as a construction worker, prevocational assessment will be undertaken to determine alternatives.
  f. Functional skills. John is independent in most self-care activities. He has adapted easily to performing essential self-maintenance skills with one hand. He demonstrated some difficulty with cutting meat, managing soap in the shower, buttoning small buttons, and carrying large heavy objects such as a carton or tray. Assistive devices were recommended to increase independence.
  Client is able to drive a standard car with power steering and automatic transmission.
2. Problem identification.
  a. Muscle weakness, resulting in loss of normal function of right hand
  b. Sensory loss
  c. Loss of vocational role
  d. Difficulty adjusting to inactivity
  e. Changed leisure roles
  f. Changes in body image
3. Assets.
  Intelligence
  Family support
  Financial support
  Good prognosis
  Good potential for reemployment
  Motivation
  Age
  Vocational skills

E Specific OT objectives	F Methods used to meet objectives	G Gradation of treatment
Acute phase of treatment		
Given a hand splint deformity will be prevented and muscles will be maintained at normal length	Static resting splint in functional position to be worn at night and periods of inactivity	Decrease amount of use as hand function increases
Through positioning and passive ROM exercises edema in the hand will be prevented or will remain minimal	Overhead sling attached to headboard of bed, which supports forearm and hand in elevated position; allow some movement to increase blood circulation; gentle passive ROM exercises to thumb, fingers and wrist after sufficient healing of nerve has occurred to allow some traction on the nerve; teach client ROM exercises and proper positioning of hand[17]	Decrease then eliminate use of overhead sling when active rehabilitation program commences

SAMPLE TREATMENT PLAN—cont'd

E Specific OT objectives	F Methods used to meet objectives	G Gradation of treatment
Acute phase of treatment—cont'd		
Through appropriate activities client will be more relaxed and less depressed, resulting in tolerance for hospital routines and social interactions	Isometric exercises for shoulder and elbow muscle groups; isometric resistive exercises for unaffected extremities; supportive approach to client, positive reinforcement for participation in activities: puzzles, games (cards, checkers, chess, dominoes, Atari television sports games), reading (sports magazines)	Decrease extrinsic motivation and initiation of activities; increase number of persons participating with client; elicit ideas on improving physical arrangement of clinic; draw up plans and material list
Given assistive devices client will perform personal hygiene and eating activities independently	One-handed rocker knife, rubber placemat for stability of plate, plate guard, suction soap holder to fix soap to wall, wash mitt, built-up handle on razor for shaving	Decrease use of assistive devices as right hand function increases
Rehabilitation phase of treatment—6 weeks after surgery		
Through therapeutic exercise full ROM of all joints of hand and wrist will be preserved	Passive ROM exercise to each joint motion 5 to 10 repetitions twice daily; active ROM of each joint motion	Decrease passive exercise; increase active exercise as strength improves
Through exercise and activity to affected wrist and hand muscles strength of affected muscles will increase from poor to good	Active exercise to wrist flexors, thumb flexors, finger abductors and adductors; thumb abduction; opposition; construction of small jewelry box with mosaic tile top; ceramics—pinch pot or coil project; therapeutic putty exercises	Increase resistance as F+ muscle grades are attained; commence PRE program
Given adequate recovery of muscle strength and hand function feasibility for return to same or related job will be explored	Construction of a large wood chest or book shelf; client is to plan and perform all operations; activities should be performed standing; purposes are to evaluate handling and use of hand tools, safety awareness, standing tolerance, and physical endurance; engage client in construction of closet or shelves for health care facility under direction of maintenance supervisor, as a job trial; aspects of the actual construction duties can be simulated in the clinic; weighted objects similar to construction materials will be lifted, carried, and manipulated and will be graded according to gained strength and endurance	Increase weight of loads and requirements for bending, lifting, and carrying large objects

Continued.

SAMPLE TREATMENT PLAN—cont'd

H. Special equipment.
  1. Ambulation aids.
     None required
  2. Splints.
     Static resting splint in functional position to be worn at night and during periods of inactivity in acute phase of treatment
  3. Assistive devices.
     One-handed rocker knife for meat cutting
     Rubber placemat to prevent plate slipping

Plate guard to prevent food spills
Suction soap holder to stabilize soap in shower
Wash mitt to eliminate need to manipulate washcloth and soap
Built-up handle on razor to accommodate weak grasp
Elastic material for sling to wear while taking a shower, to support hand in elevated position while bending and reaching

---

REVIEW QUESTIONS

1. Describe the components of the lower motor neuron system.
2. Describe the pathology and major clinical findings of poliomyelitis.
3. Compare and contrast poliomyelitis with Guillain-Barré syndrome.
4. List some treatment strategies for Guillain-Barré syndrome.
5. List at least six clinical manifestations of peripheral nerve injury.
6. Describe the sequential signs of recovery following peripheral nerve injury.
7. Describe some evaluations to determine sensory loss.
8. Identify the classic deformities associated with the radial, ulnar, and median nerves.
9. Describe some treatment strategies for peripheral nerve injuries.
10. List some contraindications when treating peripheral nerve injuries.

REFERENCES

1. Barr, M.L.: The human nervous system, ed. 2, New York, 1974, Harper & Row, Publishers, Inc.
2. Bateman, J.: Trauma to nerves in limbs, Philadelphia, 1962, W.B. Saunders Co.
3. Bradshear, R.H.: Shand's handbook of orthopedic surgery, ed. 9, St. Louis, 1978, The C.V. Mosby Co.
4. Chusid, J.G.: Correlative neuroanatomy and function neurology, ed. 16, Los Altos, Calif., 1976, Lange Medical Publications.
5. Clark, R.G.: Clinical neuroanatomy and neurophysiology, ed. 5, Philadelphia, 1975, F.A. Davis Co.
6. Drupp, M.A., and Chatton, M.J.: Current medical diagnosis and treatment, ed. 16, Los Altos, Calif., 1977, Lange Medical Publications.
7. Farber, S.: Sensorimotor evaluation and treatment procedure for allied health personnel, ed. 2, Indianapolis, 1974, The Indiana University Foundation, Purdue University at Indianapolis Medical Center.
8. Gardner, E.: Fundamentals of neurology, ed. 6, Philadelphia, 1975, W.B. Saunders Co.
9. Hopkins, H.L., and Smith, H.D.: Willard and Spackman's occupational therapy, ed. 5, Philadelphia, 1978, J.B. Lippincott Co.
10. International Poliomyelitis Conference: Papers and discussion on poliomyelitis, Philadelphia, 1955, J.B. Lippincott Co.
11. Larson, C.B., and Gould, M.: Orthopedic nursing, ed. 9, St. Louis, 1978, The C.V. Mosby Co.
12. Laurence, T.N., and Pugel, A.V.: Peripheral nerve involvement in spinal cord injury: an electromyographic study, Arch. Phys. Med. Rehab. 59:309-313, 1978.
13. Morrison, D., Pathier, P., and Horr, K.: Sensory motor dysfunction and therapy in infancy and early childhood, Springfield, Ill., 1978, Charles C Thomas, Publisher.
14. Nichols, H.F.: Manual of hand injuries, Chicago, 1955, Year Book Medical Publishers, Inc.
15. Noback, C.R., and Demarest, R.J.: The nervous system introduction and review, ed. 2, New York, 1977, McGraw-Hill, Inc.
16. Phelps, P.E., and Walker, C.: Comparison of the finger wrinkling test results to establish sensory tests in peripheral nerve injury, Am. J. Occup. Ther. 31:565-572, 1977.
17. Rathenberg, E.: Dynamic living for the long-term patient, Dubuque, Iowa, 1962, Wm. C Brown, Co., Publishers.
18. Robinault, I.: Functional aids for the multiply handicapped, New York, 1973, Harper & Row, Publishers, Inc.
19. Schmidt, R.F.: Fundamentals of neurophysiology, ed. 2, New York, 1978, Springer-Verlag New York, Inc.
20. Schumacher, B., and Allen, H.A.: Medical aspects of disabilities, Chicago, 1976, Rehabilitation Institute.
21. Trombly, C.A., and Scott, A.D.: Occupational therapy for physical dysfunction, Baltimore, 1977, The Williams & Wilkins Co.
22. Vasudevan, S., and Melvin, J.L.: Upper extremity edema control: rationale of the techniques, Am. J. Occup. Ther. 33:520-524, 1979.
23. Walter, J.B.: An introduction to the principles of disease, Philadelphia, 1977, W.B. Saunders Co.

Chapter 12

Spinal cord injury

Spinal cord injuries are caused by trauma from automobile accidents, gunshot and stab wounds, falls, sports, and diving accidents. The most common cause is the automobile accident that results in forced flexion and hyperextension of the neck or trunk, causing fracture and dislocation of the vertebrae.[19] Spinal cord functions may also be disturbed by diseases such as tumors, myelomeningocele, syringomyelia, multiple sclerosis, and amyotrophic lateral sclerosis. Some of the treatment principles outlined in this chapter may have application to these conditions. However, the emphasis will be on rehabilitation of the individual with traumatic injury.

RESULTS OF SPINAL CORD INJURY

Spinal cord injury results in quadriplegia or paraplegia. Quadriplegia is the paralysis of the four limbs and trunk musculature. There may be partial UE function, depending on the level of the cervical lesion. Paraplegia is paralysis of the lower extremities and possibly of some trunk musculature, depending on the level of the lesion.

Spinal cord injuries are referred to in terms of the regions (cervical, thoracic, and lumbar) of the spinal cord in which they occur and the numerical order of the neurological segments. The level of spinal cord injury designates the last fully functioning neurological segment of the cord, for example, C6 refers to the sixth neurological segment of the cervical region of the spinal cord as the last fully functioning neurological segment. Thus in this instance all muscles innervated by segments below the C6 neurological level will be paralyzed.

Complete lesions result in total dysfunction of the spinal cord below the level of the injury. Incomplete lesions may involve several neurological segments, and some spinal cord function may be partially or completely intact, which allows for some function below the level of the injury.

A lower motor neuron lesion that results in flaccid paralysis is present in muscles innervated at the level of the lesion. An upper motor neuron lesion that results in spastic paralysis is present below the level of the lesion. The reason for this is the destruction of the anterior horn cells and reflex arc at the level of the lesion, although these remain intact but are divorced from higher centers of control below the level of the lesion. Therefore the person who has quadriplegia usually has predominantly flaccid paralysis of the upper extremities and spastic paralysis of the lower extremities.[23]

After spinal cord injury the victim enters a stage of spinal shock that may last as long as 3 months but usually lasts less than 24 hours. This spinal shock phase is a period of areflexia, or the cessation of all reflex activity below the level of the injury.[14] During this phase there is loss of all sensation and voluntary motor function below the level of the injury, which results in complete flaccid paralysis. Bladder, bowel, and sexual functions are no longer under voluntary control. The bladder and bowel are atonic or flaccid. Deep tendon reflexes are decreased, and sympathetic functions are disturbed. This disturbance results in decreased constriction of blood vessels, low blood pressure, slower heart rate, and absence of perspiration.[8,24]

As spinal shock declines, the after shock phase commences and reflexes return to a hyperactive state. There is continued loss of motor function, but muscles that are innervated by the neurological segments below the level of injury usually develop spasticity. Deep tendon reflexes become hyperactive, and clonus may be evident. Sensory loss continues, and the bladder and bowel usually become spastic in patients whose injuries are above T12. The bladder and bowel usually remain flaccid or atonic in lesions at L1 and below. Sympathetic functions become hyperactive. Spinal reflex activity (mass muscle spasms) become evident in the limbs. Reflex erections may develop in patients with thoracic and cervical injuries but usually do not occur in clients with lumbar and sacral injuries since the essential reflex arc is usually interrupted in these individuals.

Prognosis for recovery

Prognosis for significant functional recovery after spinal cord injury is generally poor. In complete lesions if there is no sensation or return of motor function below the level of lesion 48 hours after the injury occurs, then no motor function return is expected. Return of function to one spinal nerve root level below the fracture is the usual gain and occurs in the first 6 months after injury.

In incomplete lesions progressive return of motor function is possible.[8,24] Perianal sensation, toe flexion, and sphincter control are evidence of an incomplete lesion where there is some neural transmission across the site of injury. With incomplete lesions prognosis is uncertain. When improvement begins immediately and return of muscle function appears consistently, prognosis for recovery is better than if return of motor function occurs sporadically and inconsistently several months after the injury occurred.[14,24]

MEDICAL-SURGICAL MANAGEMENT OF THE PERSON WITH SPINAL CORD INJURY

After a traumatic event in which spinal cord injury is a possibility, the conscious victim should be carefully questioned about cutaneous numbness and skeletal muscle paralysis before being moved, if possible. Careful palpation of the spinal axis should also take place before moving the victim. The victim should be moved from the accident site with extreme caution. Flexion of the spine must be prevented during the transfer procedures. A firm stretcher or board to which the victim's head and back can be strapped should be procured before moving him. After transferring the victim to the stretcher or board, while maintaining axial traction on the neck and preventing any flexion of the spine and neck, the victim is strapped to the board or stretcher and transferred carefully, avoiding bumping, to the hospital emergency room.

Careful examination, stabilization, and transportation of the person with spinal injury may prevent a temporary or slight spinal cord injury from becoming permanent or more severe.

Initial care in the hospital is directed toward preventing further damage to the spinal cord and reversing neurological damage if possible by stabilization or decompression of the injured neurological structures.[10,14] A careful neurological examination is carried out to aid in determining site and type of injury. This is done with the patient in a supine position with the neck and spine immobilized. A catheter is placed in the patient's bladder for drainage of urine. Anteroposterior and lateral x-ray films may be taken, with the patient's head or spine immobilized, to obtain a rough idea of the type of injury. A myelogram may be required for further evaluation.

In early medical treatment the goals are to restore normal alignment of the spine, maintain stabilization of the injured area, and decompress neurological structures that are under pressure. Spinal realignment and stabilization can be achieved through rest on a well-padded frame or a hospital bed with a fracture board and positioning pillows and rolls, in some cases. In more severe fractures traction is applied to the spine while the patient rests in bed or on a Stryker frame. In recent years the halo and halo brace have been widely used with success for cervical spine injuries that require skeletal traction and immobilization. If on a bed or frame the patient's position must be changed every 2 hours to prevent pressure sores.

Open surgical reduction with plating, wiring, and spinal fusion or laminectomy is sometimes carried out. The goals of surgery are to decompress the spinal cord and achieve spinal stability and normal bony alignment. The laminectomy has been performed much less frequently in recent years and only under special circumstances, as outlined by Pierce and Nickel.[14]

Complications and concomitant problems

Pressure sores or decubitus ulcers. Sensory loss enhances the development of pressure sores. The patient cannot feel the pressure of prolonged sitting or lying in one position or pressure from splints or braces. Pressure causes loss of blood supply to the area, which can ultimately result in necrosis. The areas most likely to develop pressure sores are bony prominences over the sacrum, ischium, trochanters, elbows, and heels. It is important for rehabilitation personnel to be aware of the signs of developing pressure sores. At first the area reddens and blanches when pressed. Later the reddened area becomes blue or black and does not blanch when pressed. This indicates that necrosis has begun. Finally a blister or ulceration appears in the area and it may become infected. If allowed to progress these sores may become very severe, and bony prominences may become uncovered and may eventually be destroyed.

Pressure sores can be prevented by relieving and eliminating pressure points and protecting vulnerable areas. Turning in bed, special mattresses, foam "booties" to protect the heels, and shifting weight when sitting are some of the methods used to prevent pressure sores.

The use of hand splints and other appliances can also cause pressure sores. The therapist must inspect the skin, and the patient must be taught to inspect the skin, using a mirror, to watch for signs of developing pressure sores. Reddened areas can develop within 30 minutes, so frequent shifting, repositioning, and vigilance are essential if pressure sores are to be prevented.[14,24]

Decreased vital capacity. Decreased vital capacity will be a problem in persons who have sustained cervical and high thoracic lesions. Such individuals will have markedly limited chest expansion and decreased ability to cough. This can result in proneness to respiratory tract infections. The reduced vital capacity will affect energy, tolerance level for activity, and dressing potential. This problem may be alleviated by methods of assisted breathing and by teaching the client glossopharyngeal, or "frog," breathing. Strengthening of the sternocleidomastoids and the diaphragm and deep breathing exercises are helpful. Manually assisted coughing and mechanical suctioning of chest secretions may be required if there are excess secretions or respiratory tract infection. These measures are usually carried out by physical therapy, respiratory therapy, and nursing services.[14,24]

Osteoporosis of disuse. Because of disuse of long bones, particularly of the lower extremities, osteoporosis is likely to develop in patients with spinal cord injuries. A year after the injury the osteoporosis may be sufficiently advanced for pathological fractures to occur. Pathological fractures usually occur in the supracondylar area of the femur, proximal tibia, distal tibia, intertrochanteric area of the femur, and neck of the femur. Pathological fractures are not seen in the upper extremities. Daily standing helps to prevent or delay the osteoporosis that underlies these fractures by placing the weight load on the long bones of the lower extremities.[14,24]

Postural hypotension. Postural hypotension results in fainting or blackouts. It is due to the pooling of blood in the abdominal and LE vasculature from lack of movement and poor venous return of blood to the heart. It occurs when the patient is brought to the upright position following a period of bed rest. It is a normal reaction and should be dealt with immediately in a matter-of-fact manner by locking the wheelchair brakes and tilting the chair back to elevate the feet above the level of the heart. If the patient is on a tilt table, it should be returned to the horizontal position. Abdominal binders, corsets, and leg wraps may relieve or eliminate this problem by giving support to paralyzed abdominal muscles and can aid in breathing as well.[24]

Autonomic dysreflexia. Autonomic dysreflexia is a phenomenon seen in persons whose injuries are above the T4 to T6 levels. It is due to reflex action of the autonomic nervous system in response to some stimuli, such as a distended bladder, fecal mass, bladder irrigation or rectal manipulation, thermal and pain stimuli, and visceral distention. The symptoms are perspiration, especially of the forehead; goose bumps; nasal congestion and obstruction; paroxysmal hypertension; pounding headache; and fast, then, slow pulse.

Autonomic dysreflexia is treated by placing the patient in an upright position to reduce blood pressure. The bladder should be drained by unclamping the catheter or tapping over the bladder if there is an automatic bladder. The patient should be returned to the nursing station at once, and the physician should be alerted for the administration of appropriate prophylactic measures and medication. The patient should not be left alone. Any person with a spinal cord injury who complains of headache should have a blood pressure reading to determine if there is autonomic dysreflexia.[1,14,24]

Spasticity. Spasticity is an increase of stretch reflexes below the level of injury that results from lack of inhibi-

tion from higher centers. Patterns of spasticity change over the first year, gradually increasing in the first 6 months and reaching a plateau about 1 year after the injury. A moderate amount of spasticity can be helpful in the overall rehabilitation of the patient with a spinal cord injury. It helps to maintain muscle bulk, assists in joint ROM, and can be used to assist during wheelchair and bed transfers and mobility. During the first year spasticity should be controlled by maintaining joint ROM; icing the skin, followed by stretching contractures; and using relaxant drugs.

Severe spasticity that interferes with function must be treated more aggressively. Surgical procedures that involve cutting or lengthening spastic muscles and peripheral and spinal nerve blocks designed to paralyze the spastic muscles may be used to eliminate problems of severe and disabling spasticity.[14,24]

Heterotopic ossification. Heterotopic ossification is the deposition of osseous material, usually in the muscles around the hip and knee but also at the elbow and shoulder. The first symptoms are heat, pain, swelling, and decreased joint ROM. The ossification may progress to ankylosis of the affected joint. Treatment is the maintenance of joint ROM during the early stage of active bone formation to keep breaking up the depositions of new bone and develop pseudoarthroses in the ossified area.

If the ossification progresses to ankylosis and severely limits function because of joint immobility, surgical intervention may be pursued if necessary criteria and conditions are met.[11]

SEXUAL FUNCTION

At the time of injury there is a complete loss of sexual function for any level of injury. As spinal shock subsides, variable degrees and types of sexual function may be recovered by a significant number of persons with spinal cord injuries. In clients with thoracic and cervical lesions the reflex arc from the penis or glans clitoris to the spinal cord is intact.[7] Therefore reflexogenic erections are possible in approximately 60% to 90% of persons with lesions at these levels.[22] The ability to effect erections often correlates with bladder function. Persons with upper motor neuron or spastic bladders usually have reflexogenic erections without ejaculations, while persons with lower motor neuron or atonic bladders are unable to have erections. This is most likely in lesions below the L1 level. There are exceptions in both instances, however.

Persons with incomplete injuries, especially those who have sacral function, may have psychogenic erections. For these men, ejaculation may accompany the erection and thus they may be capable of siring children.[24]

Reflexogenic erections may be effected by tactile and thermal stimuli or manipulation.[3] In men the quality and duration of the erection is variable and may not always be useful for sexual activity.[14] Spontaneous reflexogenic erections from exteroceptive stimuli may occur when not desired.[3,7] Successful sexual intercourse is usually possible for men who have reflexogenic erections. Alternate modes of sexual activity, described in explicit detail by Mooney, Cole, and Chilgren,[12] can be used by these persons as well as those in whom reflexogenic erections do not occur.

Fertility is disturbed in most men with spinal cord injuries because of urinary tract infections, retrograde ejaculations, testicular atrophy, and temperature changes that affect viability of sperm.[20] In women there is no appreciable decrease in fertility. The menses will not be significantly disturbed or changed after the spinal cord injury and will usually return to normal within a few months after the injury occurred. Normal pregnancy and childbirth are possible, although urological clearance should be obtained before pregnancy is considered. The distention of pregnancy may evoke autonomic dysreflexia, and labor may not be perceived by the pregnant woman. Appropriate precautions are necessary to deal with these possibilities. Birth control counseling is important for those sexually active persons who do not desire pregnancy.[14]

Women who have spinal cord injuries experience essentially the same physical and psychological responses that men who have spinal cord injuries experience. However, women possibly make a better and more rapid psychological adjustment and acceptance of changed sexual function than do men.[7]

Sensation is absent in persons with complete spinal cord transection and may be partial in persons with incomplete lesions. Sexual satisfaction is largely on a psychological level and is derived from pleasure given to the partner, full participation in intimate relationships, intimate communication with a significant partner, and development of a sense of personal worth and significance as a sexual being. These are important reasons for engaging in sexual activity that are above and beyond the sensual pleasures that can be derived. Finally, although not the least important reason for engaging in sexual activity, is the sexual expression of affection and love.[18]

Physically disabled individuals quickly sense the attitudes of professional helpers toward their sexuality. Traditionally professionals have viewed disabled persons as asexual and often communicated a sense that it was not all right to discuss sexual functioning. Professionals tended to put the topic off, whereas their clients waited for them to bring it up, granting permission for this important concern to be aired. Fortunately these tendencies and attitudes are changing, and sexual counseling and education are becoming a regular part of many rehabilitation programs for all types of physical disabilities.

Because occupational therapists are concerned with the functional aspects of their clients' lives, they are in an excellent role to provide information and counseling on sexual functioning. Staff education and attitude assessment are critical preliminaries to initiating sexual counseling and education.[13]

Some clients lack basic sex education. Others feel asexual because of their disabilities and are isolated from peers; thus they may fear any type of sexual interaction. Therefore sexual counseling must be geared to the needs of the individual client. In some instances social interaction skills will need improvement before sexual activity can be considered. Occupational therapy can play an important part in improving social skills.

It is important for the professional worker to introduce the topic and give an opening for the discussion. The disabled person and the partner should be counseled together if possible. A sense of trust must develop between the client and the counselor. It is important to use terminology that the client is accustomed to and comfortable with when discussing sexual matters and to maintain confidentiality. When counseling is introduced, safe or relatively superficial topics can be discussed first and then, as trust and comfort develop, deeper and more intimate and sensitive topics can be broached.

Sexual counseling and education may be carried out in a variety of ways. One-to-one counseling with audiovisual aids and literature is useful. Group discussions with partners present as well as experienced disabled persons may be a useful method. Neistadt and Baker[13] describe a sexual counseling program using counseling by the occupational therapist and literature. Clients opted for one or both methods, depending on individual interests and needs.

Finally clients need a time and place and permission to explore and experiment with the sexual options open to them. Home visits on weekend passes are an appropriate means to this end.

OCCUPATIONAL THERAPY FOR SPINAL CORD INJURY

The general treatment program is directed primarily to the quadriplegic client with a C5-6 level of injury because this is the most common level of injury. It may be modified for higher or lower levels of injury, using the information in Table 6 as a guide.

The long-range goals in the rehabilitation of the person with a spinal cord injury are (1) to achieve the maximum level of self-care independence possible; (2) accept the disability; and (3) resume meaningful family, social, community, vocational, and leisure roles.[19] Occupational

Table 6. Functional potential in spinal cord injury[15]

Level*	Muscles innervated	Movements possible	Pattern of weakness	Functional capabilities and limitations
C1-3 (10, 18)†	Sternocleido-mastoids Trapezius (upper) Levator scapulae	Neck control	Total paralysis of arms, trunk, lower extremities Dependence on respirator	Total ADL dependence Can drive electric wheelchair equipped with portable respirator with chin or breath controls
C3-4 (4, 5, 10, 11)	‡Trapezius (superior, middle and inferior)	Neck movements, scapula elevation	Paralysis of trunk and lower extremities	Confined to wheelchair and essentially dependent Only head-neck and some scapula movement
	‡Diaphragm (C3-5)	Inspiration	Difficulty in breathing and coughing	Respiratory assistance may be required assistance with skin inspection (patient cannot position mirrors but should inspect himself) Some activities can be accomplished through use of head wand or mouth stick (for example, typing, page turning, and manipulation of checkers, chess, and cards) Can operate electric wheelchair with mouth, chin, or breath controls Rancho electric arm can be operated by tongue microswitches to allow limited self-feeding with swivel utensils and other activities mentioned above
C5 (4, 5, 9, 11, 14, 21)	All muscles of shoulder at least partially innervated except latissimus dorsi and coracobrachialis	Shoulder extension and horizontal abduction (weak)	Weakness of shoulder movements, elbow flexion, and supination Absence of elbow extension, pronation and all wrist and hand movements	Confined to wheelchair and still essentially dependent Unable to roll over or come to sitting position independently and has no independent hand functions Need assistance of a swivel bar transfer
	‡Partial deltoids	Shoulder flexion (weak) Shoulder abduction to 90°	Total paralysis of trunk and lower extremities	
	‡Biceps brachii Brachialis Brachioradialis	Elbow flexion and supination		
	Levator scapula, diaphragm, and scaleni now fully innervated		Endurance low because of paralysis of intercostals and low respiratory reserve	
	Rhomboid (major and minor)	Scapular adduction and downward rotation (weak)		Require electric powered wheelchair with adapted arm controls
	Serratus anterior (C5-7)	Scapular abduction and upward rotation (weak)		Cannot apply own hand splints, but with standard MAS or elevating proximal arm with outside powered hand splint some functional activities are possible, such as feeding, light hygiene, applying makeup, and shaving; handwriting (sufficient for legal signature); telephoning (push-button telephone); and typing (five WPM), if set up and placed on a lapboard by an attendant

*Each level includes the muscles and functions of the preceding levels.
†The numbers in parentheses are references.
‡Key muscles.

Continued.

Table 6. Functional potential in spinal cord injury—cont'd

Level	Muscles innervated	Movements possible	Pattern of weakness	Functional capabilities and limitations
C5— cont'd	Teres major (C5, 6) Subscapularis (C5, 6)	Shoulder internal rotation (weak)		
	Pectoralis major (C5-8, T1)	Shoulder horizontal adduction (weak)		
	Infraspinatus Supraspinatus Teres minor (C5, 6)	Shoulder external rotation		
C6 (2, 5, 9, 11, 21)	All partially innervated C5 muscles now fully innervated except serratus and pectoralis major	Full (or nearly full) strength to shoulder flexion and extension, abduction and adduction, internal and external rotation, and elbow flexion	Functions of shoulder prime movers still not fully developed Absence of elbow extension Weakness of wrist extension (absence on ulnar side)	Still confined to wheelchair and essentially dependent, although he may be able to perform many activities on his own with equipment. Flexor hinge splint or universal cuff aid in self-feeding with regular utensils; personal hygiene and grooming (oral and upper body); UE dressing; handwriting; typing (15-20 WPM); telephoning; light kitchen activities; possibly driving, with equipment Roll from side to side in bed with aid of bed rails and assist in rolling over
	Supinator	Complete innervation for forearm supination	Absence of wrist flexion usually (may be present on radial side) Absence of hand functions	Sit up independently in bed by using elbow flexors to pull on rope looped about forearms and attached to foot of bed or trapeze bar
	Partial but significant innervation to serratus anterior (C5-7)	Scapular abduction and upward rotation	Total paralysis of trunk and lower extremities	
	Latissimus dorsi (C6-8)	Shoulder extension and internal rotation)	Endurance low because of reduced respiratory reserve	
	‡Pectoralis major (C5-8, T1)	Shoulder horizontal adduction and internal rotation)		
	Coracobrachialis (C6, 7)	Shoulder flexion		
	Pronator teres (C6, 7)	Forearm pronation		
	Flexor carpi radialis (C6, 7 sometimes)	Radial wrist flexion		Assist in transfers by substituting shoulder adduction and rotation for elbow extension and may be independent with aid of transfer board
	‡Extensor carpi radialis longus and brevis (C6, 7)	Radial wrist extension		Propel standard wheelchair with adapted rims (projections or friction tape) Relieve pressure independently when sitting Drive with adaptations Independent skin inspection May manage bladder and bowel care Employment possible

Table 6. Functional potential in spinal cord injury—cont'd

Level	Muscles innervated	Movements possible	Pattern of weakness	Functional capabilities and limitations
C7-8 (4, 5, 10, 11, 14, 19)	Shoulder prime movers now fully innervated, as well as the rest of the partially innervated C6 muscles	Full strength of all shoulder movements, radial wrist flexors and extensors, and strong pronation	Full strength of shoulder muscles but lack of trunk fixation for the origins of the shoulder prime movers	Essentially confined to wheelchair, but many attain complete wheelchair independence Can come to sitting position in bed Can perform transfers to and from bed and wheelchair independently or with minimal assistance
	‡Triceps brachii Extensor carpi ulnaris (C6-8)	Elbow extension Ulnar wrist extension		
	‡Flexor carpi radialis	Radial wrist flexion	Weakness of pronation and ulnar wrist flexion	Can roll over, sit up, and move about in sitting position
	‡Flexor digitorum superficialis and profundus (C7-8, T1)	PIP and DIP extension	Limited grasp, release, and dexterity because of incomplete innervation of hand intrinsics	Can dress independently and perform personal hygiene activities except changing catheter Self-feeding (usually with no assistive devices) Wrist-driven flexor hinge splint may still be helpful for some patients because of weakness of grasp
	‡Extensor digitorum communis (C6-8)	MP extension		
	Extensor pollicis longus and brevis	Thumb extension (MP and IP)	Total paralysis of lower extremities Weakness of trunk control	
	Abductor pollicis longus	Thumb abduction	Limited endurance because of reduced respiratory reserve	Can propel standard wheelchair (may need friction tape on handrims for long distances; may need assistance on rough ground) Drive with adaptations Nonfunctional ambulation may be possible for standing and short distances, but not practicable as a mode of mobility Independent bladder and bowel care and skin inspection Employment at home or outside home possible Light housework possible but best in assistant or supervisory role
C8-T1 (2, 4, 5, 9, 21)	All muscles of upper extremities now fully innervated			
	Pronator quadratus	Forearm pronation	Paralysis of lower extremities	Independent in bed activities, wheelchair transfers, and self-care and personal hygiene
	Flexor carpi ulnaris	Ulnar wrist flexion	Weakness of trunk control	Can manage standard wheelchair up and down curb
	‡Lumbricales and ‡interossei dorsales and palmares	MP flexion	Endurance reduced because of low respiratory reserve	Can move from wheelchair to floor and return Nonfunctional ambulation for standing or exercise may be possible but still not a practicable mode of mobility
	‡Interossei dorsales and abductor digiti minimi	Finger abduction		Independent bladder and bowel care and skin inspection Homebound work or work in a wheelchair-accessible environment possible

Continued.

Table 6. Functional potential in spinal cord injury—cont'd

Level	Muscles innervated	Movements possible	Pattern of weakness	Functional capabilities and limitations
C8-T1 — cont'd	‡Interossei palmares Flexor pollicis longus and brevis Adductor pollicis ‡Opponens digiti minimi ‡Opponens pollicis	Finger adduction Thumb flexion (MP and IP) Thumb adduction Opposition of fifth finger Thumb opposition		Light housekeeping can be done independently Drive with adaptations
T4-T6 (2, 21)	All muscles of upper extremities plus partial innervation of intercostal muscles and long muscles of the back (sacrospinalis and semispinalis)	All arm functions Partial trunk stability Endurance increased because of better respiration	Partial trunk paralysis and total paralysis of lower extremities	Self-care independence Independence in standard wheelchair May stand with braces and crutches and ambulate for short distances but not practical for mobility Can work at sedentary occupations and do some heavy lifting from sitting position Driving Wheelchair sports possible Independent in light housekeeping
T7-L2 (2, 21)	Intercostal muscles fully innervated Abdominal muscles partially to fully innervated (rectus abdominis, internal and external obliques)	Partial to good trunk stability Increased physical endurance	Paralysis of lower extremities	Independence in self-care, personal hygiene, sports, work, and housekeeping activities possible in well-designed environment Ambulates with difficulty using braces and crutches, but wheelchair is ambulation of choice for speed and energy conservation

therapy can make a significant contribution in assisting the client to move toward the achievement of these goals.

Evaluation

The client's muscle strength should be evaluated using the manual muscle test. This evaluation will help to determine areas of strength and weakness; establish a baseline for progress; determine need for special equipment, such as splints, MASs, and assistive devices; and determine the level of injury. The client's muscle strength is a critical factor in determining functional potential.

During the bed phase, when the client is still in traction or is wearing a cervical collar, resistance should not be applied to shoulder musculature. The client should not move the shoulders actively any further than he thinks he can. No rotary or flexion and extension movements of the spine are permitted until medical clearance is obtained.[21] During this phase of rehabilitation muscle strength testing may be limited to hands and forearms, and gross rather than specific manual muscle testing may be used to estimate strength while not jeopardizing stability of the spine. The occupational therapist should obtain the physician's approval before proceeding with a complete UE manual muscle test during the early phases of rehabilitation.[23] The muscle test should be repeated monthly during the early stages of rehabilitation for up to 6 or 8 months after the injury occurred.

Passive ROM should be measured with the same precautions for shoulder motions just described in the early stages. This evaluation is to determine potential or pres-

Table 6. Functional potential in spinal cord injury—cont'd

Level	Muscles innervated	Movements possible	Pattern of weakness	Functional capabilities and limitations
L3-L4 (2, 21)	Low back muscles Hip flexors, adductors, quadriceps	Trunk control and stability Hip flexion Hip adduction Knee extension	Partial paralysis of lower extremities; hip extension, knee flexion, and ankle and foot movements	Independent in all activities outlined above Can ambulate with short leg braces, using crutches or canes May still use a wheelchair for convenience and energy conservation
L5-S3 (2, 4)	Hip extensors— gluteus maximus and hamstrings Hip abductors— gluteus medius and gluteus minimus Knee flexors— hamstrings, sartorius, and gracilis Ankle muscles— tibialis anterior, gastrocnemius, soleus, and peroneus longus Foot muscles	Partial to full control of lower extremities	Partial paralysis of lower extremities, most notable in distal segment	Independent in all activities No equipment needed if plantar flexion is sufficiently strong for push off in ambulation

ent contractures that could limit functional potential and suggest the need for preventive or corrective splints and positioning.

Sensation is evaluated for light touch, superficial pain (pinprick), temperature, proprioception, and stereognosis. This aids in denoting areas of lost, impaired, and intact sensation. It may be helpful in establishing the level of injury. It provides information for precautions that must be taken by the therapist and the client and provides a baseline for measuring progress.

Spasticity in UE muscle groups innervated below the level of the lesion is estimated by the degree of resistance to passive movement. This can often be determined during the passive ROM measurements. Spasticity is mild if stretch reflexes and clonus are evoked during passive motion, but the part moves easily through the full ROM. Spasticity is considered moderate if resistance can be felt through the entire ROM, but it is still possible to complete the ROM. Spasticity is considered severe if resistance is felt through the ROM, and it is not possible to complete the full ROM because of strong hypertonicity in the muscles.

Performance of ADL is an important part of the occupational therapy evaluation. The client must have adequate balance and neck stability before complete ADL training can be accomplished. The purpose of the evaluation is to determine present and potential levels of functional ability. The evaluation may begin during the bed phase with light activities such as oral hygiene and feeding. In later stages it may progress to bed mobility, wheelchair mobility, transfers, toileting, bathing, dressing, and then driving.[21] Before driving evaluation is attempted, the client must meet certain criteria. These are the ability to (1) lock the elbow in extension with a substitution pattern if triceps is absent; (2) depress the shoulders; (3) flex, abduct, and externally and internally rotate the shoulders; (4) manage adapted driving equipment; and (5) maintain lateral and forward trunk stability. It is helpful if the client can transfer himself and his wheelchair to and from the car.[24] Specially equipped vans require less function for independent driving.

In addition to these specific assessments the occupational therapist should assess the client's stage of adjustment to the disability and his psychosocial functioning skills. She should obtain the medical, social, educational, and vocational histories of the client. These can be obtained from the medical record and from interviews with paraprofessionals, the client, and his family members and friends.[14] The occupational therapist should communicate with the client initially and continuously during the early phase of the evaluation process regarding needs, interests, aspirations, feelings about the disability and the hospital and its personnel, and frustrations.[19] This is an important time to establish rapport and mutual trust, which will facilitate participation and progress in later and more difficult phases of rehabilitation.

Establishing treatment objectives

It is important to establish treatment objectives in concert with the client and with the rehabilitation team. The primary objectives of the rehabilitation team are often not those of the client. Fuller participation can be expected if the client's priorities are respected to the extent that they are possible and realistic.

The general objectives of treatment for the person with a spinal cord injury are to (1) increase strength of all innervated and partially innervated muscles of the shoulders, elbows, and wrists; (2) maintain or increase joint ROM and prevent deformity; (3) increase physical endurance; (4) train in the use of special equipment, such as the MAS and flexor hinge splint and assistive devices; (5) develop maximum independence in the performance of ADL; (6) explore vocational and avocational potential; and (7) aid in the psychosocial adjustment to physical disability.

Treatment methods

Medical clearance should be obtained before occupational therapy is initiated. During the acute or bed phase of the rehabilitation program the client is still in traction or is wearing a neck stabilization device such as a cervical collar or halo brace to achieve stability of the neck. Precautions against resistive exercises and extremes of ranges of shoulder motions must be in force during this period. Flexion, extension, and rotary movements of the spine and neck are contraindicated. The therapist may provide gentle passive ROM to all UE joints to tolerance and within precautions. Active and active-assisted ROM to all joints within strength, ability, and tolerance levels should also be performed. Muscle reeducation techniques to wrists and elbows should be employed. Resistive exercises to wrists may be carried out. Some gentle resistance to elbows may be given with caution regarding resistance to the shoulders.[21] The client should be encouraged to engage in light self-care activities such as feeding, writing, and light hygiene, if possible, using simple assistive devices such as a wash mitt and universal cuff with a wrist cock-up splint. The occupational therapist can provide splints and overhead slings as needed. She may introduce avocational activities such as

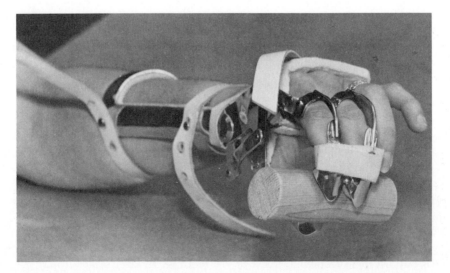

Fig. 12-1. Wrist extension is used to effect prehension through the mechanism of flexor hinge hand splint.

reading or watching television and provide the electric page turner and prism glasses so that these activities may be enjoyed while in a supine position.[19,21]

During the convalescent or wheelchair phase of the rehabilitation program, when the client can sit upright in a wheelchair, has achieved some sitting tolerance, and has stability of the neck and spine, he can participate in a fuller and more active rehabilitation program. PREs and resistive activities such as woodworking can be applied to innervated and partially innervated muscles. Shoulder musculature may be exercised with emphasis on the shoulder depressors, rotators, and adductors needed to perform sliding or loop and trapeze transfers. The biceps needed for transfers and for shifting weight to relieve pressure when in the wheelchair should be strengthened. Wrist extensors need to be exercised to power the flexor hinge splint in clients who have wrist function and will be using the splint to aid prehension (Fig. 12-1).

Active and passive ROM exercises should be continued regularly to prevent undesirable contractures. Stretching may be indicated to correct contractures that are becoming established. In clients who have wrist extension, which will be used to substitute for absent grasp through tenodesis action of the long finger flexors, it is desirable to develop some tightness in these tendons to give some additional tension to the tenodesis grasp. This will allow some clients to discard the splint and use natural tenodesis action for functional grasp. The desirable contracture is developed by ranging finger flexion with the wrist fully extended and finger extension with the wrist fully flexed, thus never allowing the flexors or extensors to be in full stretch over all of the joints that they cross[11,19] (Fig. 12-2).

The ADL program may be expanded to include independent feeding with devices; oral hygiene and upper body bathing; bowel and bladder care, such as suppository insertion and application of the urinary collection device; UE dressing; and transfers using the sliding board. Communication skills in writing and using the telephone, tape recorder, and electric typewriter with devices should be an important part of the treatment program.[19] Training in the use of the MAS, flexor hinge splint, and assistive devices is also part of the occupational therapy program.

The occupational therapist should continue to provide psychological support by allowing and encouraging the client to express frustration, anger, fears, and concerns. The occupational therapy clinic could provide an atmosphere where clients can establish support groups with more advanced clients and rehabilitated individuals who can offer their experiences and problem-solving advice to those in earlier phases of their rehabilitation.

The treatment program should be graded to increase the amount of resistance required in exercise and activity as muscle power improves, increase the amount of time spent in sitting and in activity to improve sitting tolerance and endurance, and increase the number and complexity of ADL while reducing the time it takes to perform them.

There are many assistive devices and pieces of special equipment that can be useful to the person with a spinal cord injury. The universal cuff for holding eating utensils, toothbrushes, pencils, paintbrushes, and typing sticks is a simple and versatile device that offers increased independence. A plate guard, cup holder, extended straw with straw clip, and nonskid table mat can facilitate independent feeding. The wash mitt and soap

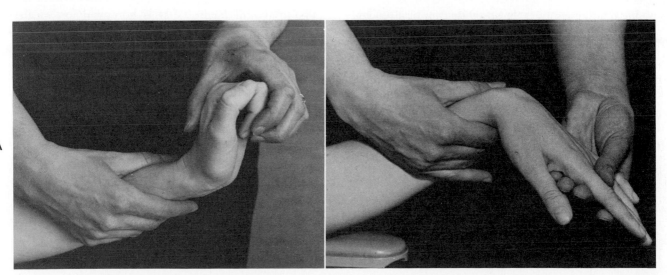

Fig. 12-2. A, Wrist is extended when fingers are passively flexed. **B,** Wrist is flexed when fingers are passively extended.

holder or soap on a rope can make bathing possible. Many persons with quadriplegia can use a buttonhook to fasten clothing. A transfer board is essential for transfers. A wrist cock-up splint to stabilize the wrist during use of the universal cuff can be useful for persons with little or no wrist extension. Clients who have quadriplegia with high cervical injuries may benefit from an externally powered flexor hinge splint or the myoelectric arm. A wheelchair lapboard may be helpful during early wheelchair use for training in feeding while using MASs, reading, and performing communication and avocational activities, such as sketching, painting, or writing. An overhead trapeze may be used by some for transfers to and from bed. A special wheelchair cushion to prevent pressure sores is essential.

During the extended phase of the rehabilitation program driving evaluation and training and home management activities may be introduced and added to the activities just mentioned. Avocational possibilities should be further explored. Activities such as checkers, chess, Scrabble, and mosaic tile work may be used. The MAS or flexor hinge splint may be needed by some to perform these skills. The use of table-based power tools, such as the jigsaw, drill press, printing press, and hand electric sander, may be feasible for many clients if they are adapted with extended handles and positioned properly. Weaving, painting, and sketching are also feasible activities if used with devices or special adaptations.[19]

The client should be introduced to home and community by the occupational and physical therapists before discharge from the treatment facility. The therapists can offer recommendations for major and minor modifications in the home, such as installation of grab bars, bathtub seats, and guardrails around the toilet. The therapists can assist in family education and adjustment by training family members that provide care or attendants in proper techniques of skin care and inspection, use of special equipment, bed mobility, positioning, transfers, dressing, and toileting activities that require supervision or assistance.

Occupational therapy services can offer valuable evaluation and exploration of vocational potential of persons who have quadriplegia. By the sheer magnitude of the physical disability vocational possibilities for these persons are limited. Clients with high intelligence have greater potential for employment than clients with low intelligence.

Many clients with spinal cord injuries must change their vocation or alter former vocational goals. Lack of intelligence, poor motivation, and lack of interest and perseverance on the part of many clients make vocational rehabilitation extremely difficult.

The occupational therapist, during the process of the treatment program and through the use of craft and work sample activities, can help to assess the client's level of motivation, functional intelligence, aptitudes, attitudes, interests, and personal vocational aspirations. The occupational therapist can observe the client's attention span, concentration, manual ability with splints and devices, accuracy, speed, perseverance, work habits, and work tolerance level. This information can be provided to the vocational counselor, who can counsel the client regarding vocational potential and future possibilities, perform specialized vocational testing, and suggest feasible educational and vocational training possibilities.[14]

The occupational therapy service can offer a work adjustment program in which work tolerance level and work habits can be developed while specific job testing and trials are under the direction of the vocational counselor.

For the person with quadriplegia who is of adequate intelligence and motivation, further education is often the solution to the vocational future. Such individuals may perform successfully in occupations such as teaching, engineering, business management, research, psychology, counseling, and sales. Adaptive equipment and a barrier-free environment may be essential to the performance of these jobs.[14]

When suitable vocational objectives have been selected, they may be pursued in an educational setting, at the treatment facility if it is equipped for vocational training, or in a work setting. This phase of rehabilitation is beyond the scope of occupational therapy.

Maximum self-care independence, personal satisfaction through avocational activities, and socialization should be the end goals of the rehabilitation program[16] for those persons who have high-level injuries or those who lack the intelligence for further education or vocational training and essential personal skills and habits for good work adjustment.[14]

SAMPLE TREATMENT PLAN

Case study

John is 17 years old. He is a C7 quadriplegic who sustained the disability in a swimming accident. He was a bright and active high school senior who had planned to go to college within a year. He enjoyed sports, art, and popular music. He was not sure what his career would be, but he was interested in forestry or the technical aspects of radio and television studio operations.

Medical problems related to bladder and bowel control are stabilized, and all precautions are in force to prevent pressure sores. He is able to sit in a wheelchair with support of a body brace and special cushion for periods up to 4 hours per day. Nursing service has reported that the client made little effort to help with daily hygiene and dressing activities.

John has demonstrated a rather flip, carefree attitude toward his problems, which seems to be an effort to cover up a deep anxiety about his physical condition and the future. Occupational therapy was ordered for this patient with aims to increase muscle strength and functional independence and aid with adjustment to disability.

Treatment plan

A. Statistical data.
   1. Name: John
      Age: 17
      Diagnosis: Traumatic injury to cervical area of the spinal cord
      Disability: Quadriplegia, C7 level
   2. Treatment aims as stated in referral:
      Increase muscle strength
      Increase functional independence
      Aid with adjustment to disability
B. Other services.
   Medical: Maintenance of general health, prescription and supervision of rehabilitation program, evaluation of physical status and progress, management of bladder and bowel problems
   Nursing: Administration of medications, bed positioning, supportive care, management of bladder and bowel training
   Social service: Family and client counseling, discharge planning, liaison with community agencies
   Physical therapy: LE ROM exercises, tilt table tolerance, transfer training, UE exercises
   Vocational counselor: Vocational and aptitude evaluation, vocational counseling, arrangements for vocational or educational training
   Psychology-Psychiatry: Facilitation of adjustment to disability, sexual counseling, psychometric evaluation
   Community social groups: Provision of peer group interaction and opportunities for socialization
   Recreation therapy: Provision of recreational and diversional activities, building of physical endurance, socialization, community outings
   Spiritual counselor: Supportive counseling, aid in acceptance of disability
C. OT evaluation.
   Strength: Test
   ROM: Test
   Physical endurance: Observe
   Involuntary movement and spasticity (spasms, clonus): Observe
   Equilibrium and protective mechanisms: Observe
   Coordination-Muscle control: Observe and test
   Sensory-Perceptual: Test
      Touch
      Pain
      Temperature
      Stereognosis
      Proprioception
   Cognitive functions: Observe
      Judgment
      Safety
      Motivation
   Psychosocial skills: Observe
      Maturity
      Interpersonal skills
      Adjustment to disability
      Reality functioning
   Prevocational potential: Observe
      Work habits
      Potential work skills
      Work tolerance level
   Functional skills: Observe and test
      Feeding
      Self-care
      Homemaking
      Community travel (public-private transportation)
D. Results of evaluation.[6]
   1. Evaluation data.
      a. Physical resources.
         (1) Strength
            Shoulder: All muscles G
            Scapula: All muscles G
            Elbow: Triceps F+, biceps G
            Forearm: Supinator F+, pronator F
            Wrist: Flexors F+, extensors F+
            Fingers: O
            Thumb: O, except for extensors: T and abductors: T

Continued.

D. **Results of evaluation—cont'd**

      (2) Passive ROM: All joints within functional to normal range, no contractures

      (3) Physical endurance: Endurance is fair; sitting and activity tolerance level up to 4 hours

      (4) Involuntary movement and spasticity: No involuntary movements observed; mild spasticity in lower extremities, no spasticity in upper extremities

      (5) Equilibrium and protective mechanisms: Trunk balance is weak; sufficient arm strength to right self

      (6) Coordination-muscle control: UE muscle control and coordination of innervated muscles is within normal limits

      (7) Hand function: Lateral prehension with difficulty, weak with tenodesis grasp

  b. Sensory-perceptual functions. All sensation below lesion (trunk and lower extremities) is absent. Touch, pain, and temperature absent from T1 dermatome down and posterior and anterior ulnar side of arm and fifth finger. Stereognosis and proprioception are within normal limits.

  c. Cognitive functions. John appears to use good judgment during wheelchair exercise and transfer training. He can anticipate results of behavior and actions. He needs some instruction in safety precautions necessary to guard desensitized areas from injury. He has a low level of motivation because of stage of adjustment to disability.

  d. Psychological functions. John's adjustment to disability is poor. He expresses a flip, carefree attitude. His expectations for recovery are demonstrated by denial of the reality and permanency of the disability. Therefore he is poorly motivated in treatment modalities that emphasize a lifelong disability, expressing interest in activities that involve lower extremities and that suggest the possibility of a total recovery.

  e. Prevocational potential. Potential work skills are limited by weakness of grasp and poor finger dexterity. Training and adaptations will increase potential. Vocational pursuits are limited because of wheelchair ambulation. Work habits are immature at present. Client needs to improve responsibility, concentration, and perseverance. Work tolerance level is potentially good. Physical endurance and sitting tolerance level should improve to allow a full day of activity. Following psychological adjustment vocational potential is good because of interests and intelligence.

  f. Functional skills. John is able to accomplish light hygiene activities independently but is poorly motivated and dependent in bathing and dressing. He currently requires moderate assistance in feeding. He relies excessively on staff and family. His potential for independence is good. John is currently unable to perform any homemaking activities independently because of poor balance, weak grasp, and poor motivation. His potential for homemaking skills is fair. He will always require moderate assistance. John has not participated in a community mobility evaluation yet but is a candidate for driving evaluation and for reaching independence in wheelchair mobility.

2. Problem identification.

  a. Muscle weakness

  b. Limited endurance

  c. Poor trunk balance

  d. Weak prehension with tenodesis grasp

  e. Sensory deficits

  f. Low motivation

  g. Poor adjustment to disability

  h. ADL dependence

  i. Limited vocational possibilities

  j. Redirection of educational goals

  k. Need for avocational outlets

  l. Restricted mobility

  m. Family adjustment

SAMPLE TREATMENT PLAN—cont'd

E Problem	F Specific OT objectives	G Methods used to meet objectives	H Gradation of treatment
a	Through a program of exercise the client's muscle grades will increase by at least ½ grade Shoulder: G to N Scapula: G to N Elbow: F+ to N Forearm: F+ to G Wrist: F to G Thumb extensor: T to P Thumb radial abductor: T to P	Wall pulleys (pulley handles are fastened around wrists to eliminate need for grasp strength) With the client's back to pulley system perform the following series of exercises to strengthen shoulder girdle and upper arm: Downward pull (scapular depression and shoulder and elbow extension): Client begins with shoulder in the fullest possible flexion and elbows extended; pulley handles are pulled from behind and overhead Forward thrust (shoulder flexors and elbow extensors): Client begins with shoulders in extension and elbows flexed; pulley handles are pulled from behind and straight forward Reach toward ceiling (scapular elevation, upward rotation, shoulder flexion, and elbow extension): Pulley handles are positioned at bottom; arm is extended down at the side of the body and pulley handles are pulled upward Bilateral midline cross (shoulder horizontal adduction, scapular abduction, and elbow extension): Client starts with shoulder in 90° abduction and elbows in slight flexion; pulleys are pulled from behind across the front of the body Bilateral horizontal abduction (shoulder horizontal abduction, scapular adduction, and elbow flexion): Client faces pulley, begins with shoulder in 90° abduction and arms crossed to reach opposite pulley handle, then pulls away from body midline into abduction With elbows flexed to 90°, resting on a table to eliminate substitutions, a cuff secured to a pulley weight system is attached around lower forearm just above the wrist; weight is medially placed for resistance to supination and laterally placed for resistance to pronation; client is instructed to perform alternations of pronation-supination[6] PRE to elbow flexors and extensors, using graded weighted cuffs on distal forearm and positioned for against gravity motion Active exercise against gravity to wrist extensors and flexors; progress to PRE as muscle strength increases Muscle reeducation to long thumb extensor and abductor; active-assisted exercise, graded to active exercise	Increase resistance Increase number repetitions of all exercises Increase resistance

Continued.

SAMPLE TREATMENT PLAN—cont'd

E Problem	F Specific OT objectives	G Methods used to meet objectives	H Gradation of treatment
d	Given a wrist-driven flexor hinge splint and training, the client will be able to use the splint for some self-care and recreational activities	Practice application and removal of splint, using arm motions and teeth to fasten straps Grasp and release practice using blocks, pegs, or common objects	Progress to holding fork for feeding and use of splint for table games such as chess or checkers
c	Through a program of activity and exercise trunk balance will increase so client can achieve maximum independence in ADL	Beach ball toss (patient to therapist), with trunk stabilization through corset, wheelchair support, or manual assistance	Vary position of therapist and client to catch ball, increase distance of toss, and increase number of repetitions
g	Through the use of therapeutic relationships, the therapeutic environment, group experiences, and activities the client will increase acceptance of physical disability so that his motivation for rehabilitation procedures and his social interactions will increase	Through patient-therapist interaction: Assist client in orientation to rehabilitation center; allow client to give up denial gradually (therapist not to condone or condemn denial); encourage ventilation of feelings and verbalization of problems; foster client-therapist relationship of warmth, responsiveness, empathy, individuality, and perception; purposeful conversation during all treatment sessions, allowing patient to consider alternatives and possibilities for the future; involve the patient in goal setting and treatment planning; encourage pride, individuality, independence, and self-esteem; facilitate problem-solving skills and needs gratification Through social interaction: Social, recreation, special interest, and expressive groups with other disabled individuals; group work focusing first on adjustment and secondly on acquisition of skills needed for success in the community;[6] group painting project with other clients with spinal cord injuries to encourage mutual sharing, accomplishment, and success experience; community outings to restaurants or public buildings first with therapist and one or two other clients	Reintroduction to family and social life should be a gradual process progressing from family to groups of friends (outside) to public situations Outings with family members and therapist; outings with nondisabled friends

SAMPLE TREATMENT PLAN—cont'd

E Problem	F Specific OT objectives	G Methods used to meet objectives	H Gradation of treatment
h	Given instruction, daily practice, and assistive devices the client will be able to feed himself without assistance and with a minimum number of assistive devices	Eating aids and assistance: Initially a suction mat stabilizing a plate with plate guard and a universal cuff may be used (progress to use of the flexor hinge splint for holding utensils); plate with plate guard is still used and regular utensils are used, if tenodesis grasp is developed and client chooses not to use flexor hinge splints	Patient progresses from easy-to-eat to more difficult-to-eat foods; eating speed increases
	Given instruction, daily practice, and assistive devices dressing will be performed in 45 minutes or less	Teach dressing techniques described by Runge[16] Donning and removing: Shirts Trousers and undershorts Socks Shoes	Practice UE dressing first, progress to LE dressing if feasible
	Given instruction and daily practice, the client will protect his own skin from pressure sores so that there is no evidence of their development	Shifting weight in wheelchair: Every 10 minutes client leans to one side, then the other side of the wheelchair by flexing elbow around wheelchair handle on that side and pulling body weight, using elbow and shoulder muscles or client pushes himself up on the wheelchair armrests to relieve ischial pressure Every morning and every evening, in bed, in side lying position, client inspects skin over buttock, trochanters, and heels with long-handle skin inspection mirror; while sitting in bed or in wheelchair, client inspects elbows and knees	Reminders, supervision, and assistance are gradually decreased as client becomes more responsible for his own self-care
j	Through appropriate experiences, trials, and exploration the feasibility of attending college will be determined by the client in concert with occupational therapy and vocational counselor	Writing training; training in use of electric typewriter with typing sticks if necessary; training in use of tape recorder for recording and transcribing; wheelchair mobility practice, indoors and outdoors; trial in adult education class	

Continued.

SAMPLE TREATMENT PLAN—cont'd

E Problem	F Specific OT objectives	G Methods used to meet objectives	H Gradation of treatment

k	Through a program of activity the client will explore avocational interests so that adaptive skills and personal satisfaction will increase	Painting and sketching—watercolor, oil, charcoal, or pencil—using flexor hinge splint or universal cuff or tenodesis grasp; practice and assistance in handwriting skills with splint
		Games, using flexor hinge splints:
		  Cards
		  Chess
		  Backgammon
		  Jigsaw puzzles
		  Crossword puzzles[6]
		Music (collecting and listening to records); spectator sports
			Reduce reliance on assistive devices when appropriate; increase length of time spent working on projects

I. **Special equipment.**
1. Ambulation aids.
   Active duty lightweight wheelchair with pneumatic tires and handrim projections for easy maneuverability and transfer of wheelchair into car and on soft, sandy, or rough surfaces. For energy conservation an electric wheelchair may be more practical.
2. Splints.
   Wrist-driven flexor hinge splint
3. Assistive devices.[17]
   a. Soap holder
   b. Bath bench
   c. Hand-held shower
   d. Razor holder
   e. Sliding transfer board
   f. Button hook
   g. Zipper pull
   h. Suppository insertion device
   i. Electric typewriter
   j. Tape recorder
   k. Dressing sticks
   l. Skin inspection mirror
   m. Long-handle bath sponge

REVIEW QUESTIONS

1. List three causes of spinal cord injury. Which is most common?
2. Describe the patterns of weakness in quadriplegia and paraplegia.
3. Describe the functional and prognostic differences between complete and incomplete lesions.
4. When reference is made to "C5" in quadriplegia, what is meant in terms of level of injury and functioning muscle groups?
5. What are the characteristics of spinal shock?
6. What physical changes occur following the spinal shock phase?
7. What is the prognosis for recovery of motor function in complete lesions and incomplete lesions?
8. What are the purposes of surgery in management of spinal injury?
9. What are some medical complications, common to patients with spinal cord injuries, that can limit achievement of functional potential?
10. How should postural hypotension be treated?
11. How should autonomic dysreflexia be treated?
12. What is the role of the occupational therapist in the prevention of pressure sores?
13. Why is vital capacity affected in patients with spinal cord injuries?
14. What effect will reduced vital capacity have on the rehabilitation program?
15. Which level of injury has full innervation of rotator cuff musculature, biceps, and extensor carpi radialis and partial innervation of serratus anterior, latissimus dorsi and pectoralis major?
16. What additional muscle power does the patient with C6 quadriplegia have over the patient with C5 quadriplegia? What is the major functional advantage of this additional muscle power?
17. What are the additional critical muscles that the patient with C7 quadriplegia has, as compared to the patient with C6 quadriplegia?
18. What additional functional independence can be achieved because of this additional muscle power?
19. What is the first spinal cord lesion level that has full innervation of UE musculature?
20. Which evaluation tools does the occupational therapist use to assess the patient with a spinal cord injury? What is the purpose of each?
21. List five goals of occupational therapy for the patient with a spinal cord injury.
22. How is wrist extension used to effect grasp by the patient with quadriplegia?
23. How does the patient with C6 quadriplegia substitute for the absence of elbow extensors?

24. What is the "contracture" that is encouraged in patients with spinal cord injuries? Why? How is it developed?
25. What is the splint that allows the C6 quadriplegic to achieve functional grasp?
26. What are some of the first self-care activities that the patient with a C6 spinal cord injury should be expected to accomplish?
27. List four assistive devices commonly used by persons with quadriplegia, and tell the purpose of each.
28. Describe the role of occupational therapy in the vocational evaluation of the client with a spinal cord injury.

REFERENCES

1. Anonymous: Autonomic dysreflexia for staff, San Jose, Calif., 1969, Santa Clara Valley Medical Center. Mimeographed.
2. Anonymous: Functional goals in spinal cord lesions, Downey, Calif., Physical Therapy Department, Rancho Los Amigos Hospital. Mimeographed.
3. Bors, E., and Comarr, A.E.: Neurological disturbances of sexual function with special reference to 529 patients with spinal cord injury, Urol Surv. 10:191-222, 1960.
4. Chusid, J.G.: Correlative neuroanatomy and functional neurology, ed. 15, Los Altos, Calif., 1973, Lange Medical Publications.
5. Daniels, L., and Worthingham, C.: Muscle testing, ed. 3, Philadelphia, 1972, W.B. Saunders Co.
6. Fodera, C., and Olsen, K.: Treatment plan for spinal cord injury, unpublished paper presented in partial fulfillment of the requirements for the course O.T. 167, San Jose, Calif., May 1979, Department of Occupational Therapy, San Jose State University.
7. Geiger, R.: Sexuality in the handicapped, lecture to Crippled Children's Services Conference, Oakland, Calif., March 1973.
8. Hamilton, R.: Spinal cord injury: medical and surgical management, lecture in course O.T. 135, San Jose, Calif., 1973, Department of Occupational Therapy, San Jose State University.
9. Long, C., and Lawton, E.: Functional significance of spinal cord lesion level, New York, 1954-58. Mimeographed.
10. Malick, M.H., and Meyer, C.M.H.: Manual on management of the quadriplegic upper extremity, Pittsburgh, 1978, Harmarville Rehabilitation Center.
11. McKenzie, M.W.: The role of occupational therapy in rehabilitating spinal cord injured patients, Am. J. Occup. Ther. 24:257-263, 1970.
12. Mooney, T.O., Cole, T.M., and Chilgren, R.A.: Sexual options for paraplegics and quadriplegics, Boston, 1975, Little, Brown, & Co.
13. Neistadt, M., and Baker, M.F.: A program for sex counseling the physically disabled, Am. J. Occup. Ther. 32:646-647, 1978.
14. Pierce, D.S., and Nickel, V.H.: The total care of spinal cord injuries, Boston, 1977, Little, Brown & Co.
15. Reedy, J.: Spinal cord level chart, unpublished paper presented in partial fulfillment of the requirements for the course O.T. 135, San Jose, Calif., November 1974, Department of Occupational Therapy, San Jose State University.
16. Runge, M.: Self-dressing techniques for patients with spinal cord injury, Am. J. Occup. Ther. 21:367-375, 1967.
17. Sammons, F.: Be OK: self-help aids, professional and institutional catalog for 1978, Brookfield, Ill., 1978, Fred Sammons, Inc.
18. Sidman, J.M.: Sexual functioning in the physically disabled adult, Am. J. Occup. Ther. 31:81-85, 1977.
19. Spencer, E.A.: Functional restoration. In Hopkins, H.L., and Smith, H.D., editors: Willard and Spackman's occupational therapy, ed. 5, Philadelphia, 1978, J.B. Lippincott Co.
20. Talbot, H.S.: The sexual function in paraplegia, J. Urol. 73:91-100, 1955.
21. Trombly, C.A., and Scott, A.D.: Occupational therapy for physical dysfunction, Baltimore, 1977, The Williams & Wilkins Co.
22. Tsuji, I., et al.: The sexual function in patients with spinal cord injury, Urol. Int. 12:270-280, 1961.
23. Venegas, N., and Del Pilar-Christian, M., editors: Proceedings of the workshop "Occupational therapy for patients with physical dysfunction," Puerto Rico, 1967, Occupational Therapy Department, University of Puerto Rico.
24. Wilson, D.J., McKenzie, M.W., and Barber, L.M.: Spinal cord injury: a treatment guide for occupational therapists, Thorofare, N.J., 1974, Charles B Slack, Inc.

SUPPLEMENTARY READING

Alexander, B., and Reid, E.: A drainage valve for urinary leg bags, Am. J. Occup. Ther. 28:619-620, 1974.
Craver, P.: Typing splints for the quadriplegic patient, Am. J. Occup. Ther. 29:571, 1975.
Dailey, J., and Michael, R.: Nonsterile self-intermittent catheterization for male quadriplegic patients, Am. J. Occup. Ther. 31:86-89, 1977.
Donovan, W., Macri, D., and Clowers, D.E.: A finger device for obtaining satisfactory voiding in spinal cord injured patients, Am. J. Occup. Ther. 31:107-108, 1977.
Feinberg, J.: Writing device for the quadriplegic patient, Am. J. Occup. Ther. 29:101, 1975.
Gilkeson, G.E.: Method of suspension for a urethral catheter drainage bag, Am. J. Occup. Ther. 32:240, 1978.
Gurgold, G.D., and Harden, D.H.: Assessing driving potential of the handicapped, Am. J. Occup. Ther. 32:41-46, 1978.
Heard, C.: Occupational role acquisition: a perspective on the chronically disabled, Am. J. Occup. Ther. 31:243-247, 1977.
Mann, W., et al.: The use of group counseling procedures in the rehabilitation of spinal cord injured patients, Am. J. Occup. Ther. 27:73-77, 1973.
McKenzie, M.: The ratchet handsplint, Am. J. Occup. Ther. 27:477-479, 1973.
McKenzie, M., and Rogers, J.: Use of trunk supports for severely paralyzed people, Am. J. Occup. Ther. 27:147-148, 1973.
Rogers, J.C., and Figone, J.J.: Psychosocial parameters in treating the person with quadriplegia, Am. J. Occup. Ther. 33:432-439, 1979.
Sinha, A.K., and Schaffer, F.J.: External urinary collecting device for the incontinent male, Am. J. Occup. Ther. 32:238-239, 1978.
Smith, B.: Adapted bed controls and the quadriplegic patient, Am. J. Occup. Ther. 32:322, 1978.
Taylor, D.: Treatment goals for quadriplegic and paraplegic patients, Am. J. Occup. Ther. 28:22-29, 1974.
Wittmeyer, M.B., and Stolov, W.C.: Educating wheelchair patients on home architectural barriers, Am. J. Occup. Ther. 32:557-564, 1978.

Chapter 13

Cerebral vascular accident

Cerebral vascular accident (CVA), commonly referred to as a stroke or shock, is a complex dysfunction caused by a lesion in the brain. It results in an upper motor neuron dysfunction that produces hemiplegia or paralysis of one side of the body, limbs, and sometimes the face and oral structures that are contralateral to the hemisphere of the brain that has the lesion. Thus a lesion in the left cerebral hemisphere will produce hemiplegia on the right side of the body and vice versa. When referring to the client's disability as *right* hemiplegia, however, the reference is to the paralyzed body side and *not* to the locus of the lesion.[17]

Accompanying the motor paralysis may be a variety of other dysfunctions. Some of these are sensory disturbances, perceptual dysfunctions, visual disturbances, personality and intellectual changes, and a complex range of speech and associated language disorders.[21]

EFFECTS

The outcome of the CVA will depend on which artery supplying the brain was involved in the vascular disease process.

Involvement of the *middle cerebral artery* (MCA) is the most common cause of CVA.[14] The general symptoms caused by occlusion of the MCA include contralateral hemiplegia with greater involvement of the arm, face, and tongue; sensory and perceptual disturbances; contralateral homonymous hemianopsia; and aphasia, if the lesion is in the dominant hemisphere.[8,17,19] Occlusion of the *anterior cerebral artery* (ACA) usually results in contralateral hemiplegia, with leg involvement greater than arm involvement; sensory deficits; mental confusion; apraxia; and aphasia, if the lesion is in the dominant hemisphere.[8,17] Signs of *posterior cerebral artery* (PCA) occlusion include contralateral hemiplegia and homonymous hemianopsia; hemisensory deficits; and receptive aphasia, if the dominant hemisphere is involved. Ataxia, rigidity, tremors, and choreiform movement may also result less often.[8,17]

The cerebellar and basilar arteries may also be involved in vascular disease that produces stroke. *Cerebellar artery* occlusion results in ipsilateral ataxia, contralateral loss of pain and temperature sensitivity, ipsilateral

facial analgesia, and contralateral hemiparesis.[8] If the *basilar artery* is involved, results could include dysfunction of cranial nerves 3 to 12, cerebellar dysfunction, loss of proprioception,[17] hemiplegia, quadriplegia, and sensory disturbances.[8,19]

Etiology

CVA is caused by an interruption of the blood supply to the brain because of thrombus, embolus, or hemorrhage.[5,6,12,17] Cerebral anoxia and aneurysm can also result in hemiplegia.[5,6,17] Some of the treatment approaches outlined in this chapter may be applicable to hemiplegia that results from causes other than CVA or stroke, such as head injuries, neoplasms, and infectious diseases of the brain.[5]

Vascular disease of the brain can result in a completed CVA with the full clinical picture just described or can cause transient ischemic attacks (TIAs) because of temporary vascular insufficiency. These attacks result in temporary neurological symptoms (less than 24 hours' duration) that disappear. They signal the probability of complete CVA sometime in the future.[17] If they are due to extracranial vascular disease, surgical intervention to reestablish patency of arteries may be effective in preventing the CVA and the resultant disability.

Predisposing factors. Some of the factors that predispose an individual to the possible onset of CVA are arteriosclerosis, hypertension, obesity, diabetes, smoking, or congenital vascular weakness that results in aneurysm.[17]

Medical management[5]

It is the physician's responsibility to make the diagnosis and apply the early lifesaving measures. These may include ordering appropriate nourishment and hydration and establishing an airway. The physician also prescribes medication to treat or prevent infection or concomitant medical problems.

During the acute illness the need for urinary drainage should be determined and catheterization carried out, if necessary. The physician should also order early mobility, adequate diet and fluids, and use of suppositories and medication to prevent or treat fecal impaction.

The physician should see that appropriate measures are instituted to prevent contractures. This means writing orders for appropriate positioning, splints, and passive exercise in the early phases of rehabilitation. Bedsores should be vigilantly guarded against through early mobilization, frequent repositioning in bed or chair, excellent hygiene, and skin inspection. The physician is responsible for ordering these measures, seeing that they are carried out, and inspecting the patient's skin on a regular basis.

It is important for the physician to not overlook the possibility of disability of unaffected parts because of disuse and immobility. The physician should see to it that the patient is involved in physical activities and exercises that are commensurate with his medical status and abilities as early as possible in the rehabilitation program.

Evaluating the residuals of the CVA, writing orders for the rehabilitation therapies, and reevaluating the patient's progress are the responsibilities of the physician, who supervises the rehabilitation program.

MOTOR DYSFUNCTION AFTER CVA

Bobath[4] outlines four major factors that interfere with normal motor performance in adult hemiplegia: sensory disturbances, spasticity, disorder of the normal postural reflex mechanism, and loss of selective movement patterns.

The degree of sensory involvement will have a profound influence on the degree of spontaneous motor recovery and the results of treatment. All movement is in response to some sensory stimuli acting on the CNS from the external and internal environments.[4,7] These sensory stimuli progress through the CNS and are integrated at the cortical level, where they produce an effective, coordinated motor response to meet the demands of the environment. Sensations arising from the movement response serve to guide it through its course,[4] determine its effectiveness, and give cues for the need for any revision of the movement response. Fig. 13-1 shows a schematic diagram of the sensorimotor process.

Because of this critical sensory-motor relationship and interdependence, it is important to think of the sensorimotor cortex as one functional unit of the brain.[4] The sensory disturbance in patients with hemiplegia aggravates the motor dysfunction even in the absence of severe spasticity. The patients lack the urge to move[4] probably in part because they cannot sense and interpret the environmental stimuli that normally evoke movement.

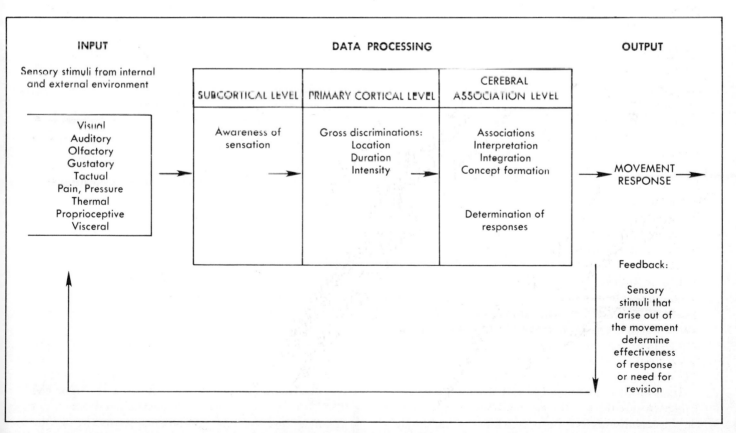

Fig. 13-1. Sensorimotor process.

Characteristics of the motor disturbance after CVA

After CVA there is upper motor neuron paralysis that follows a one-sided distribution and includes musculature of the trunk and limbs on the affected side. The muscles of the face and mouth may also be involved. The paralysis is usually characterized by increased muscle tone or spasticity. There may, in some cases, be apparent hypotonicity or flaccidity. Even in these instances some spasticity may be evoked in the finger and wrist flexors and the ankle extensors, if prolonged and strong stretch stimuli are applied. In cases where apparent flaccidity persists indefinitely, it is usually combined with severe sensory loss, and active motion is impossible.[4]

Coordination or control of smooth, rhythmical movement is lost. Rather the spasticity occurs in gross patterns of flexion and extension called *synergies* (Chapter 4). Synergies are released when cortical control of motion is interrupted. All muscles in the synergy are neurophysiologically linked, and when one of the movement components of the synergy is performed, some or all of the movement components are likely to occur simultaneously.[6,12]

Normal postural reflex mechanisms are disturbed after CVA. Normal righting, equilibrium, and protective reactions (Chapter 2) are lost on the hemiplegic side.[4] This affects the client's ability to maintain and recover balance and make the normal postural adjustments that accompany movement and activity. Primitive reflexes (Chapter 2) may be released so that changes of the position of the head and body in space will have an abnormal influence on muscle tone.

Bobath[4] describes the loss of "adaptive changes of muscle tone as a protection against the forces of gravity." This is the ability to control slow, unresisted movements in the direction of gravity. For example, in lowering the upraised arm the antigravity muscles contract and hold while their antagonists relax. The person with hemiplegia has lost this mechanism of automatic control on the affected side. He will tend to compensate for the loss with the automatic reactions of the unaffected side. He will not initiate movement with the affected side, will not support himself on the affected arm and hand, and will bear little weight on the affected leg.

Because of the spasticity and release of abnormal synergistic movement patterns, there is a loss of selective, discriminative, and isolated movement after CVA. This loss is most apparent in the arm and hand,[4] probably because of the nature of the normal function of this part. However, selective movement is also lost in the leg and foot and is evident in the inability to dorsiflex the ankle and toes regardless of the position of the hip and knee or in the inability to flex the knee while the hip is extended.[4] In function this is evidenced by the gait pattern, which is usually performed with the leg held in stiff extension or in the extensor synergy pattern. The individual with hemiplegia lacks ability to perform a wide variety of movement combinations to effect normal motor performance.[4]

Characteristics of synergistic movement

The flexor synergy dominates in the arm, and the extensor synergy dominates in the leg. Performance of synergistic movement, either reflexly or voluntarily, may be influenced by the primitive postural reflex mechanisms. When the client performs the synergy, the strongest of its components are often most apparent, rather than the entire classic patterns, as discussed in Chapter 2. By the same token the resting posture of the limb, particularly the arm, is usually characterized by a position that represents the strongest components of both flexor and extensor synergies, that is, shoulder adduction, elbow flexion, forearm pronation, and wrist and finger flexion. However, with facilitation or voluntary effort the more classic synergy pattern can usually be evoked.[6]

The recovery process

The stages of recovery as described by Brunnstrom[6] were outlined in Table 3 (Chapter 4). The recovery follows an ontogenetic process. It is usually proximal to distal so that shoulder movement can be expected before hand movement. Flexion patterns occur before extension patterns in the upper limb. Reflex motion occurs before controlled, volitional movement, and gross movement patterns can be performed before isolated, selective movement.

Recovery may cease at any stage, and the amount of recovery attained varies widely from person to person. Motor recovery is influenced by many factors such as sensation, perception, motivation, affective states, and concomitant medical problems or general health.[12] Few patients make a very good recovery of arm function, and the greatest loss is usually in the wrist and hand.

It should be noted that no two patients are exactly alike. There will be much individual variation on the characteristic motor disturbances and the recovery process among patients. The motor behavior and recovery process described represent common characteristics that may be observed in a majority of persons after CVA occurs.[6]

Prognosis for recovery of arm function.[20] The physician and therapist may wish to estimate the potential for recovery of arm function for planning rehabilitation goals. Some of the factors that are considered to be good prognostic signs are (1) good sensation and perception, (2) intact body scheme, (3) minimal spasticity, (4) functional ROM, (5) attempts at spontaneous use of the affected arm in bilateral activities, and (6) development of some isolated motion. Conversely, poor prognostic signs include such factors as (1) severe sensory and perceptual impairments, (2) moderate to severe spasticity, (3) body scheme and motor planning deficits, (4) limited ROM, (5) no attempts at spontaneous use of the affected arm during bilateral activities, and (6) inability to perform controlled movement.

Recovery period. Spontaneous neurological recovery that results in improvement of motor performance occurs primarily in the first 3 months after the onset of the CVA. Recovery may continue to the sixth or seventh month after the onset.[12] Slight, continued recovery is sometimes seen up to 1 year and in rare instances is seen somewhat longer. This does not imply that motor behavior cannot be influenced by appropriate therapy after a year, however.

Functional use of the affected arm. Therapy aimed to improve arm function is often frustrating to the client and the therapist unless realistic goals and expectations have been set. Progress should be judged by the amount of spontaneous use of the affected arm, rather than by comparing it to the normal one as a standard for progress or as a goal to be reached. Realistically few clients will recover full function of the arm. The client may use the hand and arm only when needed and perhaps then not by choice. He may use the affected arm only to assist the unaffected arm in activities that require stabilization of objects. The stage of recovery limits how the affected arm can be used. The arm that has little or no voluntary motion, but has good sensation, may be used as a passive stabilizer. If there is voluntary control of the flexion synergy with gross grasp and good sensation, the arm can be used for grasping and pulling. Voluntary control of the flexor synergy, elbow extension, grasp, active release, and good sensation may render enough function for grasping, pushing, pulling, and releasing. If isolated movements or gross movement combinations that deviate from the synergy patterns are possible, and there is good sensation, the arm can be used to perform some gross movements and activities with combined movements. If the highest recovery stages are achieved and there is normal shoulder, elbow, and forearm movement, good sensation, and limitations only in fine hand movements, the arm can be used to perform all normal daily activities except for those that require fine manipulation and motor speed.[22]

CONCOMITANT DYSFUNCTIONS

Therapists have placed much emphasis on the evaluation and treatment of the motor dysfunction. They should also be aware of and be able to evaluate and treat the total disability. On the basis of a comprehensive evaluation realistic rehabilitation goals, considering all aspects of the disability, may be planned with the client.[21]

Sensory disturbances

Disturbances in the senses of touch, pain, temperature, pressure, and vibration may occur as a result of CVA. Such disturbances prohibit the sensory feedback that is so important to the perceptual-motor functioning of the individual and thus may be one cause of disuse of the affected extremities, even when motor recovery is apparently good.[21]

Somatic perceptual dysfunctions

Loss of proprioception. The loss of the ability to perceive position and motion of body parts[1] will affect use of those parts. Impaired proprioception is a common deficit seen in patients who have CVA. Such patients are likely to leave the affected arm in a state of disuse, drop things, and not be aware of the position and movement of the arm. The arm may have a sensation of heaviness.[21]

Tactual perception. Tactual perception is the ability to recognize, localize, and make discriminations about touch stimuli to the skin surface. It includes the ability to recognize and localize light touch stimuli, ability to recognize symbols "written" on the skin (graphesthesia), ability to recognize two stimuli in close proximity (two-point discrimination), ability to recognize two simultaneous stimuli, and ability to identify common objects and geometric forms through manipulation, without the aid of vision (stereognosis). The inability to perceive the tangible properties of an object tactually (astereognosis) interferes with perceptual-motor functioning of the patient in that he receives no sensory feedback about the objects he is manipulating unless he uses his vision to compensate for the sensory loss. This compensation is often ineffective, since it is difficult to visually supervise the hand performing an activity while trying to watch the activity and focus on its goal.[21]

Body scheme disorders. Body scheme disorders are disturbances in the neurological function that includes knowledge of body construction, its anatomical elements, and spatial relationships; ability to visualize the body in movement and its parts in different positional relationships; ability to differentiate right from left; and ability to know body health or disease.[1] Body scheme disorders are found frequently enough in patients with hemiplegia to make routine evaluation for the presence of this dysfunction advisable. Since knowledge of the body scheme is basic to all motor function, a disturbance in body scheme will have a profound effect on the success of the patient's rehabilitation. Patients with body scheme disturbances will have difficulty with ADL, especially self-care and dressing activities that require a good knowledge of the body. They may have difficulty following directions related to their own bodies. They may be unable to correctly localize body parts, recognize right and left, or visualize and plan how to move their bodies to accomplish a given activity.[21]

Apraxia. The disturbance in praxis, or the ability to plan motor acts, is often intimately associated with the body scheme disorder.[1] To dress, for example, one must not only have a good knowledge of the body scheme but must also be able to plan the motions necessary to put the garment on the body. When there is apraxia, the individual often cannot formulate a plan of movement to accomplish an act.[21] He may be unable to imitate movements of the therapist in demonstrated instructions or carry out a purposeful movement on command. These problems characterize ideomotor apraxia. If there is ideational apraxia as well, the patient will not be able to carry out routine activities such as combing his hair when given a comb and told to use it.[12]

Visual-perceptual dysfunctions

Visual field defect—homonymous hemianopsia. Homonymous hemianopsia is blindness of the medial half of one eye and the lateral half of the other. The affected side of the body corresponds to the paralyzed side of the body. A patient with left hemiplegia with left homonymous hemianopsia cannot see things in the left visual field unless he turns his head toward the affected side to compensate for the deficit. In practical activity he may not see things placed on his left side. Instructions, demonstrations, and conversation given from the left side may be ignored. Objects moving toward him from the left may startle him. The patient may bump into things on the left when walking. Many patients with hemiplegia compensate for this deficit quite automatically, whereas others do not seem to make this adjustment and must be trained to use the intact visual field to compensate for the visual loss.[21]

Visual inattention. Visual inattention refers to defect in reception of and reaction to visual stimuli. It manifests itself in defective scanning of the visual field, difficulty in shifting gaze from one object to another, slowed eye movements, loss of the fixation point, and difficulty in shifting attention.[21]

Spatial relationships. The ability to recognize the relationship between one form and another in spatial areas[11] may be lost as a result of CVA. Disturbances in the perception of visual-spatial relationships are particularly common among patients with left hemiplegia. The result is a disorganization of constructional abilities such as in drawing or constructing three-dimensional objects and designs. The patient with this deficit will have difficulty or failure with tasks involving spatial analysis. Dressing failures are common.[21] Problems in body scheme and apraxia may be severe enough to prohibit the learning of dressing skills, but the problem may be compounded by the patient's inability to perceive the shape and relationship of the clothing to his body. Tasks such as matching parts in a sewing or woodworking project are impossible, as is matching puzzle parts or block designs.

Verticality. The perception of vertical lines and elements in the environment is verticality. Patients with hemiplegia often have difficulty making visual judgments of what is vertical or horizontal. Patients with left hemiplegia tend to misjudge verticality in a counterclockwise direction. Since visual orientation to verticality is important to the optical righting reactions that help in the maintenance of upright posture, directional disturbances in perception of vertical and horizontal may interfere with balance and ambulation.[21]

Figure-background perception. Figure-background perception is the recognition of forms hidden within a gestalt[11] and the ability to attend to a relevant visual stimulus while separating it from and ignoring background stimuli. Some patients with hemiplegia have difficulty distinguishing a figure from its background. The result is that they cannot always select the most relevant visual cue to which to respond.[21] The patient may appear distractible when, in truth, he is responding to many irrelevant visual stimuli. He may have difficulty selecting items from cabinet or refrigerator, because he cannot perceive the desired object as separate from the surrounding objects that constitute its background.

Visual sequencing. Visual sequencing is the ordering of visual patterns in time and space and involves temporal concepts such as first, second, and third and spatial ordering such as top to bottom, left to right, and around.[2] A disturbance in sequencing skills may affect the patient's ability to plan steps and anticipate consequences of tasks and activities that require ordering of objects and steps in a procedure.

Intellectual and cognitive dysfunctions

Since CVA may interfere with integrative processes of the brain, and intelligence and cognitive abilities depend on the integrative functions of the brain, some patients with hemiplegia will show impairment of specific intellectual functions. These may be demonstrated by a drop in intelligence test scores and an overall change in organization, mental abilities, and ability to do abstract reasoning.[12]

Memory. The ability to recall various details of recent and past visual and auditory stimuli[2] may be disturbed as a result of CVA. Memory disturbance will retard rehabilitation efforts. The patient may have difficulty recalling persons, objects, and procedures learned from day to day.

Retrieval of information may be reduced, and learning

ability may be impaired. Patients with right hemiplegia are likely to have impaired memory for language and numbers, whereas patients with left hemiplegia have impairments involving tasks of position and movement.[19]

Patients with deficits in memory will require much repetition of activity before training can be retained. The therapist needs to discover each patient's best mode of sensory learning and provide the necessary sensory and perceptual cues and methods of instruction to suit the individual.

Judgment. Poor judgment may be easily detected or may be masked by good social or verbal skills. The patient may be unable to abstract the future and make judgments about the consequences of certain behaviors. He may not be able to judge, for example, that not locking his wheelchair may have grave consequences.

Abstract thinking. Abstract thinking and reasoning may also be impaired. These patients will be very concrete, dealing best with the realities of concrete objects and situations than with ideas and speculations about them. They may not be able to generalize learning from one situation or therapist to another and may be unable to comprehend the abstract ideas conveyed in humor or idioms.[21]

Personality and emotional changes

Regression. In regression the patient does not appear to use his full adult capacities to deal with his difficulties. He seems to regress to a lower level of emotional maturity. This is not an uncommon reaction to illness and may be due in part to sensory loss.[3]

Rigidity. Rigidity is an inability to be flexible or adapt to change. The patient seems to feel most secure in a familiar and unchanging environment. This phenomenon manifests itself in the inability to function in a changed time schedule, disturbance at lack of symmetry or change in personnel, and a tenacity to old and familiar methods of performing familiar activities.[21]

Denial. Denial is an unawareness of the hemiplegia and a denial of the defective performance of the paralyzed side. It manifests itself when the patient neglects the affected side. He may move the normal side and claim he is moving the affected arm or leg. He may declare that his arm belongs to someone else or may regard it as an object. This phenomenon may be a psychological reaction to an unbearable truth or may be due to sensory and perceptual dysfunctions.[3]

Perseveration. Perseveration is the meaningless, nonpurposeful repetition of an act. The patient does not stop unless someone or something intervenes. It becomes particularly apparent during activities that are repetitive by nature such as sanding wood but can manifest itself in ADL as well. Perseveration may be exhibited in buttoning, stirring foods, and sponge bathing, for example.

Depression. Depression is usually a reaction to a catastrophic illness. The patient may feel inadequate in dealing with his problems and may be overwhelmed by them. He has a sense of loss and must mourn for his loss. He may feel rejected and out of control of his own affairs as well as his own body. The depression usually lifts and rehabilitation progresses as the patient rediscovers his assets and gains confidence and self-esteem.[3]

Emotional lability. The patient with CVA may lose the cortical control of emotional responses and thus may manifest loss of emotional control more easily than he did formerly. Emotional lability may exhibit itself in automatic laughing or crying that seems inappropriate. Situations of stress often provoke crying. The patient is embarrassed by these outbursts and requires the reassurance and understanding of family and rehabilitation workers.[3]

Amorality (reduction in behavioral and evaluative standards). The patient demonstrating amorality may exhibit a reduced level of aspiration. He may seem satisfied with shoddy performance. His pride and perseverance in working toward goals may be poor. Inadequate performance and poor products may be acceptable to the patient in contrast to his standards before the illness occurred. This problem may be organic in origin but is enhanced by inactivity and the psychological trauma of the illness.[9]

Motivation. Many patients with hemiplegia manifest an apparent defect in "intrinsic" motivation, or the inner drive to act spontaneously. This is likely to be organic in origin and should not be regarded as something the patient can modify at will. This lack of motivation may cause rehabilitation workers to overestimate the disability. It may cause workers to regard the patient as "stubborn" or "unwilling to try" and may reduce their motivation to help the patient. The problem may be related to the patient's readiness to deal with the overwhelming problems of the disability and to the tremendous amount of energy it takes every day for these patients to put their all into everything they attempt to do. Therapists must approach this problem with patience and perseverance. Patients need encouragement, reassurance, praise for success, and a lot of "extrinsic" motivation in prodding, cuing, and the planning of activities by therapists and caretakers.

Frustration tolerance. Patients with hemiplegia are likely to have a reduction in ability to tolerate stress and frustration.

Speech and language disorders

CVA may result in a wide variety of speech disorders and disturbances in the ability to deal with symbols and may vary from mild to severe. These dysfunctions occur most frequently in right hemiplegia, or damage to the left hemisphere of the brain, but may also occur in left hemiplegia. All persons with CVA should be evaluated by the speech pathologist for the presence of speech and language disorders. The speech pathologist can provide valuable information to other members of the rehabilitation team regarding the best ways to communicate with a particular client. The occupational therapist should carry over the work of the speech therapist in her treatment sessions, as it is appropriate. This may occur in reinforcing communication techniques that the client is learning; presenting instruction in ways that the client is able to integrate; and instructing and practicing writing, which often is the responsibility of the occupational therapist.

When reading the descriptions of the specific speech and language dysfunctions that follow, the reader should remember that they can exist in mild to severe form and in combination with one another.

Aphasia. The loss of ability to speak or understand the spoken word is known as *aphasia*. If there is greater difficulty with expression than with comprehension, the patient is said to have *expressive aphasia*. If there is greater difficulty with comprehension than with expression of speech, the patient is said to have *receptive* or *sensory aphasia*. Aphasia is a dysfunction in the ability to deal with spoken or written symbols. Patients with expressive aphasia may be able to produce automatic speech such as singing, praying,[19] or using profanity. It is rare for an aphasic patient to be completely speechless. A few words can usually be produced.[5]

Dysarthria. Patients with dysarthria can understand and express symbolic language.[19] However, there is an articulation disorder because of a dysfunction of the CNS mechanisms that control speech musculature. This results in paralysis and incoordination of the organs of speech that make it sound thick, sluggish, and slurred.[5,19]

Associated dysfunctions. Associated dysfunctions include *anomia*, or the inability to remember the names of persons or objects; *agraphia*, or the loss of the ability to write, which is often associated with expressive aphasia; *alexia*, or the inability to read;[18] and *acalculia*, or the loss of the ability to deal with mathematical calculations and symbols.

Communication with patients. Horwitz[13] describes principles for communication with aphasic patients. She states that they respond best to intelligent and sympathetic understanding from professional staff and family members who are interacting with them. Here are some useful principles for facilitating communication and meaningful interaction with aphasic patients:*

---

*Adapted from Horwitz, B.: An open letter to the family of an adult patients with aphasia, Chicago, 1964, National Society for Crippled Children and Adults, Inc.

1. Talk to the patient naturally, using short, simple, and concrete sentences.
2. Encourage, but do not pressure, him to respond in whatever way he can.
3. Never ridicule the patient or insist that he respond accurately and articulately.
4. Do not increase volume of voice when speaking to aphasic patients. They are *not* deaf.
5. Do not talk about the patient in his presence. He can understand part or all of what you say. Include him in conversations about him, if he is present.
6. Create an air of relaxation by your mannerisms, patience, and attitude of acceptance.
7. Include him in family activities and help him maintain his former role in the family.
8. Professional staff may explain to the patient what has happened to him, carefully, and simply.
9. Keep instructions and explanations simple. The best way to know that he has understood you is by observing the way he carries out instructions.
10. Do not confuse the patient with rapid, complicated speech or too many people speaking at once. Do not use esoteric and abstract words.
11. Ask direct questions requiring one-word answers. Some patients may say "yes" when they mean "no" and vice versa.
12. Do not answer for the patient if he is capable of responding independently.
13. Use routine daily living activities (for example, eating and dressing) as opportunities to encourage simple speech.
14. Encourage the use of words of greeting and simple social exchanges.
15. If the patient can write and spell, he should be encouraged to write responses.
16. Encourage the use of gestures to communicate.
17. Accept bizarre, inaccurate use of language and profanities without amusement or anger.
18. Aphasic patients often cannot remember the names of people and objects. Reassure the patient that this is part of his disability and does not mean he is "losing his mind."

Contrast between right and left hemiplegia

There is an apparent difference between the performance and learning styles of persons with right hemiplegia and those with left hemiplegia. This contrast is related to the difference in hemispheric functions.

The right cerebral hemisphere (left hemiplegia) is responsible primarily for perception. It discriminates form, position, weight, distance, and visual-spatial relationships.[19] Left hemiplegia may be characterized by (1) disorganization of tasks such as construction or drawing, (2) failures on tasks that involve spatial analysis, (3) frequent failures on tasks that require maintenance of spatial orientation, and (4) apraxia for dressing. There is a significant correlation between extremely poor performance on perceptual organization tasks and failures in dressing and grooming.[15] The patient with left hemiplegia may retain good verbal skills, which may tend to mask the perceptual dysfunction and give the impression of good performance. The therapist needs to require performance evaluation of self-care skills and not rely on the interview as a means of determining the patient's ability to function.

The primary responsibilities of the left cerebral hemisphere (right hemiplegia) are analysis, logic, understanding of symbolic language, and conceptualization. Even in the absence of aphasia problems in these functions may exist. The patient with right hemiplegia has little or no difficulty with visual-spatial tasks but may have difficulty with written or oral instructions. Demonstrations and pantomime may be necessary to convey information and instruction. The patient may perform very slowly and methodically in an effort to be correct.[19] He is usually more successful in achieving self-care independence earlier than his counterpart with left hemiplegia.

Conclusion

When the patient has some or all of the perceptual and psychological problems discussed, the traditional rehabilitation goals for motor and functional retraining may be more than he can master. Rehabilitation goals cannot be based on the motor evaluation alone. Rather, the total scope of the disability must be considered, including sensory, perceptual, psychological, emotional, and intellectual impairments and the patient's social and family situation. If evaluation of the patient is inadequate, and inappropriate goals are set for him, the result will be frustration for the therapist, patient, and family.

Therapists must evaluate for and observe the effect of all of the concomitant dysfunctions as well as the motor dysfunction. If the limitations of the patient are clearly recognized and identified, realistic rehabilitation goals may be set. Retraining to the degree possible can be achieved, and the therapist, patient, and his family will feel a sense of achievement rather than failure in the rehabilitation program.[21]

OCCUPATIONAL THERAPY FOR CLIENTS WITH CVA

The role of the occupational therapist in the treatment of CVA that results in hemiplegia revolves around facilitating motor function and use of the affected side and restoring the client to his maximum level of independence.

Each client must be evaluated for his residual abilities and disabilities. A treatment program must be especial-

ly tailored to the client's particular needs, since the range of possible motor, sensory, perceptual, and cognitive dysfunctions after CVA is wide. The selection of treatment objectives and treatment methods will depend on factors such as stage of motor recovery, sensory-perceptual status, cognitive functions, age, date of onset, concomitant illness, social and economic factors, and potential for further recovery.

The occupational therapist may be involved in the acute care of the client and the early mobilization aspects of treatment. Later occupational therapy may be a primary service in extended rehabilitation when the emphasis is on achieving self-care independence and performance skills for work or leisure activities.

The role of occupational therapy

Evaluation.[5,20,23] The occupational therapist begins the program with a thorough evaluation of the client's deficits and assets to establish a baseline for progress. The evaluation process is continuous, beginning with the evaluation of motor and sensory status and simple self-care skills and progression to perceptual, cognitive, and more complex performance evaluations.

Motor functions. Degree of spasticity is estimated by evaluating the amount of resistance to passive movement (Chapter 7). This is usually performed by passively moving the elbow, wrist, and fingers through their ROMs. Quick motion is more likely to elicit the stretch reflex in clients who appear to have predominantly flaccid limbs. The stage of motor recovery can be estimated using Brunnstrom's test (Chapter 2). Abnormal movement patterns, presence of primitive reflexes, and equilibrium reactions should be evaluated. These may be the responsibility of or performed in conjunction with the physical therapist. Joint ROM is measured or estimated for limitations. Ability to perform isolated movement should be evaluated and coordination should be observed when the client has some control of voluntary movement.

Sensory-perceptual functions. Senses of touch, superficial pain, temperature, and pressure should be tested, using the methods described in Chapter 2. Olfactory and gustatory sensation may be tested using common household food items, since these senses are disturbed in some clients and are often overlooked. Stereognosis, proprioception, body scheme, and motor planning should be routinely evaluated. Visual perception, including tests for hemianopsia and visual-spatial relationships, should be included in the battery of evaluation procedures.

Cognitive functions. Memory, attention span, judgment, reasoning, abstract thinking, ability to follow instructions, motivation, and affect should be observed or tested.

Psychosocial factors. Through observation and inter-

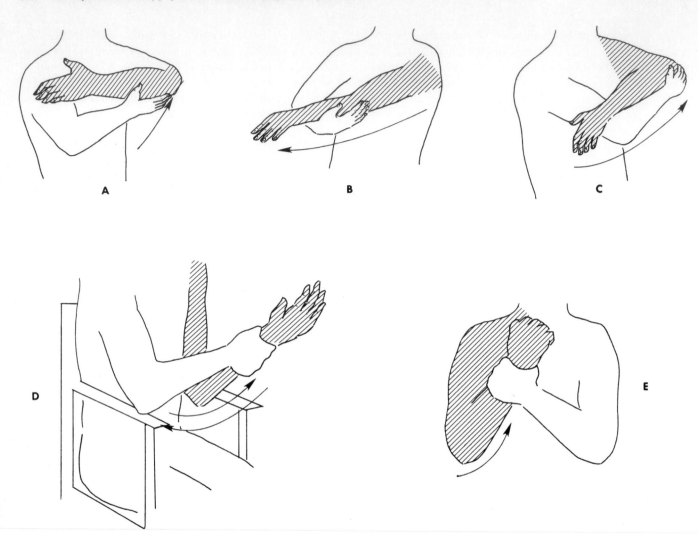

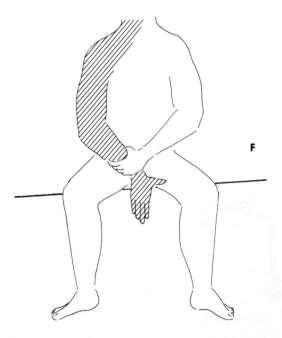

Fig. 13-2. Self-administered ROM procedures for person with hemiplegia. **A,** Affected arm is supported by unaffected arm and lifted into shoulder flexion to touch forehead. **B,** Affected arm is supported by unaffected arm to achieve adduction. **C,** Affected arm is moved to side to achieve shoulder abduction. **D,** Upper part of affected arm is stabilized between chest and wheelchair armrest. Unaffected arm moves affected arm into external and internal rotation. **E,** Unaffected arm flexes affected elbow. **F,** Unaffected arm brings affected arm down between legs to achieve elbow extension. **G,** Unaffected arm turns affected forearm into supination. **H,** Unaffected hand turns affected forearm into pronation. **I,** Unaffected hand flexes affected wrist. **J,** Unaffected hand extends affected wrist. **K,** Affected fingers are passively flexed into palm to achieve full flexion of MP and IP joints. **L,** Fingers are gently extended. If resistance is felt, they should be flexed once more and again extended, avoiding sudden stretch of finger flexors if there is spasticity.

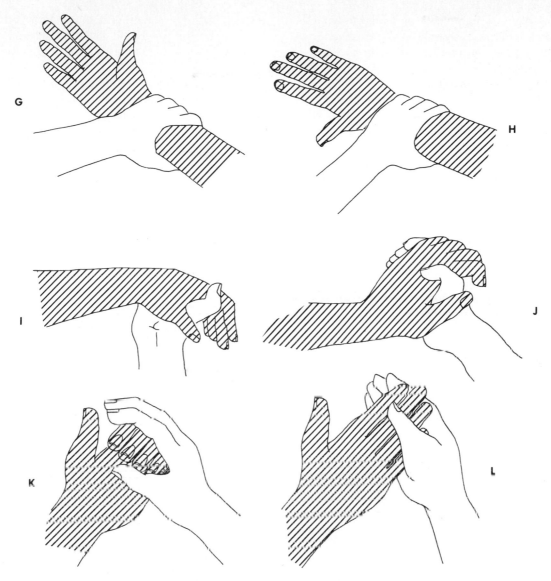

Fig. 13-2, cont'd. For legend see opposite page.

view of the client, family members, friends, or other rehabilitation team members, the occupational therapist should ascertain the client's vocational and recreational histories, role in the family and community, amount of family support, adjustment to disability, and frustration tolerance and coping skills.

Performance skills. Performance skills should be evaluated by interview and, more importantly, by actual performance of test items. Self-care and home management skills, mobility and transfer techniques, physical endurance, and work-related activities, if appropriate, should be included in the performance evaluation. It may take several weeks to complete the performance evaluation, which is an ongoing part of the treatment program.

Observation and periodic reevaluation should be carried out to record objective evidence of progress.

Treatment

Motor dysfunction. The occupational therapy program may include one or a combination of the sensorimotor approaches to treatment (Chapter 4) for the purposes of facilitating movement and use of the affected side, developing more normal postural reflex mechanisms, and inhibiting abnormal reflexes and movement patterns.

Therapists who do not use these approaches may use more traditional forms of therapeutic exercise, adapting them to the level of skills and movement of the client. Skateboard exercises are commonly used and can be adapted to use some of the patterns of motion suggested by Brunnstrom.

The maintenance of joint ROM and prevention of deformity is an important early goal in the treatment program and should be continued indefinitely if a substantial amount of spontaneous voluntary movement is not regained. This is achieved through positioning techniques such as those recommended by Bobath[4] and passive, assistive, and self-administered ROM procedures (Fig. 13-2). Both Bobath[4] and Brunnstrom[6] caution against the traditional passive ROM exercises to the shoulder in the absence of good scapular mobility. Passive flexion, abduction, and rotation of the glenohumeral joint to extreme ranges can be more harmful than helpful. Reciprocal pulley exercises, frequently used for maintenance of shoulder ROM, are usually contraindicated since they are forced passive exercise[6] and can cause joint pain and possibly damage if there is inadequate scapular mobility.

Subluxation of the humerus from the glenoid fossa is a common problem in hemiplegia. The rotator cuff muscles are probably of primary importance in the maintenance of joint stability. The function of the supraspinatus muscle is especially important to the prevention of subluxation. Brunnstrom[6] recommends procedures to activate the muscles surrounding the shoulder joint as a means of preventing subluxation. Occupational therapists have often applied arm slings to the client for wear when the arm is in a dependent position (Fig. 13-3). The purpose was to prevent or retard the progress of shoulder subluxation by avoiding stretch of the joint capsule and rotator cuff muscles. The benefits of such a sling are questionable. Brunnstrom states that such a sling, if properly fitted and worn, could hold the humeral head in the glenoid fossa but is of no value in activating mus-

cles. Bobath,[4] on the other hand, maintains that subluxation cannot be prevented if the muscles are weak and that slings only contribute to poor positioning, pain, and swelling.

Flexor spasticity in the hand musculature can result in wrist flexion and a fisted position, which can progress to contracture and deformity if not prevented. Resting splints in the functional position have been used to avoid the position of deformity. However, there is a lack of agreement about the benefits of various types of splints. Volar splints are thought to provide cutaneous stimulation to the flexor muscles, thus contributing to an increase of spasticity. Constructing splints that are applied to the dorsal surface of the forearm and hand provide sensory stimulation to the extensor surface and thereby are thought to enhance extensor tone, which is a desirable effect.[19] Techniques to facilitate relaxation of spastic wrist and finger musculature followed by gentle passive ROM, which is done to avoid stretch of the relaxed musculature, may be adequate to prevent the flexion deformity of the hand, if done regularly.

Some occupational therapists use a broad wheelchair armrest to support the arm when the client is inactive and is sitting or moving about in the wheelchair. These armrests are commercially available or may be custom made at the treatment facility. They fit on the regular wheelchair armrests and are removable. The client's arm should be stabilized in the trough of the armrest by straps, or the trough should have a fence on the lateral side to prevent possible injury to the arm and hand if they bump into walls and furniture. These armrests are usually padded and some have positioning devices to maintain the hand in a functional position. Rubber balls

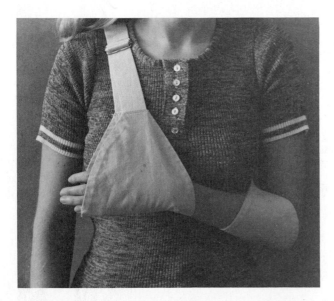

Fig. 13-3. Double loop arm sling for hemiplegia.

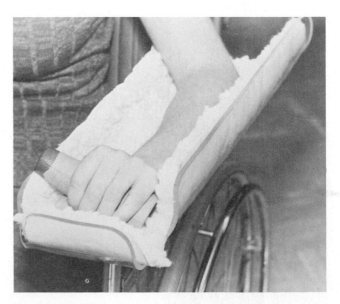

Fig. 13-4. Wheelchair armrest with yarn spool positioned in hand.

or other soft objects such as a wadded washcloth should *not* be used for this purpose. Soft objects tend to increase flexor spasticity, which is an undesirable effect, whereas it is thought that firm pressure over tendons has an inhibitory effect. Therefore grasping a hard object may have a more beneficial effect in inhibiting spastic muscles. A cone made of a thermoplastic material or from a large spool of yarn can be used to enhance the functional position of the hand. It should be positioned with the wide end on the ulnar side of the hand.[19] (Fig. 13-4).

The occupational therapist should use therapeutic activities as early as possible. These will enhance development of alertness, interest, and motivation and will provide opportunities for socialization and communication. In addition they should be selected to accommodate for use of the affected extremities. In the earliest phases of recovery the affected arm may be used as a passive stabilizer of objects or materials. As recovery progresses, the affected arm can take an increasingly active role in bilateral activities. Examples of some therapeutic activities that have been used effectively to include the affected upper extremity are weaving, leather lacing, braid weaving, sanding and other woodworking processes, and letterpress printing. When planning therapeutic activities the therapist needs to take into account the client's sensory, perceptual, and cognitive dysfunctions. It is important for the client to be successful at accomplishing the tasks. This can only be achieved if the tasks chosen are within his capabilities.

Performance skills. Training in ADL is a primary function of the occupational therapy service. Specific procedures are described in Chapter 4. Early in the rehabilitation process this may include wheelchair mobility and transfer skills (Chapter 5) and simple self-care activities, such as feeding and oral hygiene. Training in more complex bathing and dressing skills might be added later. As the client progresses in independent performance of the skills of self-maintenance, evaluation and training in appropriate home management activities should be included in the ADL program.

Unless there is adequate, spontaneous function of the affected arm, these skills should be learned using one-handed methods. Activities that require skill and safety such as ironing and using the stove and appliances and those that should be relaxing and pleasurable such as eating should be performed with the unaffected arm.

Coordination and skill training in one-handed performance is an important part of both the therapeutic activities and ADL programs. This is especially valuable if it is the dominant upper extremity that has been affected and if a change in dominance must be accomplished.

The client must learn methods of stabilizing objects and equipment for one-handed performance. He must learn to use assistive devices and equipment adapted to ease functioning with one hand. It is the role of the occupational therapist to acquire the necessary assistive devices and train the client in their use.

Some activities that can be adapted to one-handed performance and that can train in coordination are leather crafts, oil painting, mosaic work, minor woodworking, and some needlecrafts (Fig. 13-5).

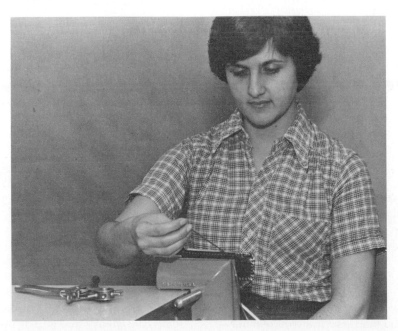

Fig. 13-5. Leather lacing is craft that can be one-handed skill if small bench vise is used to stabilize project.

In some cases one-handed performance may be necessary as a temporary measure, and in many others it will be a permanent mode of functioning. Usually the unaffected extremities will perform the primary and more complex motor functions required in activities, and the affected limbs will play an assistive role.

Sensory retraining. Occupational therapy may include sensory reeducation and techniques to compensate for sensory, perceptual, and cognitive dysfunctions.

Techniques of sensory retraining have met with limited success. Therapists have used increased sensory stimulation in the form of cutaneous stimulation to the affected parts with terry cloth,[12] proprioceptive stimulation in the form of joint approximation, and weighting of the extremities to increase the proprioceptive feedback. A technique to improve stereognosis is described by Ferreri[10] for adults with hemiplegia resulting from cerebral palsy. This involved comparing two dissimilar objects or forms, first with the unaffected hand and then with the affected hand. The therapist verbalized about the characteristics of the objects or forms during the manipulation process. The same training item was used for each session until the subject achieved five successive correct responses in the test portion of the session. Then a new training object was substituted. The investigator met with some success in improving stereognostic function of the subjects of the study.[10] This technique could be applied to adult clients with CVA. Visualization of the training objects could be used to facilitate the perception of tactual and proprioceptive qualities of the training objects.

Teaching compensation for sensory losses through vision is a common approach to dealing with sensory deficits. The client must be trained to monitor the location and position of the extremities. The therapist may do this by frequently reminding him to watch for the position of the limbs and helping him to include this visual monitoring as a regular part of the routine of moving and by adjusting position.[19] Success in teaching visual compensation is limited. If the client has disturbances such as homonymous hemianopsia, denial of the affected side, body scheme disorder, or memory deficits, it may not be possible for him to compensate in these ways. In addition, even for those who are alert enough and who do not have the added disturbances, it is difficult to watch out for a sensory-deficient limb when actively engaging in an activity and focusing on its goal. For example, it is not possible to watch the hand to see that it is holding a spoon and also to focus on the goal of eating.

Another method used to deal with sensory, perceptual, and cognitive deficits is adapting the environment. Using color or auditory cues, working in a nondistracting environment, and special methods of instruction may be employed.[19] Instructions must be broken down into very simple and small steps and presented one at a time. The number of steps the client is expected to perform is gradually increased. Repetition of instruction is necessary. As tasks are mastered in a completely nondistracting environment, the client may be asked to perform in increasingly stimulating environments until he can perform adequately in the clinic or home environment.

Psychosocial adjustment. An important role of the occupational therapist is to aid in the client's adjustment to hospitalization and, more importantly, to disability. A patient and supportive approach by the therapist is essential. The therapist must be empathetic to the fact that the client has experienced a devastating and life-threatening illness. Sudden and dramatic changes in life roles and performance have resulted. The therapist must be cognizant of the normal adjustment process (Chapter 1) and gear approach and performance expectations to the client's stage of adjustment. Frequently the client is not ready to engage in rehabilitation measures with wholehearted effort until several months after the onset of the disability.

Many clients will dwell on the possibility of full recovery of function and will need to gradually be made aware that some residual dysfunction is very likely. The therapist may approach this by discussing what is known about prognosis for function recovery from CVA in objective terms. This may need to be reviewed many times with the client before he begins to apply the information to his own recovery. This should be done in a way that is honest, yet does not rob the client of all hope. The therapist can present the information about the usual period for spontaneous recovery. She should indicate that the final outcome, in terms of function, cannot be accurately determined until at least 1 year after the CVA onset.

The occupational therapy program should focus on the remaining skills and abilities of the client. His attention should be focused, through the performance of activity, on his remaining and newly learned skills. Therapeutic group activities for socialization and sharing common problems and their solutions can be included.

The discovery that there are residual abilities and perhaps new abilities and success at performing many daily living skills and activities that were initially thought to be impossible can have a beneficial effect on the client's mental health and outlook. The occupational therapy program can be thought of as a laboratory for real living in which skills are learned and practiced and abilities are recovered or discovered.

Home evaluation. As the client nears discharge to home and community, the occupational therapist should be involved in a home evaluation (Chapter 2), and vocational or leisure skills potential should be explored. A living situation should be recommended that accommodates the client's needs. The occupational therapist, having evaluated self-care and home management skills performance, should be the most qualified to estimate the client's potential for independent living. Clients with hemiplegia will range from those who can resume living independently to those who require continuous supervision and assistance. The outcome depends on the severity of the CVA, success in rehabilitation, mental status, and social factors.

Gradation of treatment. The manner and speed with which treatment is graded will depend on the client and the treatment approach. If the Brunnstrom approach is used, facilitation techniques should be decreased as voluntary control of motion is improved. The amount of resistance in exercise and activity should be decreased as control and coordination are gained. The difficulty of performance skills demanded can be increased as synergistic movement subsides, and isolated voluntary motion is possible.[16]

Treatment time and time spent in standing and ambulation activities can be gradually increased to improve endurance. The complexity and number of ADL can be increased as physical, perceptual, and cognitive functioning improves. The amount of assistance given during transfers and for all activities should be decreased as independence is increased.

Conclusion. The reader should consider that the degree to which the client achieves treatment goals will depend on the CNS recovery and the facilitation and utilization of that recovery by therapists, client, and family. Some clients will remain severely disabled in spite of the noblest efforts of rehabilitation workers, and others will recover quite spontaneously with minimal help in a short period of time.

SAMPLE TREATMENT PLAN

Case study

Mr. S. is a 59-year-old man who worked as a trucker until he suffered a CVA 6 weeks ago. He lives with his wife and teenage daughter in a modest, three-bedroom suburban home. He is their sole support.

Before the onset of CVA Mr. S. was a very hard worker and enjoyed working around the house doing repairs and gardening. Cooking and furniture refinishing were his hobbies.

His wife and teenage daughter are very loving but are exhibiting signs of oversolicitiousness and denial of Mr. S.'s limitations and the potential residual disability. Mr. S. is depressed and is expressing feelings of worthlessness because of the loss of his role as worker and breadwinner. He is beginning to sense his family's unrealistic attitude and feels he has to "play along" with them. He resents this and would prefer to be open and get on with the business of dealing with life adjustments.

The CVA resulted in right hemiplegia and mild expressive aphasia. Mr. S. is now able to ambulate with a quadruped cane under supervision. He walks slowly and occasionally loses his balance. He tolerates standing and walking activities up to 10 minutes. His right upper extremity exhibits beginning spasticity and some evidence of the flexor and extensor synergies, which can be elicited reflexly.

Mr. S. has been in the occupational therapy program since the first week of hospitalization for maintenance of ROM, development of sitting balance, and training in simple self-care skills. He is now referred for improvement of the function of the right upper extremity, improvement of standing balance and tolerance, increased performance of self-care skills, and aid with adjustment to the disability.

Treatment plan*

A. **Statistical data.**
 1. Name: Mr. S.
  Age: 59
  Diagnosis: Cerebral vascular accident, 6 weeks after onset
  Disability: Right hemiplegia, expressive aphasia
 2. Treatment aims as stated in referral:
  Improve function of right upper extremity
  Improve standing balance and tolerance
  Improve performance of ADL
B. **Other services.**
 Physician: Supervision of rehabilitation team and provision of care
 Nursing: Provision of nursing and supportive care; follow through in self-care skills
 Social service: Assistance in family and social adjustment
 Speech therapy: Treatment of expressive aphasia
 Physical therapy: Gait training and improvement in LE function
C. **OT evaluation.**
 Stage of motor recovery: Test
 Strength of left arm: Test
 Standing tolerance: Observe
 Standing balance: Observe
 Walking tolerance: Observe
 Touch: Test

---

*Adapted from Abrams, E., Hittle, J., Mobley, M., and Reed, C.: Treatment plan for CVA, unpublished paper presented in partial fulfillment of the requirements of O.T. 167, San Jose, Calif., November 1978, Department of Occupational Therapy, San Jose State University.

Continued.

SAMPLE TREATMENT PLAN—cont'd

C. OT evaluation—cont'd
 Pain: Test
 Temperature: Test
 Stereognosis: Test
 Proprioception: Test
 Body scheme: Test
 Visual fields: Test
 Visual-spatial relationships: Test
 Memory: Test and observe
 Motivation: Observe
 Judgment and reasoning: Observe
 Problem solving: Test and observe
 Expression: Observe
 Adjustment to disability: Observe
 Self-care: Test
 Homemaking: Test
 Attempts at use of involved extremity: Observe
D. Results of evaluation.
 1. Evaluation data.
  a. Physical resources.
   (1) Strength: Left upper extremity within normal limits; right upper extremity not tested because of spasticity
   (2) ROM: Right shoulder flexion and abduction limited to 90°; all other joints within normal limits
   (3) Standing tolerance and balance: Moderate impairment; unable to stand without cane and fatigues after 10 minutes
   (4) Sitting balance: Trunk stability sufficient to maintain sitting position
   (5) Walking tolerance: With assistive devices patient walks slowly for short distances
   (6) Stage of recovery—stage 2: Flexion synergy is slightly stronger than extension synergy. Extension synergy is stronger in lower extremity. Client exhibits proximal traction response and prone positioning for TLR, which elicits flexor tone.
  b. Sensory-perceptual functions.
   Touch: Intact
   Pressure: Intact
   Pain: Intact
   Temperature: Intact
   Stereognosis: Mildly impaired
   Proprioception: Mildly impaired
   Body scheme and praxis: Intact
   All visual tests: Within normal limits
  c. Cognitive functions.
   Memory: Intact visual memory and follows demonstrated instructions well; auditory memory and ability to follow verbal instructions slightly impaired
   Motivation: The patient is discouraged and shows a lack of motivation but responds well to praise and encouragement.
   Judgment and reasoning: Observed to be intact
   Problem solving: Intact
   Reading: Language skills seem to be intact.
   Writing: Difficult because of inability to use dominant hand
   Expression: The client has mild expressive aphasia. Speech is limited but comprehensible for communication of basic needs, opinions, and some abstract ideas. With cues, questioning, and some use of pictures, the therapist can elicit expression of Mr. S.'s ideas.
  d. Psychosocial functions. The client was a trucker and sole provider for his wife and teenage daughter. He exhibits depression and feelings of worthlessness related to loss of this role. His family denies his limitations and is overanxious to help. Before his stroke the client was a kindly, placid man, as described by his family, who enjoyed working around the house, cooking, and furniture refinishing.
  e. Prevocational potential. Mr. S. is considering the possibility that he will be forced into early retirement because of his age and disability and the nature of the work he did. He has a pension plan that includes disability benefits, and he hopes to take advantage of this. He wants to explore the possibility of performing more cooking, home maintenance, gardening, and furniture refinishing skills at home to use his retirement purposefully.
  f. Functional skills.
   Self-care: The client feeds himself independently and helps with grooming. He needs assistance with dressing and transfer skills. His mobility is limited for walking because of limited tolerance and balance. He can walk with supervision, using a quadruped cane, for short distances.
   Home management skills: Mr. S. is able to prepare a cold meal while sitting but is unable to use the range safely or perform household tasks that require standing and walking about. He can use some one-handed assistive devices and techniques for tasks such as cutting and spreading jam.
   Attempts at use of the affected upper extremity: The client exhibits attempts at use of the right arm about 50% of the time when confronted with bilateral activities. However, limited voluntary control renders

SAMPLE TREATMENT PLAN—cont'd

most of these unsuccessful at this time. The client is being encouraged to use the right arm whenever possible. He anticipates the improved motor function will make it possible to use the arm more effectively in the future.

2. Problem identification.
   a. Limited standing balance and tolerance
   b. ADL dependence
   c. Depression
   d. Limited ROM of the right shoulder
   e. Lack of voluntary control of motion
   f. Lack of skill and coordination in left hand (the unaffected, nondominant member)
   g. Changed role as financial provider
3. Assets.
   a. Realistic outlook about limitations, potential disability, and employment future
   b. Supportive and strong family unit
   c. Leisure interests
   d. Previous demonstration of good coping skills
   e. Financial security
   f. Homeowner

E Problem	F Specific OT objectives	G Methods used to meet objectives	H Gradation of treatment
f	Through instruction and practice left hand coordination will improve to the degree that Mr. S. can write his name and address legibly, with ease, and in no more than twice the time it takes to write with the dominant hand	Small leather lacing projects, stabilized in a table vise, requiring manipulation of needles and lacing with the left hand Mosaic tile trivet construction, using 1-inch tiles and a simple geometric design Writing practice, beginning with various sequences of lines, circles, and curves, as in the Palmer method, then progressing to series of letters and numerals[19]	Increase the complexity of the lacing stitch Decrease size of tiles and complexity of design Progress to words and then sentences
d	Given appropriate positioning and mobilization techniques, ROM of the right shoulder will increase from 90° of flexion and abduction to 110°, and all other upper extremity joints will be maintained at full ROM	Bed and wheelchair positioning techniques of Bobath for shoulder and shoulder girdle[4] Shoulder mobilization techniques of Brunnstrom[6] Self-administered ROM techniques with careful instruction to avoid stretching and pain; teaching techniques for relaxation of spastic hand musculature before proceeding with gentle ROM to the fingers Dowel exercises using a hand mitt with straps for bilateral exercise; left hand will guide dowel and thus right hand through ranges of shoulder motion, avoiding stretching and pain	Decrease facilitation and assistance as spasticity declines and active motion improves Grade from passive to active ROM techniques as voluntary control of isolated motion is gained
e	Given facilitation to enhance performance of the flexor and extensor synergies, on a reflex basis, the client will be able to perform these synergies at will at least 75% of the time in treatment sessions	Using Brunnstrom's movement therapy techniques flexor synergy will be elicited in the sitting position through: Rotation of head toward unaffected side (ATNR) Evoked as an associated reaction by giving resistance to below flexion on the unaffected side Proximal traction response—stretching flexors of one joint in right upper extremity to evoke flexion in all other joints	Stop use of reflexes and associative reactions as soon as the synergy patterns are fairly well established

Continued.

SAMPLE TREATMENT PLAN—cont'd

E Problem	F Specific OT objectives	G Methods used to meet objectives	H Gradation of treatment
e—cont'd		Local stimulation of biceps by rubbing or tapping[6] Facilitation will be accompanied by verbal commands to "pull your hand to your mouth" to elicit some voluntary control of the motion Extension synergy will be elicited through: Bilateral contraction of pectoralis major: therapist faces the client, supporting his arms in horizontal position, resistance is applied to medial side of normal arm as client is asked to adduct arms Head rotation toward affected side (ATNR) Stroking over triceps as elbow extension is attempted Bilateral rowing exercise against resistance Resistance to a push on the unaffected side[6] (work with extension synergy is to be emphasized so an imbalance will not occur)	Decrease other forms of facilitation as voluntary control is gained
	Given appropriate activities the client will use synergy patterns purposefully during the treatment session	The flexor and extensor synergies will be used with voluntary effort and control in: Skateboard exercises for "push" and "pull" in a diagonal plane across the body from right to left (push)	As recovery progresses, add combined movements such as arcs and figure eights on the skateboard
b	Through instruction and practice the client will be able to dress himself independently in no more than three times the time it takes a nondisabled adult to dress	Sanding, using the same push-pull pattern in a frontal plane Bilateral activities—pushing a broom or carpet sweeper, if standing and walking are adequate Leather lacing, using the extensor synergy to pull the lace Teach one-handed dressing techniques for pants, T-shirt, shirt, shoes, socks, and shorts	Sanding in a sagittal plane and leather lacing, using shoulder abduction and elbow extension to pull the lace away from the body Increase dressing speed Begin with one garment, T-shirt; progress to shirt, then shorts, socks, pants, and shoes

SAMPLE TREATMENT PLAN—cont'd

E Problem	F Specific OT objectives	G Methods used to meet objectives	H Gradation of treatment
a	Through participation in activities that require standing and walking the client's balance will improve and standing tolerance will increase to 20 minutes	While working on leather lacing, activities, client will be positioned in the stand-up table Client will begin to engage in light homemaking activities that require walking for short distances: meal preparation, table setting, and dusting Client will perform grooming activities in a standing position under supervision	Amount of support from the table will be decreased Later, client will stand at a high worktable without support Supervision is decreased as balance and stability are gained
c, g	Given twice weekly participation in an activity-oriented support group, the client will exhibit increased openness in communication of his feelings about disability and changed life roles, within the group	A group of 5 to 8 clients will meet biweekly for one and one half hours; the therapist will act as group facilitator; the group will initially be task oriented; activities such as exercises to music, simple crafts, and cooperative meal preparation will be used The group will move from the activity into discussion of the problems encountered during the activity, feelings about these, and solutions; the therapist will facilitate expansion of the discussion to include problems encountered beyond the activity and the treatment facility	Clients take increasing responsibility for planning the activities As group support and cohesiveness grows, discussion can include deeper feelings, and group members can act as facilitators

I. **Special equipment.**
 1. Ambulation aids.
   Cane: Quadruped then regular cane to provide support and balance during ambulation.
   Short leg brace: To position and stabilize the right ankle for ambulation
   Wheelchair: For early mobility before walking is feasible
 2. Splints. Dorsal resting splint: For maintaining the hand in the functional position to reduce flexor spasticity and increase extensor tone[19]
 3. Assistive devices.
   Rocker knife: For one-handed meat cutting
   Long-handle shoehorn: To facilitate donning shoes in a sitting position

   Elastic shoelaces: To eliminate the need to tie shoes
   Clip-on neckties: To eliminate the need to tie knots in necktie
   Suction brushes: One for washing left hand and fingernails, one for scrubbing vegetables
   One-handed cutting board: For slicing and peeling foods, spreading butter on bread, and making sandwiches
   Zim jar opener: For opening jars with one hand
   Pan holder: To stabilize pans on range while stirring
   Long-handle scrub sponge: For washing back and feet while bathing

REVIEW QUESTIONS

1. Define "hemiplegia."
2. List three other dysfunctions that could accompany the motor dysfunction in hemiplegia.
3. List the disturbances that are likely to result from occlusion to the ACA, MCA, PCA, and basilar artery.
4. Which artery is most frequently affected in CVA?
5. Define "transient ischemic attack."
6. Describe the dependence of motion on sensation in the normal sensorimotor process.
7. Besides the upper motor neuron paralysis of limbs and trunk after CVA, what other important motor disturbances can result?
8. Describe or draw a picture of the typical "resting posture" of the spastic upper extremity in hemiplegia.
9. List three poor prognostic signs for functional recovery of the arm, and tell how they inhibit function.
10. If recovery has progressed so that there is voluntary control of the flexion synergy and grasp, what can be expected in terms of functional use of the affected arm?
11. If recovery has progressed so that synergies no longer dominate and grasp and release can be performed, what can be expected in terms of functional use of the affected arm?
12. In which direction does return of function progress in the motor recovery after CVA?
13. What differences in performance can be expected between persons with right and left hemiplegia? What accounts for these differences?
14. What is the importance of comprehensive occupational therapy evaluation of clients with hemiplegia?
15. Describe two methods that are used to maintain ROM.
16. Compare two methods for dealing with shoulder subluxation and the rationale for each.
17. Which synergy predominates in the arm? Which predominates in the leg?
18. List three good prognostic signs for functional recovery of the arm.
19. List four activities in which patients may use the basic limb synergies. Explain how the motions required in the activity are like the synergy patterns.
20. Describe what is meant by "lability." How can it be dealt with during a treatment session?
21. Why is it contraindicated for the client to grasp a ball or another soft object?
22. How does body scheme disorder interfere with rehabilitation?
23. How would training be approached if there is a memory loss?
24. Describe apraxia. Give examples of apraxic behavior. How would it interfere with rehabilitation, and what training techniques would be useful with an apraxic patient?
25. How does aphasia differ from dysarthria?
26. Describe four suggestions for more effective communication with an aphasic client.
27. List four major elements of the occupational therapy program for hemiplegia. Describe the purposes of each.
28. How can occupational therapy assist with the psychosocial adjustment of the hemiplegic client?

REFERENCES

1. Ayres, A.J.: Perceptual motor training for children. In Approaches to the treatment of patients with neuromuscular dysfunction, Proceedings of study course IV, Third International Congress, World Federation of Occupational Therapists, Dubuque, Iowa, 1962, Wm. C. Brown Co., Publishers.
2. Banus, B.S., editor: The developmental therapists, Thorofare, N.J., 1971, Charles B Slack, Inc.
3. Bardach, J.L.: Psychological factors in hemiplegia, J. Amer. Phys. Ther. Assoc. **43:**792-797, 1963.
4. Bobath, B.: Adult hemiplegia: evaluation and treatment, ed. 2, London, 1978, William Heinemann Medical Books, Ltd.
5. Bonner, C.: The team approach to hemiplegia, Springfield, Ill., 1969, Charles C Thomas, Publisher.
6. Brunnstrom, S.: Movement therapy in hemiplegia, New York, 1970, Harper & Row, Publishers, Inc.
7. Buchwald, J.: General features of nervous system organization, Am. J. Phys. Med. **46:**89-103, 1967.
8. Chusid, J.: Correlative neuroanatomy and functional neurology, Los Altos, Calif., 1973, Lange Medical Publications.
9. Delacato, C., and Doman, G.: Hemiplegia and concomitant psychological phenomena, Am. J. Occup. Ther. **11:**186-187, 196, 1957.
10. Ferreri, J.A.: Intensive stereognostic training: effect on spastic cerebral palsied adults, Am. J. Occup. Ther. **16:**141-142, 1962.
11. Gilfoyle, E., and Grady, A.: Cognitive-perceptual-motor behavior. In Willard, H., and Spackman, C., editors: Occupational therapy, ed. 4, Philadelphia, 1971, J.B. Lippincott Co.
12. Hopkins, H.L.: Occupational therapy management of cerebral vascular accident and hemiplegia. In Willard, H.S., and Spackman, C.S., editors: Occupational therapy, ed. 4, Philadelphia, 1971, J.B. Lippincott Co.
13. Horwitz, B.: An open letter to the family of an adult patient with aphasia, Chicago, 1964, National Society for Crippled Children and Adults, Inc.
14. Larson, C.B., and Gould, M.: Orthopedic nursing, ed. 9, St. Louis, 1978, The C.V. Mosby Co.
15. Lorenze, E., and Cancro, R.: Dysfunction in visual perception with hemiplegia: relation to activities of daily living, Arch. Phys. Med. Rehab. **43:**514-517, 1962.
16. Perry, C.: Principles and techniques of the Brunnstrom approach to the treatment of hemiplegia, Am. J. Phys. Med. **46:**789-815, 1967.
17. Spencer, E.A.: Functional restoration. In Hopkins, H.L., and Smith, H.D.: Willard and Spackman's occupational therapy, ed. 5, Philadelphia, 1978, J.B. Lippincott Co.
18. Taber, C.: Taber's cyclopedic medical dictionary, Philadelphia, 1959, F.A. Davis Co.
19. Trombly, C.A., and Scott, A.D.: Occupational therapy for physical dysfunction, Baltimore, 1977, The Williams & Wilkins Co.
20. Venegas, N., and Del Pilar-Christian, M., editors: Occupational therapy for patients with physical dysfunction, Puerto Rico, 1967, University of Puerto Rico Press.
21. Williams, L.A.: Some non-motor aspects of cerebral vascular accident, unpublished paper in partial fulfillment of the requirements for the master of science degree, San Jose Calif., 1964, San Jose State College.
22. Wilson, D.: Hemiplegia, paper presented to the annual conference of the California Occupational Therapy Association, Moro Bay, Calif., 1969.
23. Wilson, D., and Caldwell, C.: Occupational therapy treatment guide, adult hemiplegia, Downey, Calif., 1968, Department of Occupational Therapy, Rancho Los Amigos Hospital. Mimeographed.

SUPPLEMENTARY READING

Anderson, E.K., and Choy, E.: Parietal lobe syndrome in hemiplegia, Am. J. Occup. Ther. **24:**13-18, 1970.
Bouchard, V.C.: Hemiplegic exercise and discussion group, Am. J. Occup. Ther. **26:**330-331, 1972.

Brunnstrom, S.: Motor behavior of adult hemiplegic patients: hints for training, Am. J. Occup. Ther. **15:**6-12, 1961.

Ferreri, J., and Tumminelli, J.: A swivel cock-up splint-type arm-trough, Am. J. Occup. Ther. **28:**6, 1974.

Haese, J.B., et al.: Attitudes of stroke patients toward rehabilitation and recovery, Am. J. Occup. Ther. **24:**285-289, 1970.

Huffman, A.L.: Biofeedback treatment of orofacial dysfunction: a preliminary study, Am. J. Occup. Ther. **32:**149-154, 1978.

Leff, R.B.: Teaching stroke patients to dial the telephone, Am. J. Occup. Ther. **30:**313-315, 1976.

Marmo, N.A.: A new look at the brain-damaged adult, Am. J. Occup. Ther. **28:**199-206, 1974.

Schwartz, R., Shipkin, D., and Cermak, L.S.: Verbal and nonverbal memory abilities of adult brain damaged patients, Am. J. Occup. Ther. **33:**79-83, 1979.

Silverman, E.H., and Elfant, I.L.: Dysphagia: an evaluation and treatment program for the adult, Am. J. Occup. Ther. **33:**382-392, 1979.

Snook, J.H.: Spasticity reduction splint, Am. J. Occup. Ther. **33:**648-651, 1979.

Stephens, L.C.: Introducing a stroke service in a general hospital setting, Am. J. Occup. Ther. **29:**418-422, 1975.

Steverson, B.T.: The Steverson sling for the flaccid hemiplegic, Am. J. Occup. Ther. **27:**44-46, 1973.

Chapter 14

Head injury in adults

BARBARA A. BAUM, O.T.R., and DIANE L. MEEDER, O.T.R.

During the evolution of rehabilitation medicine various metabolic, systemic, or traumatic injuries have come into focus. Sociological occurrences or changes in lifestyles can have a major effect on the types of disabilities that prevail. For example, with the advent of war an increased number of gunshot wounds or amputations could occur. In recent years changes in diet and exercise regime altered the attention of medical and allied health professionals to cardiac and stroke management. As society became more mobile, and the automobile developed into a necessity of life, again the focus of medical care was altered. Recently statistics on the occurrence of spinal cord injury and head trauma have forced those involved in acute and rehabilitation medicine to deal with a whole new set of concerns. The material presented in this chapter will deal only with head trauma.

The mechanism and occurrence of head injury, surgical management, and a description of the levels of recovery are briefly outlined. The patient's clinical picture, including the physical, cognitive, perceptual, functional, and psychosocial aspects, is described. The occupational therapy evaluation and treatment of these problems are also provided.

In 1975 10 million people, or 3.68% of the U.S. population, sustained a head injury significant enough to require medical attention.[10] In 1976 7.56 million Americans sustained a head injury.[13] A breakdown of the place of occurrence and severity of these injuries is presented in Tables 7 and 8. The occurrence and severity of head injury are sufficient to warrant the attention of medical and allied health personnel working in acute and rehabilitation medicine.

MECHANISM OF HEAD INJURY

Most head injuries are ". . . blunt injuries caused either by the moving head striking a static surface . . . or by the head being struck by a moving object."[21] The degree of deformation and damage sustained by the brain after the injury depends on the amount of acceleration or deceleration of the skull and its contents.[27] *Deceleration* refers to the sudden, rapid slowing of the moving head when it strikes a solid surface. *Acceleration* refers to the movement of the brain inside the skull when the

Table 7. Head injuries, 1976 (total 7,560,000)*

Place of occurrence	No. of injuries
Motor vehicle accident	1,202,000
At home	3,828,000
At play, in school, or in public domain	2,472,000
At work	196,000

*Based on data from Caveness, W.: Incidence of craniocerebral trauma in the United States with trends from 1900 to 1975, Adv. Neurol. **22:**1-3, 1979.

Table 8. Types of injury sustained, 1976 (total 7,560,000)*

Types of injuries	No. of injuries	
Superficial or minor		6,305,000
Lacerations of head	4,686,000	
Contusions of scalp, face, and neck, except eye	1,619,000	
Major		1,255,000
With concussion	644,000	
With skull fractures, extradural, subdural, or subarachnoid hematomas	611,000	

*Based on data from Caveness, W.: Incidence of craniocerebral trauma in the United States with trends from 1970 to 1975, Adv. Neurol. **22:**1-3, 1979.

☐ Barbara A. Baum, Administrative-education supervisor, Occupational Therapy Department, Santa Clara Valley Medical Center, San Jose, Calif.; Diane L. Meeder, Senior therapist—Head Injury Service, Occupational Therapy Department, Santa Clara Valley Medical Center, San Jose, Calif. The valuable contributions of Liane Michael and Linda Panikoff for their editorial assistance in the preparation of this chapter are greatly appreciated.

stationary head is struck. An additional type of head injury is a penetrating injury, which may be due to "low-velocity agents" or sharp objects or to high-velocity ballistic missiles. Low-velocity penetrating injuries generally result in local damage, whereas high velocity and acceleration-deceleration injuries will usually result in diffuse damage.

Forces can injure the brain by (1) compression (pushing the tissues together, (2) tension (tearing the tissues apart), or (3) shearing (sliding of portions of tissues over other portions). These three types of injuries can occur simultaneously or in succession.[27] Damage can occur where the blow was sustained (coup lesion) or to the intact skull opposite to where the blow was applied (contrecoup lesion).[21]

In addition to the primary damage sustained on impact, secondary events often follow that may develop a few hours or days after the onset, for example, hemorrhage, infection, and brain swelling.

For a detailed analysis and description of the mechanism and pathology of head injury, including primary and secondary damage, anoxia, and infectious encephalitis, the reader is referred to the references.* Although it is not vital that the reader have a detailed knowledge of the mechanisms of head injury, the concepts and terms used should be understood.

MEDICAL AND SURGICAL MANAGEMENT

The medical and surgical management of a person who sustains a severe head injury begins when he is rescued and brought into the emergency room. The patient with a severe head injury may experience many complications. Some of the major complications are increased intracranial pressure, wound infection or osteomyelitis, pulmonary infections, hyperthermia, shock, and associated injuries or fractures.[14]

When the patient arrives at the hospital, the first concern is to establish an unobstructed airway, and this may require suctioning, intubation, or tracheostomy. The patient may be in shock and may require intravenous fluids, plasma, blood transfusions, or vasopressor agents. The neurosurgeon then performs a neurological examination to determine the extent and severity of the head injury. The neurosurgeon may need to perform an emergency craniotomy after arteriography to reduce increased intracranial pressure and any demonstrated hematoma.[17]

Because of the patient's decreased level of awareness and decreased oral-bulbar status, nasogastric tube feedings or a gastrostomy procedure may be required to ensure that the patient gets adequate nutrition. This, compounded with a tracheostomy, will make it difficult to

---

*References 8, 12, 17, 21, 28, 30, 34.

establish the patient's oral-bulbar training as his overall level of awareness improves.

Posttraumatic seizures are also complications. These may begin as early as 1 week after sustaining a head injury in some patients and as late as 1 week to 10 years or more after injury in others.[17] In some cases seizures following head injury may never occur at all or may be controlled by medication prescribed by the physician. The patient may often be incontinent and may require catheterization; later in the rehabilitation phase, as these functions start to return, a bowel and bladder program may need to be established.

Once the patient has been medically stabilized and cleared by the physician, the occupational therapist may begin her evaluation and treatment program. It will be important for her to be aware of the medical and surgical management problems and precautions before establishing her treatment plan. Usually a patient with an open head injury will require a helmet before he gets up for the first time to protect the open skull from further brain injury in case the patient falls. Treatment should start as early as possible while the patient is in the intensive care unit but should be closely coordinated with the physician and nursing staff.

DESCRIPTION OF THE DYSFUNCTION
Recovery stages

The recovery of an individual from a severe brain injury can be extended and involve the physical, cognitive, visual-perceptual, psychosocial, and behavioral functions. The adult with head injury can regain lost functions rapidly, over a period of many years, or not at all. Moving out of coma through the rehabilitation stages to reenter the community is often a complicated and difficult process. No two patients will have the same clinical picture, problems, needs, or family support systems. There are many different methods for analyzing the stages of recovery or the changes in level of awareness that lead to a higher level of functioning. The following is an overview of some of the different methods of rating recovery in patients with head injury.

Neurological examination. In general the neurological examination performed by the physician describes the states of awareness as follows[17]:

Head injury with loss of consciousness

COMA: No response to painful stimuli

SEMICOMA: Withdrawal of a body part from a painful stimulus

STUPOR: Spontaneous movement and groaning in response to various stimuli

OBTUNDITY: Arousal by stimuli and response to a question or command; confusion and disorientation with poor judgment

FULL CONSCIOUSNESS: Recovery of orientation and memory; full recovery

Glasgow Coma Scale.[38] The Glasgow Coma Scale is the method most frequently used by the physician to categorize the levels of consciousness following a traumatic injury to the brain. This test is an attempt to quantify the severity of the brain injury and establish a baseline from which to predict the outcome of the patient. The physician using this scale assesses consciousness by three major areas: (1) motor responses, (2) verbal responses, and (3) eye opening.[38] The patient is then rated and assigned the corresponding number of points for the best response elicited.

Levels of awareness. Still another system used for evaluating a patient's level of awareness is one that was developed at Rancho Los Amigos Hospital in Downey, California. The Rancho Los Amigos scale uses the following eight levels: (1) no response; (2) generalized response; (3) localized response; (4) confused-agitated; (5) confused, inappropriate, nonagitated; (6) confused-appropriate; (7) automatic-inappropriate; and (8) purposeful-appropriate.[31]

In general the adult with head injury can be categorized as having primary or advanced head injury. The mechanism of a traumatic head injury and the resulting neurological impairment vary so much that it is extremely difficult to label or categorize the individual with brain damage. Whereas general trends for recovery can be seen in patients with head injuries, no two individuals have the same set of problems, rate of recovery, environment, disposition, or neurological deficits.

The patient at the primary level. The term *primary* is a classification used in the Head Injury Unit at the Santa Clara Valley Medical Center in San Jose, California, to describe the patient who is functioning at a very basic or low level, such as the comatose patient. The patient at the primary level may be at a low level in any one or a combination of the following areas:

1. *Severe motor impairment.* The patient may have severe spasticity, abnormal reflexes, and loss of motor control in any or all four limbs. Head and trunk control are severely impaired, and the patient is generally dependent in all self-care activities.

2. *Severe impairment of perceptual-motor skills.* The patient may have very poor gross visual skills and perceptual-motor skills that prevent him from being involved in any self-care or higher level functional activities, that is, severe motor planning problems prevent the patient from self-feeding or dressing and poor visual attentiveness and visual tracking prevent performance of the simplest ADL.

3. *Decreased functional cognition and behavior.* The patient with cognitive-behavioral deficits has extremely poor judgment, safety awareness, problem-solving abilities, and memory, which make him dependent in most functional tasks even though he may be physically intact.

Generally the patient at the primary level is very dependent or requires maximum assistance either physically, cognitively, perceptually, or in all three ways. A person may have severe motor involvement with perceptual and cognitive abilities intact. This is very frustrating for the patient at the primary level who has severe motor deficits, because he is "locked in" to his body and cannot communicate or control any aspect of his environment. On the other hand, the patient who has severe cognitive or perceptual deficits, but who has good motor skills, that is, can ambulate, may still be considered at the primary level because he cannot perform self-care activities or function safely without verbal cues and constant supervision. Memory may be so impaired that the patient shows limited carry-over in therapy from day to day. This patient is often referred to as the "walking wounded," that is, good motor function but poor cognitive abilities.

The patient at the advanced level. The term *advanced* is applied to the patient who may have cognitive, perceptual, motor, and behavioral deficits, but they are not significant enough to cause total dependence in ADL. The occupational therapist working with the patient at the advanced level must be able to correlate the physiological problems with the functional ones at this stage. The patient at the advanced level, unlike the patient at the primary level, has the potential to make an adaptive motor response and carry over learning in therapy toward achieving a functional goal. For example, the patient may now have sufficient equilibrium reactions and UE function to work on UE dressing while sitting with legs over the edge of the bed.

The overall level of awareness of the patient at the advanced level is higher, and he has a better ability to control more aspects of his environment and participate in his program. He still may have significant cognitive, perceptual, or motor deficits, but therapy can now be structured toward working on a functional goal such as feeding or dressing. It is important to assess whether the patient at the advanced level has sufficient memory and understanding to benefit from repetitive, structured training. The general aims of treatment for a patient at the primary level will be discussed later in this chapter and should help to clarify the distinguishing characteristics of the two levels.

Clinical picture

Physical aspects. The physical deficits encountered in patients with head injury can be quite severe and complex. One may see motor involvement of one to four extremities; decreased total body function, oral-bulbar status, sensation, coordination, balance, endurance, and ROM; abnormal reflexes, motor patterns, and muscle tone; muscle weakness; and poor isolated muscle control. The occupational therapist must have a good theoretical knowledge of these physical deficits to remedy them during sensorimotor and functional activities.

An injury to the brain from a traumatic insult has a different clinical picture from that typically seen in CVA. Bilateral motor involvement is frequently seen in head injury because the insult may occur at the brain stem or midbrain level, thus blocking impulses from being sent to the higher brain centers, or from lesions occurring in both the right and left hemispheres.[16]

Limitation of joint motion. Loss of ROM that results in contractures is a frequent problem. During the coma or acute rehabilitation phase patients can develop decorticate or decerebrate rigidity or posturing.[9] The failure of the brain to control or inhibit abnormal postural reflexes and hypertonicity may cause joint deformities and contractures. The prolonged immobilization of the comatose patient or patient with primary head injury, with severe spasticity enhances the development of possible joint ossification and calcification. It is extremely important in the early period after the onset to become aware of and start to control potential loss of ROM. In head injury a patient may start out with flaccid muscles and may very rapidly develop severe spasticity and deformities.

Muscle weakness. Most adults with head injury do not have muscle weakness. Rather, there is severe spasticity or excessive abnormal muscle tone. The patient without close to full isolated muscle control cannot have the muscle tested, for resistance applied to a spastic muscle would only set off the stretch reflex and would not truly test muscle strength.

Abnormal reflexes and tone. Abnormal postural reflexes are a common problem after head injury. Postural reflexes regulate the degree and distribution of muscle tone. The brain, depending on the site of the lesion, can no longer inhibit certain reflexes that were integrated at an earlier developmental stage.[7] The most common abnormal reflexes and reactions found are ATNR, STNR, and TLR; associated reactions; positive support reaction; extensor thrust; and decreased equilibrium, righting, and protective reactions. These abnormal reflexes and reactions affect ROM, muscle tone, and selective movements. Unless prevented or controlled through reflex-inhibiting postures and NDT, they may prevent the patient from making even basic physical and functional gains. Table 9 was developed to help define the abnormal postural reflex mechanism by giving (1) an observation of the problem, (2) the reflex underlying the problem, (3) the reflex-inhibiting posture or treatment, and (4) the possible functional implications. Specific reflex

testing must be performed to establish which abnormal reflexes are present. This table is not meant to imply that a mere observation of an abnormal pattern means that the abnormal reflex is present.

Patterns and isolated muscle control. The components of the flexor and extensor patterns have been described in Chapter 4. Patients with head injury will usually have severe flexor patterning of the upper extremities and extensor patterning of the lower extremities. Often a patient has a combined flexor-extensor pattern in the upper or lower extremities. The patient, for instance, may have spasticity in both the triceps and biceps. The muscle with a greater degree of hypertonicity has the stronger action. Until the patient's gross motor skills develop, he will not perform well in fine motor activities. Development of controlled movement usually progresses from proximal to distal, although at times it can occur segmentally. For example, without good, selective shoulder control, hand function and coordination will be limited. Gross grasp and release usually return in the adult with head injury before prehension.[7]

Many patients may have deficits in coordination at the trunk, head, and hips, as well as that typically seen in the upper and lower extremities. The origin of the incoordination must be analyzed to establish an effective treatment plan.

Ataxia. Ataxia is an abnormality of movement and a disordered muscle tone that is seen in patients with damage to the cerebellum or the sensory pathways to result in a cerebellar or sensory ataxia. A patient may have ataxia of the total body, trunk, or upper or lower extremities or may have gait ataxia. The normal flow of a smooth voluntary movement is destroyed by errors in the direction and speed of movement.[26] Ataxia ranges from mild to severe and can be a significant impediment to achieving a functional goal. The therapist must carefully assess the joints most affected by ataxia to control it and reduce its limitation on function.

Spasticity. Spasticity is one of the most frequent and damaging physical problems encountered in head injuries. Spasticity is the activation of a hyperactive stretch reflex with resultant hypertonicity.[40] It ranges from minimal to severe in any particular muscle or muscle group. Spasticity may occur in combined flexor and extensor patterns, thus making its inhibition more complicated. Usually flexor spasticity predominates in the upper extremities, and extensor spasticity predominates in the lower extremities.

Loss of sensation and perception. The most common sensory and perceptual losses seen are decreased proprioception, response to deep pain, superficial pain, touch, and stereognosis; and diminished temperature sense, two-point discrimination, and kinesthesia. The patient may also have impaired senses of taste and smell,

Table 9. Abnormal postural reflex mechanisms

Observation	Reflex	Reflex-inhibiting posture and treatment	Functional implication
Severe plantar flexion, clawing of toes, inversion of ankle	Positive supporting reaction—extensor tone predominates	Dorsiflexion of toes to shift weight to heel (hips and knees will want to flex) Foot wedge and mini foot splint for dorsiflexion of toes	Cannot bear weight without facilitating extensor pattern; poor balance reactions with rigid limb, small base of support for foot
Neglect of one side and head off to right or left	ATNR—increased extensor tone on jaw (preferred) side and increased flexor tone on skull (neglected) Rule out visual-perceptual deficits	Head and neck in midline; turning and tracking to skull side Head devices, neck collars, turning to auditory stimulus or getting neck rotating during feeding training	Prevents reach, grasp, and midline activity; imbalance of muscle tone, decreasing selective movement, mostly in upper extremities
Severe flexor spasticity of upper extremities, severe extensor tone of lower extremities	STNR—flexed head increases flexor tone of upper extremities and extensor tone of lower extremities and vice versa	Extend head-neck to increase extensor tone of upper extremities and flexor tone of lower extremities Consider key points of control to decrease spasticity, not just reflex Other methods—heat, cold, casting	Will affect coordination, reciprocal movements, total body function; can develop contractures; decreased ability to bear weight on upper extremities in transfers
Severe extensor spasticity and adduction of lower extremities when supine in bed	TLR—extensor tone predominates in supine and flexor tone in prone (depends on position of head in space)	Key points of control In supine position abduct hips and flex knees In sitting position hip flexion works to break pattern Knee abductor, seat wedge	Cannot roll over, that is, bend leg to roll or bring shoulder forward to roll; decreased mobility, sitting, and transfers; cannot bear weight on lower extremities
Increased spasticity in arm while ambulating	Associated reactions—increased spasticity in some part of the body produced by forceful activity of another part	Must take care in using resisted activity in spastic conditions even of sound limb, as it can cause associated reaction	Functional activities such as writing and dressing and other purposeful movements of sound hand can increase flexor spasticity of affected hand

depending on the cranial nerves involved. The primary-level patient's response to pinprick or deep pain can help to establish his level of awareness. Evaluation of a patient at the primary level is discussed later in this chapter.

Abnormal posturing. Along with the abnormal reflexes and hypertonicity, postural problems can develop. Frequently kyphosis and scoliosis are seen in patients with head injuries because of the imbalanced muscle tone that puts an unequal pull and stress on the skeletal system, thus pulling the body into several possible abnormal postures. It is important to know the biomechanics of the body and prevent deformities rather than to try to deal with them after the poor posture has developed.

Decreased physical capacity. Decreased vital capacity, endurance, and general tolerance for an exercise or activity are common problems of head injury. Having gone through medical complications such as pneumonia, prolonged bed rest, or immobilization, the patient with head injury who suddenly starts getting up in a wheel-

chair will be easily fatigued or overloaded. The comatose patient or patient at the primary level must be closely monitored for changes in blood pressure and vital signs the first few times he gets up.

Loss of total body function control. Total body function skills include head and trunk control, sitting and standing balance, reaching, bending, stooping, and functional ambulation. At the acute phase of the patient's recovery, decreased head and neck, trunk, and hip control are encountered along with the upper and lower extremity losses. Sitting balance and the ability to support oneself with the legs over the edge of the mat or the bed are poor. The patient at the primary level has a tendency for excessive forward flexion of the neck or too much hyperextension. The patient at the advanced level exhibits such problems as poor sitting or standing balance and difficulty bending and stooping and reaching to high or low areas. Total body function skills are necessary for performing higher level functional skills, such as functional ambulation during a kitchen activity.

Cognitive-behavioral aspects. As previously described, there are several levels of awareness that the patient with head trauma may exhibit. As he begins to progress out of a semicomatose state, he will be able to tolerate more formal cognitive testing. At this stage the therapist may begin to realize how severely impaired the patient may be. In most rehabilitation facilities the speech pathologist or psychologist performs the structured cognitive evaluations. It is necessary, however, for all members of the rehabilitation team to have a working knowledge of the cognitive problems that may appear and how to deal with these problems in the most effective way for the patient.

The occupational therapist should direct attention to areas that may affect the patient's functional status. Some problems that are frequently seen may be disorientation; decreased level of attention, safety awareness, and insight into disability; impaired memory, sequencing, judgment, and problem-solving skills; and decreased ability to process information accurately and think abstractly.

Reduced attention level and concentration ability. Reduced level of attention and the ability to concentrate may seriously affect functional independence. Most normal individuals find it difficult to concentrate on reading while the radio or television is on or people are talking nearby. One has to be able to tune out nonessential stimuli in the environment. One must also be able to attend to stimuli that are important to the task at hand. Patients with head trauma may be unable to distinguish those stimuli that are pertinent to successful performance. The patient with head injury often loses not only the ability to filter out distraction, but also his ability to concentrate for any length of time may become severely limited.

Impaired sequencing. Sequencing is the ability to accurately process information in steps or sequentially. One does this automatically primarily through the visual and auditory modes. Because of the extensive disruption of CNS functions, these skills may be severely disturbed in the patient with a head injury. He may be able to process information presented visually, but not information presented audibly. He may be able to process the information through both systems, but with extreme delay. For example, the patient may understand a request even though there may be significant time lag before the message has been processed, and a response is made. At times he may be able to process information only when it is presented in the simplest manner. Instructions involving long explanations, specific sequence of direction, or complex, unfamiliar vocabulary may hinder performance. It is vital for the occupational therapist to know exactly what the patient's processing abilities are to establish an appropriate treatment approach.

Decreased safety awareness. The patient with head injury often displays unsafe behavior. This may be a result of impulsiveness, decreased insight into his disability, impaired judgment, or a combination of all of these. Decreased insight, disorientation, and impaired memory can contribute to the patient's inability to recognize his limited abilities for specific situations or analyze the consequences of his actions. It is therefore imperative that all members of the treatment team assist the patient in structuring his environment and understanding his limitations to maximize relearning of appropriate, safe behavior.

Impaired memory. Impaired memory is probably one of the most devastating problems that the patient with head injury must face. There are several types of memory impairments, ranging from the inability to recall a few words just heard to remembering events that occurred a few months or years before the injury. Although the degree of severity differs with each patient, the majority of patients with head injuries will have some level of impaired memory. This manifests itself in the inability to learn and carry over new tasks and contributes to confusion and inability to participate in the environment.

Impaired intellectual functions and abstract thinking. An additional aspect of impaired cognition is that of reduced intellectual functioning. The patient has lost the ability to solve problems, analyze information presented, and come up with appropriate solutions. He is unable to structure his own thoughts and may require external structure from those around him. He may be able, with some assistance, to recognize his errors but may be unable to resolve the errors without external cuing. Patients with head injury tend to analyze problems in concrete terms, interpreting all information at the most literal level. The ability to think abstractly and generalize knowledge and experience is usually significantly impaired. Functional independence demands the mastering and manipulation of basic cognitive and academic skills such as categorizing, calculating, and generalizing experiences. The occupational therapist must consider and incorporate these critical cognitive skills into the treatment plan.

Aberrant behavior. Common aberrant behavior that the patient with head injury displays includes distractibility, agitation, combativeness, emotional lability, inappropriate affect, and socially unacceptable behavior. The patient who is unable to filter distractions will become agitated in a noisy environment. The patient with limited insight will become frustrated and at times combative when unable to perform simple tasks. Most patients with head injury are unable to process and respond to excessive stimulation, and as a result, a turning off, or shutdown of systems, occurs. When this happens, he is no longer able to participate effectively.

Depending on the area of the brain affected, the patient may show an inability to control his emotions. He may show inappropriate outbursts of anger, tears, or laughter. He may be socially inappropriate in his behavior, shouting obscenities or making indiscriminate sexual advances. At the other extreme he may display flat affect or passivity or may lack initiative, interest, or participation in his environment. This lack of participation may be interpreted as poor motivation on the patient's part when in fact this apparent lack of responsiveness is the result of organic damage. It is important to recognize that the behavior exhibited by the patient with head injury correlates significantly with his level of cognitive function.

Cognitive and behavioral aspects of head injury are vast and complicated. This constitutes an overview of areas that pertain to occupational therapy. For a detailed analysis of cognitive functions as they relate to head injury, the reader is referred to the references.[18,24] Practical remediation techniques are discussed in the treatment section of this chapter.

Perceptual-motor aspects. The ability to accurately perceive and respond to people and objects within the environment is necessary for successful, independent function. Disruption of various pathways within the CNS can cause the patient with head injury to have difficulty with a multitude of perceptual-motor skills that were previously taken for granted. Depending on the nature and extent of damage, the impairment may involve gross visual-perceptual or perceptual-motor skills.

Impaired gross visual-perceptual skills. Gross visual skills involve basic abilities such as visually attending to a task or effectively scanning the environment. The patient with head injury is often unable to focus on an object for more than a few seconds. When asked to follow a moving object with his eyes, incomplete scanning and jerky eye movements may be present. Inattentiveness and impaired scanning may be further complicated by the presence of either homonymous hemianopsia or visual-spatial neglect. Homonymous hemianopsia can be described as "blindness of right-sided or left-sided fields of both eyes."[35]

Apraxia. The ability to determine the appropriate type and sequence of movement to perform a task is praxis or motor planning. Despite intact sensation, motor power, or coordination, the patient with head injury may exhibit impaired motor planning skills, or apraxia. One or more types of apraxia may be apparent. The patient may be able to carry out tasks that involve one limb and at the same time may be unable to perform tasks that involve total body movement. He may be unable to blow out a match but can cut paper with scissors. If asked to pantomime, some patients are unable to demonstrate how a task is performed unless allowed to use the necessary objects. For example, at the most concrete level a patient may be unable to show you how he would drink water from a glass unless provided with a full glass of water when he happens to be thirsty. The

presence of any of these motor planning impairments, combined with additional cognitive problems, can be a source of extreme frustration for the patient. His apraxia is often unjustly interpreted by members of the team as uncooperative behavior. It is vital therefore for the occupational therapist to accurately assess the patient's motor planning abilities to avoid unreal expectations and mislabeling of the patient's behavior.

Constructional apraxia is "the inability to produce designs in two or three dimensions by copying, drawing or constructing, upon command, or spontaneously."[35] The patient with a head injury with damage to the right side of the brain may show a lack of perspective and poor spatial relations. Those patients with damage to the left side of the brain may show a tendency toward simplicity of design and difficulty in the execution of the requested tasks. There has been considerable documentation on the relationship between constructional praxis abilities and the ability to dress.[23,43] Because of this high correlation between abilities the occupational therapist must include a constructional praxis evaluation in her perceptual-motor testing.

Impaired body scheme. Impaired body image and impaired body scheme are related but are not identical perceptual disorders. Body image is the "visual and mental memory image of one's body."[35] A patient's body image, often tested by the Draw a Man test, reveals his feelings and perceptions about himself. Body scheme relates to the ability to perceive one's body position and the relationship of body parts. To deal effectively with objects within the environment, the patient must develop an internal awareness of his body and its parts.[33] The patient with impaired body scheme will not know how to move around in his environment effectively.[1]

Impaired figure-ground perception. The ability to distinguish an object from its background visually is figure-ground perception. The patient with figure-ground impairment may have difficulty locating an item on a supermarket shelf or finding an item in a cluttered drawer. A white facecloth placed on the white sheets of his bed may be missed. Severe figure-ground impairment can obviously have a dramatic effect on function.

Impaired position-in-space perception. Position-in-space perception is the ". . . ability to understand and deal with concepts of spatial position such as up-down, in-out, right-left, before-behind."[35] The therapist who is treating the patient with impaired position-in-space perception must carefully analyze how she instructs the patient to follow commands. For example, the patient may not be able to conceptualize a command such as "Get your toothbrush, which is behind your comb." Taken at its extreme the patient with severely impaired perception of position in space may be unable to make a sandwich, because he cannot place the lunchmeat "in between" two slices of bread. Some remaining areas of impaired perception that may appear in the patient with head injury are form and size discrimination, part-whole visualization, and depth perception. A classic example of impaired form perception is the patient who mistakes his water pitcher for a urinal.[35] The patient with impaired part-whole perception, when presented visually with only part of an object, may not be able to synthesize the parts to identify the object correctly. A hair dryer may be mistaken for a telephone. Impaired depth perception will affect the patient's ability to ambulate on stairs or on uneven surfaces such as the ground.

• • • •

From this summary of perceptual problems found in patients with head injury, the reader may be led to believe that impairments occur in an isolated manner. This is rarely the case. Rather, the therapist is usually presented with a patient who has a constellation of problems. The therapist's job is to carefully observe the patient's behavior and interpret the reasons or impairments underlying abnormal responses.

Psychosocial factors. The psychosocial aspects of head injury are frequently overlooked but can be key components to the success of the patient's recovery process. It is important to know the family and social history along with previous personality characteristics, for as the patient's level of awareness improves, these traits will start to appear again, possibly in an exaggerated way.

Family support is an important concept when dealing with head injury. It can be a determining factor in the patient's level of motivation to achieve functional independence. Family and friends are an integral part of the rehabilitation process, especially in the beginning stages, since they may be able to elicit a response from the patient when no one else can.

Family role alterations and the patient's coping mechanisms for dealing with these role changes must be considered. The patient may go from being an extremely independent individual to being totally dependent, and this is very frustrating and degrading for him. It will be difficult for both the patient and the family members or significant others to cope. No matter how cognizant the family and the patient are of the disability, it disrupts the family structure. It is often difficult for family members to understand the uncontrolled behavior they observe in their loved one.

Mood and affect can have frequent swings, with the patient being unable to control these variations in how he feels. He may be inappropriately friendly and indiscriminate in his affections. As the patient becomes more aware of himself and his environment again, he may be depressed by a sense of loss. He may suddenly start to perceive the confinements of his current world and begin to face the fact that he is no longer what he used to be.

The alteration of sexual functioning and the ability to deal with sexual needs and feelings can occur. The patient may lack the impulse control to keep from making sexual advances toward others. These impulsive advances may be coupled with verbal abuse, and often the patient is not cognitively aware of what he is doing. Memory deficits further complicate this problem. He may not remember that the woman he is making advances toward is his therapist or nurse.

Previous educational status and values play an important part in the patient's progress toward independence. These factors must be incorporated into the long-term treatment plan. Eventual discharge plans must be set up to meet the needs of the patient. For example, a patient who had a learning disability before his head injury and always had difficulty in school may not benefit from a traditional college program but rather from a disabled students' program, directed toward the specific problem areas, at a community college.

A lack of insight into the disability can be a serious problem affecting adults with head injury. The patient may not even be aware of his deficits or why he should be working on a certain functional activity or exercise. He may be embarrassed by performing a certain task or may simply refuse to do it. In general the psychosocial aspects of the patient with head injury go hand in hand with the cognitive and behavioral aspects and contribute to or retard recovery throughout the overall rehabilitation process.

Functional limitations. A patient with head injury may have problems in all performance skills. Possible areas of deficit are listed below.

Self-care	Communication
Feeding	Speech
Dressing	Symbolic language
Hygiene	Transportation
Grooming	Public modes
Bathing	Driving ability
Toileting	Community function
Mobility	Shopping
Bed	Street safety
Wheelchair	Community facilities
Transfer skills	Work skills
Functional ambulation	Prevocational activities
Home management	Work activities
Kitchen tasks	Leisure activities
Housekeeping	Social activities
Child care	Sports and games
Marketing	Hobbies

The functional disabilities cannot be separated from the cognitive, perceptual, sensory, motor, or behavioral problems. A problem in one of these areas can cause or contribute to the functional deficit. In other words, visual perception, sensation, motor ability, cognition, and psychosocial skills are all the basic building blocks to

ADL, each playing an integral part at various levels of task performance. For instance, a kitchen activity requires a combination of skills such as UE function, wheelchair mobility, figure-ground and form perception, scanning, sequencing, direction following, memory, safety awareness, and judgment. It is easy to forget how complex such a task is and take for granted the skills required, because it has become automatic to the nondisabled person. The individual with head injury struggles to put even the most basic components of the process together in some meaningful and ordered fashion.

Another example of a functional task that can be analyzed for areas of function that interact for effective performance is feeding ability. If there is decreased feeding ability, improvement in some or all of the following areas is the necessary building block to independent functioning: oral reflexes, level of awareness, oral sensation such as hypersensitivity, head and trunk control in sitting, UE function, and cranial nerve functions.

It becomes extremely important, then, for the therapist to identify the underlying components that relate to the functional deficit so that the best treatment approach can be established. She must have good observational skills and the ability to do formal testing to help pinpoint how the functional task should be broken down into steps and structured to gain optimal results in performance.

EVALUATION

Joint measurement, muscle testing, evaluation of reflexes and equilibrium reactions, sensory testing, ADL, home management, and home evaluations are described in Chapter 2. Evaluation for degree of spasticity is described in Chapter 12. All of these assessments may be applicable to the patient with head injury.

GUIDELINES FOR EVALUATION OF THE PATIENT AT THE PRIMARY LEVEL
Position and posture

TEST POSITION: Note whether the patient is supine, sitting, or upright in a wheelchair. The response may vary with proprioceptive, kinesthetic, labyrinthine, and visual input. The best response usually occurs when the patient is optimally positioned and sensory input is more normalized.

POSTURAL REFLEXES: Note symmetry between the two sides of the body and check for any abnormal postural reflexes. Note tonus changes and differences from one position to another, and estimate ROM and spasticity. Note if there is decorticate or decerebrate posturing or rigidity.

DECEREBRATE RIGIDITY: Note clenching of the jaw and extension of all four limbs (upper extremities more than lower extremities). Upper extremities are adducted and internally rotated, shoulders elevated, and feet plantar flexed. Basically it is a postural extensor synergy. Wrists and fingers are flexed.[9]

DECORTICATE RIGIDITY: Note triple flexion of upper extremities, that is, they are adducted, elbows and wrists severely flexed, and fists clenched. Lower extremities are hyperextended. Simultaneous hyperactivity of extensor muscles in upper extremities can also occur.[9]

Motor picture

Observe ROM, spasticity, flaccidity, and contractures. Note if there are any spontaneous movements and if the patient can move a limb (1) spontaneously (lowest level), (2) to a stimulus, (3) with sensory input and imitation, (4) to imitation only, or (5) on command. Note also if the movement is (1) reflexive, for example, withdrawal to pain; (2) automatic; or (3) voluntary.

Sensorimotor picture

PAIN: Evaluate for response to pinprick on upper and lower extremities and face. Is the response generalized or localized? Assess whether the response is away from, toward, delayed or absent.

DEEP PAIN: Either pinch the patient on the leg, arm, or neck and note response (same as for pain), or put pressure on fingernail with a hard object like a pen.

ORAL AREA: Refer to testing of oral reflexes. If patient is prone to seizures, placing ice on lips can set off seizures.

OLFACTORY: See if the patient can be aroused with noxious odors. Watch out for rebound phenomenon. Noxious stimuli have an arousing effect, whereas pleasant odors have a calming effect. Various smells may be used to arouse the patient before a treatment session.

GUSTATORY: Check out response to taste. This can be used as a stimulation technique or for working on the oral feeding mechanisms, for example, sour tastes help with lip pursing, which in turn helps with sucking. This area is mentioned because the patient may need to be aroused to truly assess level of awareness.

AUDITORY: Use a bell, jingle keys, clap hands, or simply talk to the patient to see if he responds to sound. Note if the patient turns his head or eyes toward the sound or if there is merely a startle response. Note if there is a generalized, localized, delayed, or absent response. Abnormal postural reflex mechanisms may prevent the patient from responding. Positioning should be optimal.

TACTILE: Note if there is any response to touch, rubbing, vibration, or different textures. Response could be the same as for auditory. Fine tactile discrimination cannot be assessed with the patient with head injury at the primary level, but responses can be observed to combine with observations of other responses to come up with a clinical picture.

Gross visual skills

TEST POSITION: Patient should be sitting with his head upright for testing visual skills.

ATTENTIVENESS: See if the patient can attend to a bright object or to the therapist. Be sure to measure attentiveness in terms the amount of time it takes for response so that future tests can be measured against this baseline to show progress. Keep a flow sheet record, noting the time that it takes to respond.

TRACKING: See if the patient can track a large, bright object side-to-side or up-down. Note the specific quality of the movement, that is, jerkiness, nystagmus, convergence, completeness, or delay. Also note and be aware of any other clues that you are giving to the patient to get him to track the object, such as verbal, auditory, or by standing on one side of patient. Keep a flow sheet of the kind of cuing used and the length of the delay from introduction of stimulus to the response. Tracking requires attentiveness.

NEGLECT: It is not possible to test specifically for field deficits or visual-spatial neglect in a patient with a head injury at the primary level, but generally it can be noted if the patient tends to neglect one side or responds better on the other side. The therapist may want to work initially on the more responsive side and then on the neglected side to facilitate head turning and body awareness.

Head and total body control

TEST POSITION: Evaluate the patient with another person to assist him over the bed edge.

BALANCE AND CONTROL: Check for sitting balance, trunk control, head control, and any balance reactions. After looking at all these areas together, evaluate head and trunk control separately in the wheelchair after hips and lower extremities are properly positioned. Head and neck control will develop along with visual skills. Measure head control by the amount of support required. This will help determine the type of device needed to support the head. The length of time that the head can be held erect by itself or during an activity, num-

ber of times per day without head device, and length of time without head device are also important to note for assessing improvement. Set up a flow sheet to keep a record of progress.

Summary

In general it is important to provide consistent sensory input to evaluate the quality of the motor output. It is best to structure the environment or task to demand a motor response after sensory stimulation. Keep track on a flow sheet of which sensory stimulation is being used, its frequency, duration, sequence, and combinations. Then on the flow sheet, note the response after specific stimulation techniques. Keep track of progress by consistency (how often) and by timing (how long) the various responses. Most of all, record observations to note the quality of the response. Is the response spontaneous, to a specific stimulus, with sensory input and imitation, to imitation only, or to command?

For the patient with head injury at the primary level note if there is a delay in processing, and be sure to allow time for the delay. The patient needs time to make the adaptive response and therefore increase his level of awareness.

Oral reflexes

Oral functions of the adult with head injury may be affected and have an influence on the ability to eat, drink, swallow, and speak. The oral reflexes and procedures for their evaluation are outlined in Table 10.

Table 10. Oral reflexes

Reflex	Age	Function	Stimulus	Response
Rooting	0 to 3 mo	Assists in locating food source	Touch corner of lip or cheek	Head turns toward stimulus with slight tongue protraction
Sucking-swallowing	0 to 3-5 mo	Initial intake of food; sucking followed by swallowing	Nipple or unbreakable object into mouth	Sucking with buccinator and orbicularis oris compressing; followed by swallowing
Bite	0 to 3-5 mo	If hyperactive cannot introduce food; leads to chewing	Double-pad tongue blade or toothbrush between teeth	Jaws clamp shut
Soft palate elevation	0 to life	Weak or absent elevation allows food to escape to nasal cavity	Light touch on lateral portion of soft palate	Soft palate elevation
Gag	0 to life	Hypoactive—no swallowing mechanism triggered and there is aspiration of food Hyperactive—food expelled and patient cannot feed himself	Apply pressure two thirds of way back on tongue	Gag—simultaneous head and jaw extension with rhythmical protrusion of tongue and contraction of pharynx
Swallowing	0 to life	Food intake of solids and fluids—nutrition	Stretch digastric and geniohyoid muscles Depress spoon or tongue blade one half of way back on tongue Introduce eyedropper full of fluid	Swallowing
Coughing	0 to life	Prevents aspiration	Observe for voluntary or spontaneous coughing	Coughing

Perceptual-motor evaluation

In evaluating perceptual-motor impairments in head injuries, care must be taken to do so in an orderly, progressive, and complete manner. Gross visual skills must be assessed before higher level visual-perceptual skills such as figure-ground or position in space. Motor planning skills must be evaluated early to ensure that problems noted in higher level skills are not a result of apraxia but are truly difficulties in the function being tested. For examples of complete, progressive cognitive-perceptual-motor evaluations, the reader is referred to the references.[33,42]

Cognition

In most facilities it is not the role of the occupational therapist to administer formal cognitive evaluations. It is within her role, however, to observe, interpret, and apply methods in treatment to remedy or compensate for the areas of cognition or behavior that are affecting the patient's functional status.

Hand function

After muscle tone, ROM, muscle strength, and selective movements have been assessed, hand function can be examined. The therapist must analyze first if the hand has isolated control for (1) gross grasp and release, (2) lateral pinch, (3) palmar prehension, and (4) fingertip prehension. A good test used for this purpose is the Quantitative Test of Upper Extremity Function by Carrol[11] (Chapter 2). Higher level skills are assessed only if full isolated muscle control is possible. Manipulation of objects and fine finger dexterity are examples of these skills.

It is also important to assess speed of movement and any other complicating clinical signs such as ataxia or shoulder weakness, for these will affect hand function. A test frequently used is the Jebsen-Taylor Test of Hand Function.[20] This test assesses speed and coordination by timing the patient as he performs a variety of simulated functional tasks, such as writing, feeding, and fine prehension activities. It is extremely important for the occupational therapist to assess hand function through the application of standardized tests, for then she can begin to correlate objective improvement with that seen in gains made in performance of daily living skills.

Total body function

It is important for the occupational therapist to assess total body function to relate it to ADL. For the patient with head injury at the primary level, one of the first things the therapist should evaluate is head and trunk control when the patient is sitting over the edge of the bed, along with total body patterning to see what kind of wheelchair is appropriate. Next the therapist should assess sitting balance when unsupported, noting equilibrium and protective reactions. As the patient progresses, the therapist will need to assess standing balance when unassisted and standing balance while performing an upper extremity activity, such as bending or reaching for an item in a kitchen cupboard. It is one thing to ambulate, for instance, forward and backward in the parallel bars, but it is much more complex to maneuver in tight spaces when performing an activity. Functional ambulation needs to be assessed in various settings, such as kitchen, bathroom, and community. It is essential that the therapist know what perceptual-motor skills are significant to total body function so that she can break them down and work on the deficit areas. A patient may be able to climb stairs, but the coordination, speed, and perception needed to step on a city bus or get on an escalator in a shopping center are considerably more complex.

Kitchen evaluation

The patient's ability to be safe and independent in the kitchen may determine his future living place. In evaluating the patient with head injury in the kitchen, his cognitive status is of the utmost importance. Adapting utensils and equipment and adapting and structuring the environment may be necessary to improve the patient's safety, judgment, and problem-solving skills. The components of the kitchen evaluation used for the patient with head injury are not very different from those used with other patient populations. The major difference is the need for the occupational therapist to closely evaluate the amount and type of supervision and structuring required in these tasks and the degree of physical assistance required.

Prevocational evaluation

Before a formal prevocational evaluation is administered, it is important to assess the patient's overall physical capacity. This evaluation will reveal areas that may pose problems in future job training and placement. The wheelchair-bound patient should be assessed for indoor and outdoor mobility, reaching height, ability to retrieve items from the floor, and sitting tolerance. The ambulatory patient must be evaluated for the ability to alternately stand and sit, stoop, crouch, carry objects, and maintain standing balance. Patients classified at either primary or advanced levels should be evaluated in communication skills, unilateral and bilateral strength and coordination, and overall endurance. Some tests that can be used for measuring hand function and coordination and speed in performance are the Purdue Pegboard,[32] the Bennett Hand Tool Test,[5] and the Minnesota Rate of Manipulation Test.[29]

After the occupational therapist has completed a comprehensive disability evaluation, including overall physical capacity, structured prevocational evaluations can be administered when appropriate. Possible tools for evaluation are the TOWER,[39] Micro-TOWER,[2] and Valpar[41] systems. Although these and other standardized systems of evaluation are extremely useful, the patient with head injury is often unable to follow the exact test procedures. When this happens, it is up to the evaluating therapist to modify and structure the test for optimal success. By doing so she will be unable to use the standardized methods of scoring but instead can describe the patient's performance and how the testing was altered to get a general picture of his skills. It is also advisable that the patient with head injury be evaluated separately from other patient populations. In this way the therapist can provide special guidance, structure, and support, which the patient may require, without causing him embarrassment and frustration.

Driving evaluation

The first step in the driving evaluation of the patient with head injury is a complete disability evaluation. The patient's visual, cognitive, and perceptual status is extremely important, because the task of driving requires complex visual functions, and vision influences more than 90% of the decisions of the individual while driving.[3]

In addition to the previously mentioned perceptual tests, it is helpful to use specific visual-perceptual exercises that depict various street scenes and driving situations. These can be indicative of a previous driving style and can demonstrate some problem solving abilities.

Before the patient attempts the actual driving task, in addition to the complete disability evaluation, the therapist must have a complete patient history and information about previous driving record, medication, seizure history, and the type of car the patient may drive. The Department of Motor Vehicles in California does not have a specific ruling regarding a time period to be seizure free, since one case differs from the next. (Section 2572 of California Administrative Code Title 17 defines the policy of the Department of Motor Vehicles regarding this issue.) Therapists should check for similar regulations in each state.

After the history and disability evaluations are completed and it has been determined that the patient is a candidate for driving, then an "on-the-road" evaluation is initiated. Ideally this should be done by both the occupational therapist and an adaptive driving instructor. The actual driving phase should progress from a quiet residential area to more congested areas, including highways. It should be noted that there is very little training done at this stage. It is more observational, with minimal instruction given on problem areas to determine the pa-

tient's rate of relearning and degree of compensation. Level of alertness and ability to concentrate in varied driving situations are carefully assessed. Conversing with the patient may occur during this assessment to examine abilities to maintain simultaneous attention to the driving task. Although the patient with visual field defect or visual neglect may demonstrate lane positioning difficulties, he is assessed in his potential to compensate with some cuing from the instructor.

Various pieces of adaptive equipment can also be used to improve vehicle control, such as a steering device for one-handed steering, signal level extensions, left foot accelerator, or hand controls, if necessary.

Each problem is assessed separately during the evaluation as well as in training. Sometimes it may prove to be too early for a client to drive. If so, he should be seen for a reassessment at a later time.

Although each patient is different, the fundamental principle behind the evaluation and training is the ability to drive defensively. No matter what the patient's major problems are, he must be able to compensate for them by planning ahead, maintaining good vehicle control, and driving defensively.

GENERAL PRINCIPLES OF OCCUPATIONAL THERAPY INTERVENTION

The occupational therapist who will be working with patients with head injury must be committed to improving the quality of life for a difficult, complicated, and, more often than not, frustrating patient population. Since there are no clear-cut localized lesions, as seen in stroke patients or patients with spinal cord injury, the therapist is often dealing with unknown long-term expectations for level of recovery and prognosis. Additionally, she will come to realize that each patient has a different set of problems that forces her to use clinical observation and creative problem-solving skills and make unique judgments and treatment plans in each case.

Although there is no set of magic answers to the treatment of patients, certain principles and guidelines for occupational therapy intervention can be generalized for most patients with head injury. All patients require structured, normalized sensory input from their environment. For example, the semicomatose patient must not remain indefinitely in bed but must be placed upright and positioned to inhibit abnormal muscle tone. As a result, he can begin to perceive his environment from the proper perspective and consequently may display an increased level of awareness. During treatment of the patient at the primary level the therapist should assume that at least some information is getting through to him. In approaching all patients with head injury, the therapist should not relate to them in a condescending manner. They are adults and as such deserve respect. They will not respond any better if they are yelled at or patronized.

The occupational therapist treating patients with head injury must constantly observe, reevaluate, interpret behavior and response, and alter treatment accordingly. This patient population demands a great deal of flexibility and astute observation skills from the treating therapist.

When establishing a treatment plan, the therapist is faced with a long list of problems regarding the patient's physical, cognitive, perceptual, psychosocial, and ADL functioning. She must place these problems in order of priority and set up realistic goals for the patient. She must analyze the treatment tasks and activities she chooses and structure the treatment sessions to facilitate maximum function. Treatment strategies for each problem can vary, and she must decide which is best for her as well as for the patient. Common impairments already discussed can be treated functionally with tabletop activities for perceptual retraining or using sensorimotor approaches. However, most therapists who treat this population feel that any combination of methods may be the most beneficial. To minimize patient confusion and agitation and facilitate carry-over of learned tasks, there must be constant communication among team members. If the nursing staff is instructing a patient in one type of transfer, and the occupational therapist is instructing him in another type, the patient will become confused and show limited progress. A consistent, repetitive, and appropriately structured approach to the patient by all members of the treatment team will yield optimum results.

General aims and methods of treatment

Patients with head injury at the primary level. The general aims of treatment for the patient at the primary level are fundamental to increasing the patient's level of response and overall awareness. Input must be well structured, timed, and broken down into simple steps, and enough time must be allowed for a response, since response will often be delayed during this phase of treatment.

Sensory stimulation program. After the patient has been evaluated, a baseline for treatment is established. Treatment of the patient at the primary level should start as soon as the patient is medically stable. Often the patient may still be comatose or semicomatose. The goal of treatment is to increase the patient's level of awareness by trying to arouse him with controlled sensory input. The occupational therapist needs to provide visual, auditory, tactile, olfactory, and gustatory stimulation. In addition to these, it will be important to start getting the patient up in a wheelchair to normalize sensory input through the kinesthetic and labyrinthine systems.

Many patients who appear semicomatose when lying supine in bed suddenly respond when sitting erect in a wheelchair. The therapist is changing the position of the body in space and placing the patient in a position where be can start to visually perceive his environment. Once the patient is up, the therapist will start to work on gross visual skills, starting first with visual attentiveness. The goal is to try to get the patient to attend to an object and people in the environment. Next it will be important to try to elicit visual tracking by using a bright object and sometimes the additional input of an auditory stimulus. The different levels or ways and analysis of the patient's response should be noted according to guidelines given in the preceding section on evaluation.

Auditory and tactile stimulation are used to see if the patient can localize the specific stimulus given. Even when working with a comatose patient with head injury, the therapist should talk to him as if he can understand her. Even if the patient is not responsive, verbal commands that are clear and simple should be given. Examples of auditory stimuli are ringing a bell, clapping hands, cassette tape recordings of familiar sounds, or the therapist's voice. The goal is to get the patient to localize the sound or respond to it voluntarily. Usually the automatic responses, such as turning the head toward a loud noise, will occur before the voluntary responses. Tactile stimulation includes superficial pain (pinprick), deep pain (pressure on the fingernails), rubbing an affected limb with cloths of various textures, and stroking body parts while giving verbal cues to increase overall body awareness.

Olfactory and gustatory stimulation are important but are often overlooked for arousal of the comatose or semicomatose patient. Generally, noxious odors such as onion have a facilitory effect, and pleasant odors have a calming or inhibitory effect.[15]

Vestibular stimulation. The use of vestibular stimulation and sensory integrative therapy for the adult with head injury is essential to the patient's progress. The vestibular system, that is, the vestibular pathways running throughout the brain stem and cerebellum,[4] has a major influence on posture and equilibrium responses. By providing vestibular stimulation via slow spinning, rocking, or inverting the head during developmental activities on the mat, tone in the antigravity muscles can be reduced, followed by muscle co-contraction.

There are three major roles of the vestibular reflexes: (1) The body acts to oppose or compensate for changes in the direction of the force of gravity (negative geotrophic movement); (2) through kinetic action the muscles co-contract to maintain equilibrium and ocular stability during movement; and (3) the vestibular reflex activity helps maintain posture and regulate muscle tone.[4] Therefore the vestibular system can be used to reduce or inhibit abnormal muscle tone or spasticity, facilitate equilibrium and righting reactions, and enhance gross visual skills. "The maintenance of body equilibrium and posture and appreciation of spatial orientation in everyday life are complex functions involving multiple receptor organs and neural centers in addition to the labyrinths. Visual and proprioceptive reflexes in particular must be integrated with vestibular reflexes to insure postural stability."[4]

It is important that the occupational therapist use a neurophysiological basis for the treatment of head injury. The goal is not to develop specific or splinter skills or simply learn to compensate for a visual or motor problem but to try to reintegrate or redevelop the impaired function. For example, asking a patient to lift his foot may be ineffective, because it is a cortical level approach to treatment. The problem must be approached from a lower level of the brain for its integration there, if the skill is to be mastered. Rood stated that the cortex is not the highest control center of motor activity. Rather she believes that treatment should be aimed at the cerebellum and basal ganglia to gain effective and long-lasting results.[33]

An example of vestibular stimulation is through the use of a scooterboard up and down inclines to get an inverted position of the head. It is important to monitor the patient's vital signs closely during mat activities that provide vestibular stimulation, such as when the patient is inverted over a bolster while bearing weight on the upper extremities or is rocking on an equilibrium board. In some cases continued vestibular stimulation can cause seizures, nausea, fatigue, dizziness, blood pressure changes, and associated reactions. The patient's level of awareness is an important factor. The patient at the primary level may not be able to voluntarily give cues to the therapist when he has had enough stimulation. The therapist should communicate closely with the physician, nursing staff, and other members of the rehabilitation team before, during, and after vestibular stimulation has been initiated in the treatment program to determine and monitor its effects on the patient.

Rood stated that once co-contraction has been established through the use of the inverted position, stability in space is gained, and this is the basis for kinesthetic figure-ground perception. Kinesthetic figure-ground perception serves as a foundation for orientation of the body in the dimensions of space and time. Once a person can separate figure from ground internally, then he can begin to deal with the external environment. He can begin to gain bilateral integration and proper body image.[33]

The use of vestibular stimulation in conjunction with NDT is an important tool for changing and maximizing the patient's response. Ayres states that the primary cerebellar function is that of an integrating and regulating servomechanism whose action has been frequently linked to motor output.[33] As in any type of sensorimotor

stimulation, it is important to demand a motor response, after giving the stimulation, to help facilitate CNS integration. It is important in the treatment of the patient with head injury to provide stimulation in a structured and goal-oriented way and help regulate the response toward the desired outcome. At all times during treatment application, precautions and contraindications to specific treatment modalities should be kept in mind.

The use of vestibular stimulation in the treatment of adults with head injury is important to the patients' recovery. However, this area of treatment is complex and requires specific study and training before it is used. The beginning therapist *should not* attempt to incorporate vestibular stimulation into the treatment program unless supervised by an experienced therapist.

Oral-bulbar problem facilitation. Treatment of oral-bulbar problems must follow the developmental sequence outlined in Table 10. The therapist should have special training in appropriate facilitation-inhibition techniques for improving oral-bulbar status before attempting to treat a client. The general progression of training is from oral facilitation-inhibition to feeding by the therapist to self-feeding.

The most common problems found in the patient's oral-bulbar status can stem from the presence of abnormal reflexes. The problems usually seen are oral hypersensitivity, poor sucking ability, decreased swallowing mechanism, hypoactive gag reflex, drooling with poor lip closure, and poor tongue movements.

Sucking occurs before swallowing and may be impaired or absent in the patient with head injury. Sour tastes or ice in the mouth, given in small quantities, can help to elicit a sucking response. Nipple spoons are used to elicit sucking ability. Applying ice around the mouth should be used with precautions, since it may set off a seizure in a person with a seizure disorder.

When working on swallowing it is best to start with pureed foods, since they are safer and easier to swallow. The therapist may need to start with a small amount of food on a nonbreakable spoon, depending on how depressed the swallowing ability is.

A hypoactive gag reflex is one of the more dangerous feeding problems encountered, since the patient can aspirate a piece of food. The patient with a hypoactive gag reflex should never be given chunks of food that require chewing or should never be left unsupervised. Stimulation of the gag reflex is facilitated by pressure applied two thirds of the way back on the tongue.

Tongue lateralization and, in general, tongue and lip control are necessary functions for moving food in the mouth and for stabilizing food for chewing. An ice popsicle is good for working on sucking and lip control. A patient can work on tongue movements by trying to lick jelly or peanut butter off the corners of his mouth.[15]

Since the patient's mouth and gums may be hypersensitive, the therapist may have to start with desensitization techniques such as rubbing the gums with a cotton swab. Generally, facilitation of a delayed oral mechanism can be done through a quick stretch to the muscle controlling that movement, such as the orbicularis oris for lip control or sucking. The patient's oral reflexes and basic feeding mechanisms must be closely analyzed to set up the most effective treatment program. Once the patient can start to put together in sequence the mechanisms required for feeding, he can generally start to take in food of a thicker consistency. Once the patient has progressed from an oral facilitation-inhibition program to a self-feeding program, then the aspects of UE function and feeding devices can be incorporated into the training sessions.

Positioning. With the release of abnormal postural reflexes, abnormal muscle tone, and decreased isolated muscle control, it becomes very difficult for the adult with head injury to control his body or maintain good posture (Fig. 14-1). The occupational therapist must help inhibit this abnormal muscle tone and facilitate voluntary movement through proper wheelchair positioning.

The parts of the body that are affected are the head, trunk, hips, knees, and upper and lower extremities. The place to start for wheelchair positioning is the hips. Poor hip placement will disturb head and trunk alignment. A lap roll or seat wedge can be used to flex the hips and break up the total body pattern of extension. A knee abductor or side wedges can be used to control lateral hip placement.

Once the hips are properly positioned, then trunk positioning can follow. Lateral trunk supports or a chest strap is frequently used to decrease kyphosis and scoliosis. A hard seat or good firm wheelchair cushion is important to facilitate a more erect posture of the spine.

After good trunk alignment is accomplished, then upper extremity control can be commenced. The use of a lap tray to support the upper extremities will also help to support the trunk. Along with splinting, the upper extremities should be positioned out of reflex or spastic patterns. This can be done on the lap tray or with an arm trough and the use of cones or straps. To position the arms out of a flexor pattern, the arms must be flexed forward and rotated externally at the shoulders, elbows extended, forearms supinated, and wrists and fingers extended with the thumbs abducted[22] (Fig. 14-2). A stretch splint and a bivalved elbow cast can be used in conjunction with the positioning device such as a wheelchair arm trough to break up the total pattern.

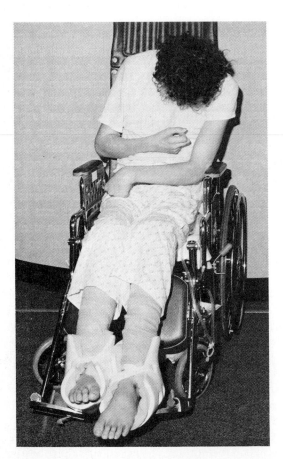

Fig. 14-1. Abnormal reflexes and postural tone result in poor control of posture in wheelchair.

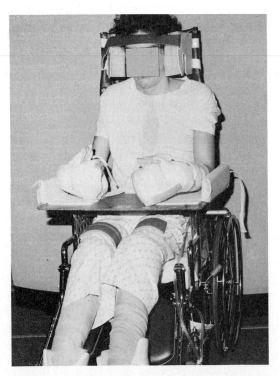

Fig. 14-2. Improved posture and trunk alignment is achieved with splints and positioning devices.

Head positioning is one of the most difficult tasks for the therapist. The patient with poor head control usually needs to be in a recliner wheelchair that is in the upright position. The head extension found on the recliner wheelchair is a good base from which to work when making the head device. The head should be kept in midline, and the force used to keep the head erect is best applied over the forehead and the chin. The sterno-occipital mandibular immobilizer (SOMI) brace is a commercially available head device.[37]

LE positioning is done to break up abnormal postural patterns or reflexes, most commonly the positive support reaction. To inhibit this reflex a foot wedge is attached to the wheelchair footrests that equally distributes the weight throughout the foot, taking the pressure off the ball of the foot. Straps can be attached to the elevating leg rests to help keep legs that are in flexor pattern pattern in extension.

Positioning the patient is a key factor to normalized sensory input from the environment. Positioning goes hand in hand with developmental techniques done on the mat and with other sensorimotor integration techniques. Devices are removed gradually as the patient starts to control his body and manipulate the environment more. It is important to make a schedule of use of a head device, for example, so that the patient learns to control his head and does not merely rely on the static device for support. Positioning is done in a progression, or graduated sequence, which must be closely monitored at all times.

Reality orientation. Reality orientation is an important concept in the rehabilitation of the adult with head injury. With the disorientation, confusion, and decreased memory that the patient may experience, the therapist must consistently provide structure and familiarize the patient with his environment, himself, and current events. A reality orientation group is held every morning at the same time for patients with head injury at the Santa Clara Valley Medical Center and provides a good means to assess improvement. A patient will not benefit from such a group unless he has sufficient attentiveness, level of awareness, controlled behavior, and potential for carry-over of learning from day to day. As in all treatment techniques used with patients with head injury, the treatment plan must be structured and the patient must start on the next phase of treatment only when it is appropriate and when he will truly benefit from it.

Splinting and casting. Splinting and casting for the spastic upper or lower extremities are effective means of reducing muscle tone, preventing contractures, increasing ROM and coordination, and complementing mat activities. The most frequently used splints and casts for the upper extremity are the elbow cast (Fig. 14-3), stretch splint, stretch splint-cast, cock-up splint, and cock-up cast. For the lower extremities the posterior knee shell, foot splint, foot cast, and long leg cast are used. The elbow cast is usually fabricated to break up an upper extremity flexor pattern and increase ROM. Serial casting of the elbow should be done every 24 to 48 hours to progressively stretch out the flexor muscles.

The stretch splint is used to break up the UE flexor pattern by placing wrist and fingers in maximum extension with the thumb radially abducted (Fig. 14-4). A stretch splint can also be used during weight-bearing activities, such as mat work or bed mobility. Maintained stretch accomplished through splinting or casting changes the muscle bias and therefore facilitates muscle relaxation.[40] If a patient's wrist and finger flexors are so tight that ROM is severely limited, the therapist may have to start out with a resting hand splint that is changed or adjusted for progressive stretching. For cases of severe spasticity a bivalved stretch splint-cast was

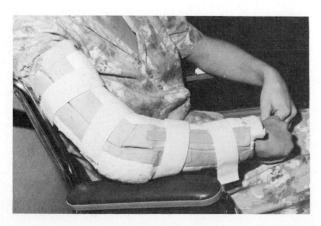

Fig. 14-3. Elbow cast.

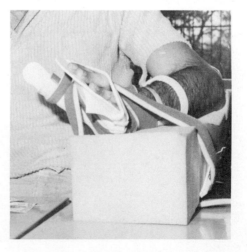

Fig. 14-4. Stretch splint.

developed at Santa Clara Valley Medical Center to provide equal pressure over the dorsal and volar surfaces to minimize skin breakdown and maintain a fuller static stretch. Bivalved means that a cast is sawed in half and the edges are lined with moleskin so that it may be strapped on and taken off easily at any time (Fig. 14-5).

Once selective hand movements have started to develop, a cock-up splint or cast can be used to promote hand skills such as prehension. A cock-up splint is also useful in cases where ataxia or intention tremors are present at the wrist. It has a stabilizing effect, thus giving finer motor control.

LE splinting or casting is usually done to break up an extensor pattern or a positive support reaction. The goal is to extend the knee and place the ankle in midline with the foot dorsiflexed to neutral. In cases where there is severe plantar flexion, serial casting should be used in conjunction with foot wedges to distribute the weight equally from the ball of the foot to the heel. LE casts may also be bivalved.

It is important to establish a splint schedule for the nursing staff to follow, with regular splint checks for any potential pressure areas. In cases of severe spasticity the initial splint schedule may only be 2 hours on and 2 hours off until the patient can tolerate it for longer periods. The patient should never be locked up in his splints, casts, or positioning devices all the time, for they are only static tools to help the patient become more mobile. Splinting and casting for patients with head injury and severe spasticity must at all times be done in a progression, from initially breaking up the abnormal pattern to eventually aiding the individual to improved UE function and coordination.

Communication systems. As a result of head trauma, there may be severe language impairment (Chapter 13) and inability to communicate.[17,19] Communication involves many different modalities such as speech, writing, and sign language. There are several communication systems available to the adult with head injury to compensate for nonfunctional speech.

Communication systems range from simple to complex. There are three major approaches to consider when developing a nonoral communication system: direct selection, scanning, and encoding.[36] By direct selection a patient would directly select his desired choice. For example, the patient might directly select pictures or letters to spell a word on a communication board. The occupational therapist must work closely with the speech pathologist in adapting the communication system to allow for a maximal response based on perceptual and motor abilities.

When a scanning system is used, the patient signals when a desired choice is present or directs an indicator toward the choice.[36] Various control systems, such as the puff and sip mechanism, may be adapted to be a scanner system so that a light scans across a row of letters or symbols until the desired choice is reached. At that time the patient signals the light to stop.

The third kind of system is the encoding system in which the patient indicates his choice by a code of input symbols,[36] such as Bliss symbols.[6] This system, because it is much more complex, requires a higher level of cognitive functioning.

The inability to communicate needs to others is one of the most frustrating problems that the adult with head injury faces. It is extremely important for the therapist to assess the patient's level of awareness, gross visual skills, visual perception, and motor status before working on adapting a communication system. The communication system allows the patient to interact again with his environment and should be geared to the patient's level of function. For example, a patient who could respond yes and no to questions by nodding may not be able to do so until good head control is developed or proper head positioning is provided.

It is essential that the therapist uses good observational skills along with her evaluation to help solve the communication problem. There was one dramatic example of a patient examined at Santa Clara Valley Medical Center, 5 years after the head injury occurred, who had severe motor impairment involving his whole body, except for his head. He did not orally communicate nor interact with his environment at all on admission because of severe motor deficits. A mouth stick set was fabricated for the patient, and he was able to type, pick

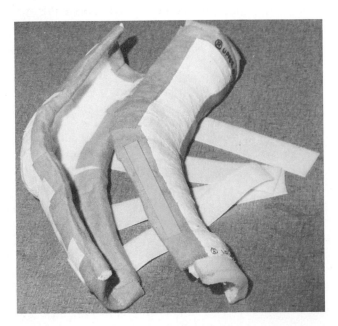

Fig. 14-5. Bivalved elbow cast.

up small objects, draw, and engage in avocational activities. He learned to type, and the first thing he ever wrote was that he loved his wife. It cannot be emphasized enough that the potential for communication may be lying dormant within the patient and can be used, if only it can be tapped.

Patients with head injury at the advanced level. The patient at the advanced level has progressed to a point where he is able to tolerate formal evaluations and full treatment sessions. Obviously the evaluation results, specific to each patient, will outline which areas are priorities for treatment. Usually the patient will have some degree of deficit in all major categories. The following is a description of the areas that may require treatment and the general principles of occupational therapy interventions for these.

Self-care. When the patient begins to enter a more advanced stage, the therapist can begin to analyze his ability to manipulate and effectively use familiar objects. With this in mind, light hygiene and early dressing activities can be initiated. Not only is this an effective means of identifying possible difficulty in motor planning, but it is also an avenue to increase the patient's functional independence and improve body image.

Because of the patient's cognitive status, hygiene or dressing activities must be broken down into segments and done repetitively in the same way. Depending on the patient's balance and total body function, training in dressing should progress from in bed to the wheelchair to the bed edge to standing. During training it is necessary to decide which techniques to use. The therapist must be aware of techniques that increase functional independence but cause the reinforcement of abnormal motor patterns. She must constantly assess the techniques at each stage in recovery with other team members and decide if the goal is normalization or compensation. For example, teaching the patient to place his unaffected leg under his affected leg to enable him to remove his legs from the bed improves his functional independence but reinforces an abnormal pattern of movement.

Feeding. To reinforce the neuromuscular facilitation techniques used in oral-bulbar training, as well as to increase the patient's functional independence, training in feeding is initiated when appropriate. There are numerous factors to consider when feeding the patient who has CNS dysfunction. The following are just suggestions that will assist in feeding patients with a few specific types of impairments. The reader is referred to the references for additional resources.

When feeding the patient who has head injury he should be upright with his head and neck in the neutral position or slightly flexed. Use a small spoon and small amounts of food; do not use a plastic spoon with patients who have a bite reflex. Remove the spoon as soon as lip closure has occurred and avoid scraping teeth. If the patient with a bite reflex clamps down on the spoon, do not attempt to pry his mouth open. Either wait until he relaxes or push up on the jaw to facilitate opening. Be sure to wait for swallowing to occur before presenting the next bite.

When feeding the patient who has tongue thrust or lack of lateralization of the tongue, food should be deposited in the corners of the mouth. Place the food in the molar region of the mouth, applying pressure on the tongue as the food is deposited. As the patient improves with increasing lateralization and decreasing thrust, food can be placed in the more frontal, midposition of the tongue.

Milk and sweet fluids will increase the flow of saliva; therefore when working with the patient who has difficulty swallowing secretions, liquids such as beef broth are preferred, because they will thin the saliva.

Mobility. Mobility training can be subdivided into bed mobility and transfer training, including functional ambulation and wheelchair mobility.

When working on *bed mobility* the occupational therapist must aim for improving independence while using the sensorimotor approaches to improve sensory and motor function. It is not to the patient's benefit to simply teach him to compensate for a loss of function or develop splinter skills. The bed mobility skills that the patient with head injury may need to work on include scooting in supine position, rolling, bridging, moving from supine to sitting position, long leg sitting, sitting over the bed edge, and sitting balance.

The occupational therapist must have a good theoretical knowledge of treatment to reduce spasticity, for example, in the upper extremities, to incorporate this goal into a gross motor activity such as bed mobility. The following example of using a Bobath (NDT) technique when working with the patient sitting over the edge of the bed is provided to clarify the application of theory to practice. The affected spastic arm and hand are extended, outwardly rotated, and used for support. It is important to decrease flexor spasticity and use protective extension to prevent falling. The shoulder girdle should be held back. Wrist and fingers should be extended with thumb abducted. A stretch splint is good for this bed mobility activity. It is important to keep the shoulder girdle level and practice weight shifts from side to side with the upper extremities back slightly behind the patient. Joint approximation can be given to the shoulder in this position, or the patient can bear weight on an elbow by leaning on it to the side. The patient should learn how to go from supine to sitting position by pushing up from the affected elbow, with the therapist applying approximation to reduce muscle tone and ultimately improve function.[7]

Transfer training has been described in Chapter 5. Cognitive, perceptual, and physical status will affect the type of transfer used in training. Memory and limited carry-over mandate that training be consistent in type and sequence among all staff members treating the patient. When the patient has begun to master the mechanics and sequence of the bed-to-chair transfer, toilet, bathtub, and car transfers can be initiated. At this stage the therapist becomes involved with evaluating the need for equipment. Bathroom dimensions and layouts are discussed with the family, and a home visit is planned. Architectural barriers, which are a constant issue for the wheelchair-bound individual, are considered at this time. It is preferable, if possible, that transfers be practiced moving in either direction. Often a patient becomes proficient in a transfer with an approach to one side and is dismayed when entering a public bathroom only to discover that the particular approach is not possible. An additional reason for encouraging transfers to both sides is that by doing so, more normal sensory input is provided by encouraging the patient to bear weight on his affected leg and use the trunk muscles of his affected side. Thus the therapist is encouraging normalization of tone and movement, rather than compensation.

Bathtub transfers are practiced with both a dry surface and the more realistic wet surface. Generally it is safer to have the patient in the bathtub before filling it with water. On the same note the water should be emptied, and the patient should be dry before he attempts to get out of the bathtub. Bathtub mats can aid in safety by making the bathtub surface less slick. There is a variety of bathtub, shower, and toilet equipment that is commercially available. Although this equipment is often necessary, the therapist should remember that the ultimate goal is to eliminate the need for as much equipment as possible without creating a safety hazard for the patient or his family.

The car transfer is one of the most important transfers to the patient. Patient motivation for this area is rarely a problem, because this is the patient's ticket out for a day or a weekend. The patient and an appropriate family member should be cleared by the occupational therapist in car transfers before he is allowed out on a weekend pass. This depends on the patient's *functional* level and may take more than one session for the necessary arrangements, which should be made in advance. Teaching the family member car transfers is only one of the many areas with which the therapist and family are involved. This ongoing communication will alleviate many of the family's and patient's fears and lessen the change of failure during the initial visits home.

Although hopefully not a common occurrence, the patient may at some time fall to the floor. It is therefore necessary that the occupational therapist instruct the pa-

tient and his family in wheelchair mobility techniques, for example, getting from the floor back to the wheelchair. The patient will need sufficient gross motor skills and balance to be able to accomplish this task. Generally, if lying on the side, the patient will need to get himself in the all fours or kneeling position. He can use the wheelchair, if stabilized, or a sturdy piece of furniture to assist him. Next he will need to prop his elbows on the seat of the wheelchair, and bring one or both legs into position as if to stand. Then, pushing up into a bent stand–pivot position, the patient will reach for an armrest, pivot, and sit. Floor-to-wheelchair transfers can only be done with a patient who is advanced in motor skills. Any abnormal patterns that the patient might have should be kept in mind. The method described is only one general technique, and each transfer should be worked out for the individual's unique set of problems and assets.

UE function. The types of motor impairment present in the patient with head injury are numerous. Weakness, synergistic movement, spasticity, rigidity, ataxia, primary reflexes, and impaired sensation will all affect the patient's ability to perform UE activities. Treatment techniques for the patient with synergistic movements, spasticity, or the presence of primitive reflexes are described. The general aims of treatment for the upper extremity of the primary-level patient and the CVA patient were presented earlier. Ataxia is a common and frustrating problem that often develops early, persists into the late rehabilitation phase, and may remain permanently. Although various treatment methods have been tried, it is difficult to assess their ultimate long-term value. Weighting of body parts and use of resistive activities appear to improve control during performance of tasks but show inconsistent carry-over of control when the weights are removed. When applying weights to the patient, the therapist must carefully evaluate at which joint or joints the tremor originates. Applying weights to a patient's wrists when the tremor originates in the trunk or shoulder is ineffective. The amount of weight applied will also affect results. Generally 2 to 2½ pounds is the optimum weight that can be applied without causing additional tremor. Resistive bracing, in which resistance is applied at each joint throughout the ROM, has been tried at Santa Clara Valley Medical Center with some success. By adding continued resistance throughout the ROM, muscle groups are forced into co-contraction and therefore tremor decreases. Unfortunately, bracing is expensive and often is not cosmetically acceptable to the patient.

Perceptual training. Treatment approaches to perceptual dysfunction can vary, depending on the patient and the therapist. A developmental approach can be used by demanding lower level skills, thus lessening the possibility of developing splinter skills. Repetitive tabletop activities are another treatment approach with the ultimate aim being carry-over of functional tasks. Obviously a third approach is attacking the problem where it is affecting function. Often the approach that the therapist will use is a combination of the three. She must remember to keep a keen eye in observing the patient's response to isolate and monitor the most effective approach or combination of approaches for a particular patient. The reader is referred to the references for details of the treatment of perceptual dysfunction.

Home management. As the patient gains increased skills and independence in dressing, feeding, and functional mobility, treatment is expanded to include kitchen and homemaking tasks. As in other areas of treatment, kitchen training is graded to suit the patient's progress. Beginning tasks might include simple sandwich preparation. Depending on the patient's cognitive status, the therapist may place all food items on the table and have the patient verbally review the task before doing it for the first time. At the end of the session the following day's activities can be discussed. A session such as this requires simple sequencing, organizing, and memory for the task. As the patient improves, more demands are made on him until he reaches the final stages in the progression. Then he should be able to plan and cook a complete meal with no verbal cuing or structure given by the therapist.

Total body function and endurance are also important aspects of kitchen activities. Standing endurance is measured as well as ability for bending to low shelves or reaching for high shelves. Safety becomes a key issue in this setting. The patient's judgment in handling sharp utensils and using the stove can become key issues is selecting a living place after discharge.

Homemaking activities can include light housekeeping such as dusting, vacuuming, or making the bed. As in other functional training, energy conservation and work simplification are stressed.

Child care is an area of treatment that is often overlooked. Family involvement is vital if a woman is to return effectively to her role as wife and mother. Sensory overload is a common problem that must be handled. Most people would agree it is a problem even for the mother who has not sustained a head injury. One-handed diapering techniques or commercially available strollers, cribs, and child care equipment that can be handled more easily by the handicapped woman are examples of the areas that might be covered by occupational therapy services.

Community reintegration. Often in the rehabilitation process the patient with the head injury reaches his maximum level of independence in the protected and structured atmosphere of the hospital and, when discharged into the community, is faced with people, situations, and problems that he has not yet encountered and resolved.

It is therefore vital that the occupational therapist initiate a community reintegration program before discharge. The training can begin with the basic skills involved in a simple purchase, that is, handling money or communicating needs. As the patient's cognitive, perceptual, and physical status changes, the therapist can help him to progress to a more demanding activity or setting. Table 11 illustrates simple settings and the skills demanded for these. The transition of treatment from an initial setting such as a hospital gift shop to a community store not only demands skills in the areas listed but also presents new psychosocial issues with which the patient must deal. It is often of benefit for an appropriate family member to accompany the therapist and patient on a community trip. The family member can gain increased insight into the individual's level of functioning and into how the outside world views his disability. The therapist must be aware of the patient's and family's attitudes toward a community reintegration program. She may

Table 11. Community reintegration program*

Setting	Skills demanded
Vending machines	Wheelchair mobility Physical handling of money Simple computation Decision making
Hospital gift shop	*Above skills plus:* Use of elevators Orientation to location in hospital Social skills—communication of needs Exchanging money
Hospital cafeteria	*Above skills plus:* Mobility in crowds Handling food Eating etiquette Social behavior in groups
Fast-food restaurant	*Above skills plus:* Architectural barriers Safety crossing streets Use of telephone
Drug store	*Above skills plus:* More complex money management Orientation to complex spaces (store and parking lot)
Grocery store	*Above skills plus:* Nutrition Long-term planning
Shopping center (department store)	*Above skills plus:* Greater complexity in physical, perceptual, cognitive, and social skills

*Based on a program developed at Santa Clara Valley Medical Center, San Jose, Calif.

become frustrated when a cooperative patient suddenly refuses to participate in the program. He may not feel ready for the outside world to view his handicap, and it is up to the therapist to give him the support and guidance needed for the easiest transition possible.

Prevocational training and placement. Vocational training and placement of the patient with head injury are extended processes that require the involvement of an occupational therapist, vocational evaluator, and other allied health professionals usually under the co-ordination of a vocational counselor. Each professional brings to the case a different expertise that is essential to successful job placement. Many patients with head injury are not immediately ready for sheltered workshop or competitive employment, therefore it may be more appropriate for them to be involved in an adapted learning program at a local university or community college. Regular follow-up and reevaluation of the patient by the therapist and counselor will ensure changes in placement as the patient improves. When assessing different alternatives for placement, it should be considered that workshops that are geared for mentally retarded persons are often not the best choice for patients with head in-

jury. They are unable to identify with retarded persons, and the workshop staff is usually not trained to deal with the memory, cognitive, and behavioral problems that are specific to head injury.

One of the most exciting ways for the occupational therapist to use her problem-solving skills is environmental and equipment modification at the patient's job site. Employers are extremely receptive and pleased when the employee with head injury is no longer a liability but is a competitive, successful employee.

Family training and follow-up. The importance of family involvement in the patient's treatment program has already been discussed. Family involvement in treatment should occur throughout the patient's hospital stay. Constant communication between the therapist and the patient's family will aid in appropriate follow-through of important skills that the patient has learned during treatment. Before the discharge from the hospital, the family will meet with the occupational therapist to go over the patient's home program. Because the patient with head injury continues to improve over long periods, an appointment is set up for a follow-up and reevaluation.

SAMPLE TREATMENT PLAN

Case study

K.B. is a 24-year-old male who sustained a gunshot wound to the head during an altercation 4 months ago. The bullet entered the left occipital area and traversed to the right temporal-parietal area. An emergency craniotomy and decompression were performed 1 week later. Craniotomy and debridement with removal of devitalized brain tissue, foreign bodies, and bone chips were performed 3 weeks after the injury.

K.B. was living in a city about 30 miles from the rehabilitation facility and had been married for 4 years. Presently he is divorced. He has a high school education and has worked as a bricklayer for 6 years. When initially interviewed by the occupational therapist, he stated that he would be returning to work "in a couple of weeks."

K.B. was referred to occupational therapy for evaluation and appropriate treatment to facilitate maximum function and independence.

Treatment plan

A. **Statistical data.**
  1. Name: K.B.
     Age: 24
     Diagnosis: Traumatic injury to the head
     Disability: Motor, sensory-perceptual-cognitive dysfunction

  2. Treatment aims as stated in the referral:
     Evaluation
     Facilitate maximum function and independence
B. **Other services.**
  Physical therapy: Ambulation, mat mobility, strengthening exercises
  Nursing: Nursing care, reality orientation
  Speech: Cognitive skills, language retraining
  Psychology: Intelligence, memory testing
  Social service: Counseling, community placement, financial arrangements
  Educational program: Academic skills retraining
C. **OT evaluation.**
  ROM: Measure
  Spasticity: Test, observe
  Abnormal movement: Test, observe
  Selective movement: Test
  Sensation: Test
  Hand function: Test
  Perceptual-motor skills: Test, observe
  Self-care, mobility: Test, observe
  Cognitive skills: Observe
  Behavior: Observe
  Home management: Observe
  Community skills: Observe
  Prevocational: Test, observe
  Driving evaluation: Test, observe
  Physical capacities: Test, observe

SAMPLE TREATMENT PLAN—cont'd

D. Results of evaluation.
  1. Evaluation data.
    a. Physical resources.
      (1) Strength: There is isolated motion and normal strength in the right upper extremity. In the left upper extremity there is a mild flexor pattern, with moderate spasticity in horizontal adduction, elbow extension, pronation and finger flexion. Minimal spasticity is present in the wrist and elbow flexors.
      (2) Selective movement: With the left upper extremity the patient is able to perform the following selective movements with difficulty: shoulder flexion to 90°, hand behind back, and hand to opposite shoulder. Incomplete motion is possible when performing hand behind head and wrist flexion and extension with the elbow relaxed.
      (3) ROM: ROM is within normal limits for both upper extremities.
      (4) Hand function: The right hand functions normally. With the left hand the patient can perform gross grasp and lateral prehension, but these are weak. The patient is unable to effect and put the prehension patterns to functional use. He is also unable to perform any fine manipulative skills with the left hand.
    b. Sensory-perceptual functions. All sensory modalities are intact in the right upper extremity. In the left upper extremity there is impairment of superficial pain (pinprick) sensation. Proprioception and stereognosis in the left upper extremity are absent. Visual attentiveness is intact. Visual scanning is impaired, that is, slow, jerky, and decreased to the left. There is an apparent left homonymous hemianopsia or neglect of the left visual field, but it is difficult to assess. There is a severe impairment in praxis, visual figure-ground perception, and perception of position in space. There is an impairment in right-left discrimination, body scheme, and three-dimensional spatial orientation. There is also a unilateral neglect of the left side of the body.
    c. Cognitive functions. K.B. is generally cooperative, in spite of his difficulty in following simple commands. Impaired safety awareness, judgment, and limited insight into his disability are apparent. He becomes extremely frustrated when unable to perform simple tasks.
    d. Functional skills.
      (1) Self-care: K.B. requires minimal physical assistance for all dressing, hygiene, and grooming activities. He has a severe dressing apraxia, that is, he would put on his shirt upside down or backwards or put his shoes on the wrong foot, unless given cues by the therapist. He requires assistance with all fastenings. For feeding he requires assistance for opening containers and cutting meat.
      (2) Transfer skills: Bed, chair, and toilet transfers require moderate physical assistance and verbal cues to compensate for apraxia, difficulty with sequencing the steps of the transfer, and decreased perception of position in space.
      (3) Bed mobility: Moderate physical assistance and verbal cues are required for rolling over, coming to sitting from supine position, scooting, and managing legs. The cues are required because of decreased motor planning skill (praxis) and impaired perception of position in space.
      (4) Wheelchair mobility: The patient is dependent for wheelchair propulsion and management of footrests and armrests because of sensory dysfunction, decreased coordination of the left arm, and perceptual-motor impairments just outlined.
  2. Problem identification.
    a. Self-care dependence
    b. Dependence for functional mobility transfers, that is, bed mobility and wheelchair management
    c. Sensory impairments
    d. Lack of selective control of the left upper extremity
    e. Decreased hand function on left side
    f. Deficit in postural mechanism and equilibrium
    g. Visual perceptual dysfunction
    h. Apraxia
    i. Body scheme disorder
    j. Cognitive deficits
  3. Assets.
    a. Good function of right upper extremity
    b. Good motivation
    c. Intact memory
    d. Supportive family
    e. Supportive employer and possibility for reemployment
    f. Intact functional communication skills

Continued.

SAMPLE TREATMENT PLAN—cont'd

E Problem	F Specific OT objectives	G Methods used to meet objectives	H Gradation of treatment
a	Through appropriate cues, structure, and training independence for dressing and hygiene will be increased	Daily practice in dressing and hygiene activities with structure and cues from therapist Sensory stimulation before dressing activities to increase awareness of left side Try use of a mirror for visual feedback of performance Avoid print garments to compensate for visual figure-ground deficit	Increase number of activities; decrease structure and cues as independence increases
b	Through training in hemiplegia transfer techniques, patient will perform them with increased independence, until verbal cues from therapist are no longer required	Daily training in bed, chair, and toilet transfer techniques Use consistent type and sequence of transfer Patient is to explain each step of the transfer before it is performed, until verbal cues from the therapist are no longer required	Progress to bathtub and car transfers Decrease verbal cuing and structure as there is improvement
	Through NDT training independence in bed mobility will increase	Bed mobility training Rolling side to side Supine to sitting position Sitting to supine position Sitting on edge of bed NDT (Bobath) techniques to normalize sensory input and inhibit abnormal movement patterns Weight bearing on affected arm Reflex-inhibiting patterns Equilibrium reactions in sitting	Decrease supervision, assistance, and verbal cues Decrease use of techniques of facilitation and inhibition
	Ability to use a wheelchair will improve so that patient can use the chair independently in the hospital ward	Wheelchair propulsion practice, bilateral method	Functional ambulation on ward
c	Through sensory stimulation awareness of the left upper extremity will be increased	Self-applied cutaneous stimulation with rough washcloth and application of cream to left upper extremity Resistive activities for proprioceptive input, for example, clay board and bilateral sanding Tactile box for identification of common objects, using manual form perception without the aid of vision	
d	Ability to perform controlled, selective movement of the left upper extremity will be increased	Unilateral and bilateral reaching in all planes incorporated in coordination activities Weight bearing on left upper extremity while performing activities with right upper extremity during kitchen and other functional activities	

SAMPLE TREATMENT PLAN—cont'd

E Problem	F Specific OT objectives	G Methods used to meet objectives	H Gradation of treatment
e	Through activities, training, and practice, function of the left hand will improve so that the patient uses it spontaneously in bilateral activities	Theraplast exercises—pinch, squeeze, pulling Card turning Grasp and release of blocks Manipulative activities—paper collation, opening jars, and containers	Grade from large to small Grade gross to fine
f	Through exercises and activities that involve the total body the patient's postural integration, equilibrium, and protective reactions will improve	Bending Reaching Functional ambulation Obstacle courses made with chairs and tables to maneuver during ambulation Scooterboard activities—prone lying, push off walls, up or down inclines	
g	Through appropriate activities and supervised practice the patient's visual-perceptual deficits, that is, visual scanning, visual figure-ground, and position in space, will decline	Using magazine pages have client scan from left to right and cross out a given letter each time it appears in every line Spread out playing cards in random order, call out a card, and have patient select it from the group In a real or simulated market have patient select specific items from among others on the shelves Practice finding items in a cluttered drawer Figure ground tabletop perceptual activities using cards or pictures with hidden figures to be identified Leather craft	
h	During performance of activities to meet objectives outlined above, motor planning skill will be improved	Scooterboard activities Structuring tasks Obstacle course All functional tasks	
i	Given activities and sensory stimulation, body scheme awareness will increase	Practice imitation of postures Use a mirror when performing self-care, craft, and tabletop exercises for visual feedback Cutaneous and proprioceptive sensory stimulation to the left arm	
j	Through structure, support, supervision, and education functional cognition will improve ability to follow directions, insight into deficits, frustration tolerance, and ability to recognize and correct errors	Educate patient about his deficits through discussion and pointing out problems as they occur Videotape patient's performance, play back, and discuss evidence of cognitive problems Support patient when he is frustrated Structure treatment session and supervise to minimize frustration and aid in compensating for cognitive deficits	Reduce structure and supervision

Continued.

SAMPLE TREATMENT PLAN—cont'd

I. **Special equipment.**
 1. Ambulation aids.
 Wheelchair: Primary mobility
 Walker: Early ambulation

2. Splints.
 None required
3. Assistive devices.
 None required

REVIEW QUESTIONS

1. Describe what is meant by acceleration and deceleration injuries.
2. When is a gastrostomy performed?
3. Describe the major clinical signs of the primary and advanced levels in recovery from head injury.
4. What are the three major assessment areas of the Glasgow Coma Scale?
5. Name five major physical impairments that may be present in the patient with head injury.
6. What are the seven most common primitive reflexes present in the patient with head injury? How does each one function?
7. Define "spasticity" and "ataxia."
8. How does the patient's cognitive status affect his function?
9. Define the following: Visual neglect, hemianopsia, praxis, constructional praxis, body scheme, figure-ground, and position in space.
10. List four psychosocial variables that will influence the patient's behavior.
11. What are the major clinical areas that will affect function?
12. Which areas are covered in the primary-level evaluation?
13. How are gross visual skills evaluated?
14. What is included in a physical capacity evaluation?
15. What type of approach do all patients with head injury require?
16. Give examples of auditory, visual, and olfactory stimulation.
17. Describe the most common oral-bulbar problems seen in patients with head injury and the methods of intervention for these problems.
18. Where should the therapist start with wheelchair positioning? Why?
19. What are some examples of methods of reality orientation?
20. What would be the splinting-casting plan for the patient with decorticate posturing?
21. When in the treatment progression are kitchen activities appropriate?
22. How can the Bobath theory of treatment be incorporated in bed mobility tasks?
23. What are the three treatment approaches to perceptual impairment?

REFERENCES

1. Ayres, A.J.: Sensory integration and learning disorders, Los Angeles, 1972, Western Psychological Services.
2. Backman, M.E.: The development of the Micro-TOWER, New York, 1977, I.C.D. Rehabilitation and Research Center.
3. Ballard, S.S., and Knoll, H.A., editors: The visual factors in automobile driving, National Research Council, Pub. No. 574, Washington, D.C., 1958, National Academy of Sciences.
4. Baloh, R.W., and Honrubia, V.: Clinical neurophysiology of the vestibular system, Philadelphia, 1979, F.A. Davis Co.
5. Bennett, G.K.: Hand tool dexterity test, manual of directions, New York, 1965, Psychological Corp.
6. Bliss, C.K.: Semantography (Blissymbolics), ed. 2, Sydney, Australia, 1965, Semantography (Blissymbolics) Publications.
7. Bobath, B.: Adult hemiplegia: evaluation and treatment, London, 1978, William Heinemann Medical Books, Ltd.
8. Brain, L., and Walton, J.N.: Brain's diseases of the nervous system, ed. 7, New York, 1969, Oxford University Press, Inc.
9. Bricolo, A., et al.: Decerebrate rigidity in acute head injury, J. Neurosurg. **47:**680-698, 1977.
10. Bruce, D., Gennarelli, T., and Langfitt, T.: Resuscitation from coma due to head injury, Crit. Care Med. **6:**254-269, 1978.
11. Carroll, D.: A quantitative test of upper extremity function, J. Chron. Dis. **18:**479-491, 1965.
12. Cave, E., Burke, J.F., and Boyd, R.J.: Trauma management, Chicago, 1974, Year Book Medical Publishers, Inc.
13. Caveness, W.: Incidence of craniocerebral trauma in the United States with trends from 1970 to 1975, Adv. Neurol. **22:**1-3, 1979.
14. Chusid, J.G.: Correlative neuroanatomy and functional neurology, ed. 15, Los Altos, Calif., 1973, Lange Medical Publications.
15. Farber, S.: Sensorimotor evaluation and treatment procedures for allied health personnel, 1974, Indiana University Foundation.
16. Gatz, A.J.: Manter's essentials of clinical neuroanatomy and neurophysiology, ed. 4, Philadelphia, 1970, F.A. Davis Co.
17. Gilroy, J., and Meyer, J.S.: Medical neurology, New York, 1969, Macmillan Inc.
18. Groher, M.: Language and memory disorders following closed head trauma, J. Speech Hear. Res. **20:**212-223, 1977.
19. Halpern, H., Darley, F.L., and Brown, J.R.: Differential language and neurological characteristics in cerebral involvement, J. Speech Hear. Disord. **38:**162-173, 1973.
20. Jebsen, R.H., et al.: An objective and standardized test of hand function, Arch. Phys. Med. Rehabil. **50:**311-319, 1969.
21. Jennett, B.: An introduction to neurosurgery, ed. 3, London, 1977, William Heinemann Medical Books, Ltd.
22. Johnstone, M.: Restoration of motor function in the stroke patient, New York, 1978, Churchill Livingstone, Inc.
23. Lorenze, E., and Cancro, R.: Dysfunction in visual perception with hemiplegia: its relation to activities of daily living, Arch. Phys. Med. Rehabil. **43:**514-517, 1962.
24. Luria, A.R.: Higher cortical functions in man, New York, 1966, Basic Books, Inc.
25. McLaurin, R.: Head injuries, proceedings of the second Chicago Symposium on neural trauma, New York, 1975, Grune & Stratton, Inc.
26. Marsden, C.D.: The physiological basis of ataxia, Physiotherapy J. **61:**326-328, 1965.
27. Meyer, J.S.: Medical neurology, New York, 1969, Macmillan Inc.
28. Meyer, J.S.: An orientation to chronic disease and disability, New York, 1965, Macmillan Inc.
29. Minnesota Rate of Manipulation Tests: examiner's manual, Circle Pines, Minn., 1969, American Guidance Service, Inc.
30. Plum, F., and Posner, J.: Diagnosis of stupor and coma, Philadelphia, 1966, F.A. Davis Co.
31. Professional Staff Association of Rancho Los Amigos Hospital: Rancho Los Amigos Hospital Head Trauma Rehabilitation Seminar, Downey, Calif., 1977.

32. Purdue Pegboard: examiner's manual, Chicago, 1968, Science Research Associates, Inc.

33. Randolph, S., and Heineger, M.: A psychoneurologically integrated model for learning capacity, lectures on the Rood Treatment Approach, White Plains, N.Y., May 1975, Burke Rehabilitation Foundation.

34. Shires, T.G.: Care of the trauma patient, ed. 2, New York, 1979, McGraw-Hill, Inc.

35. Siev, E., and Frieshtat, B.: Perceptual dysfunction in the adult stroke patient, Thorofare, N.J., 1976, Charles B. Slack, Inc.

36. Sinatra, K.: Nonoral communication systems, lecture given at Santa Clara Valley Medical Center, San Jose, Calif., Feb. 8, 1980.

37. Sterno-occipital mandibular immobilizer: United States Manufacturing Co., Glendale, Calif. Commercially available head device.

38. Teasdale, G., and Jennett, B.: Assessment of coma and impaired consciousness, Lancet 2:81-83, 1974.

39. TOWER system: evaluator's manual, New York, 1967, I.C.D. Rehabilitation and Research Center.

40. Trombly, C.A., and Scott, A.D.: Occupational therapy for physical dysfunction, Baltimore, 1977, The Williams & Wilkins Co.

41. Valpar Component work sample series 1-16: Tucson, Ariz., 1974-1977, Valpar Corp.

42. Wall, N., et al.: Hemiplegia evaluation, Boston, 1979, Massachusetts Rehabilitation Hospital.

43. Williams, N.: Correlation between copying ability and dressing activities in hemiplegia, Am. J. Phys. Med. 46:1332-1340, 1967.

Index

□ Pages on which tables appear are indicated by t.

Rheumatoid arthritis—cont'd
  with synovial invasion of carpal bones, 221
  with synovial invasion of extensor tendons, 220-221
  with synovitis of radioulnar joint, 221
  treatment of, 222
  with wrist synovitis, 220-221
Rheumatoid factor, 217
Rhomboids, functional test involving, 39
Righting reactions, 51
  evaluation of, 52
Rigidity, 281
Rocker knife, 138
"Role disorders" accompanying disability, 1, 8
ROM, 14
  average normal, 14, 16t
  evaluation of
    form for recording, 15
    functional, 65
    by measuring
      ankle, 34-35
      elbow, 21
      fingers, 26-27
      forearm, 22-23
      hip, 30-33
      knee, 33
      lower extremity, 30-35
      shoulder, 17-20
      thumb, 28-29
      upper extremity, 17-29
      wrist, 24-25
    quick, 14
  limited, ADL techniques with, 113, 122-125
    in communication, 124, 125
    for dressing, 113, 122, 123
    for environmental hardware, 125
    for feeding, 122-123
    in home management activities, 125
    in hygiene and grooming, 123-125
    for mobility and transfer skills, 125
  procedures, self administered, 284-285
Rood, M.S., 151-152, 287, 309
  approach of, to treatment of neuromuscular dysfunction, 151-154
    definition of, 152
    general methods of treatment in, 152
    general principles of, 152
    prerequisites of practicing, 154
    sensory stimuli used in, 152
    specific techniques and precautions in, 152-154
  relaxation procedures introduced by, 152
Rooting reflex, 51
  evaluation of, 52
Rule of nines, 208, 209
Runge, M., 143, 273

S

Scapula
  functional tests of, 39
  mobilization of, rationale for, 158
Schedule, daily, 64
Scissor reachers, 122, 123
Scoop dish, 126, 127
Scott, A.D., 101, 111, 112, 199
Self-care, definition of, 110
Self-definition of clients, 7-8

Self-Dressing Techniques for Patients with Spinal Cord Injury, 143
Self-help groups, 8, 9
Self-valuation, effect of, on adjustment to physical dysfunction, 2
Semicoma, 297
Sensation, 87
  phantom, 194-195
  tests for; see Sensory testing
Sensitivity
  light touch, test for, 54, 55-56
  pressure, test for, 56
  superficial pain, test for, 53-54, 55
  thermal, test for, 56, 57
Sensorimotor approaches to treatment, 144-161
  reflex mechanisms used in, 145
  sequence in, 145
Sensorimotor process, 277
Sensory aphasia, 282
Sensory functions, 87
Sensory retraining, 288
Sensory testing, 53-56, 65
  diagnoses requiring, 53
  gross, 43
    procedures for, 53, 55
  importance of, to occupational therapy, 53
  occluding patient's vision in, 55
  recording scores on, 54
Sensory-perceptual-cognitive evaluation, 53-64
  purposes of, 53
Sequencing, visual, 260
Serratus anterior, functional test involving, 39
Sewing activities, evaluation of, 71, 120
Shock; see Cerebral vascular accident
  as stage in adjustment, 4
Shoe tying method, one handed, 137
Shoulder; see also Glenohumeral joint
  abduction of, 19
    functional test of, 39
    horizontal, functional test of, 39
  adduction of, horizontal, functional test of, 39
  and elbow, position and motion sense test of, 58, 60
  extension of, 18
    functional test of, 39
    reflex-inhibiting pattern to obtain, 158
  flexion of, 17
    functional test of, 39
    ROM for, 16t
  protraction of; see Shoulder, extension of
  rotation of
    external, 20
      functional test of, 39
    internal, 19
      alternate method of measuring, 19, 20
      functional test of, 39
  synovitis of, 221-222
Sides, right and left, testing concept of
  method of, 60
  responses for, 60
  scoring after, 62
    form for, 61
Simon, J.I., 3
Skin inspection mirror, 143
Slings, "static" and "dynamic," 252-253
Smith, H.D., 13
Soap on rope, 123, 124

W

Walker, C., 250
"Walking wounded," 298
Warmth, neutral, 152
Watanabe, S., 13
Weber, E.H., 47
Weighted cuffs, 126, 127
Wellerson, T.L., 199
Wheelchairs, 163-174
  accessories for, 165
  advantages of, 163
  with amputee frame, 164
  armrests of, 165, 286-287
  backrests of, 165
  construction of, 164
  electric, 165
  footrests of, 165
  home evaluation for, 165
  with one-arm drive, 164-165
  propulsion of, 164-165
  ramp for, 165
  and safety, 166
  selection of, 164-166
    factors influencing, 164
    life-style considerations in, 165
  size of, 163-164
  with standard drive, 164
  therapists' responsibilities regarding, 163
  tires of, 165
  transfer techniques with, 166-174
  with traveler frame, 164
  with universal frame, 164
Wheelchair lapboard, 141, 142
Willis, B.A., 212

Wood, H., 47
Words stigmatizing disabled, 3
Work adjustment, 78
Work, alternatives to, 78-79
Work evaluation; *see* Vocational evaluation
Work heights, evaluation of, 72, 121
Work skills for evaluation, 76t
Worth, intrinsic, 2
Wrinkle test for nerve regeneration, 250
Wrist
  circumduction of, evaluating, 44
  extension of
    evoking, 150
    functional test for, 40
  flexion of, functional test for, 39-40
  position sense test of, 58
  ROM of
    average normal, 16t
    measuring
      in extension, 24, 25
      in flexion, 24
      in radial deviation, 24, 25
      in ulnar deviation, 24, 25
  stabilization of
    of client by therapist, 48
    evaluating, 44
    importance of, 47
  subluxation of, 50
  synovitis of, 220-221
"Wrist drop," 251
Writing aids, 124, 125

Z

Zim jar opener, 138